# Human Sexuality
## THE BASICS

Eric Golanty
Las Positas College
Livermore, California

Gordon Edlin
Professor of Genetics Emeritus
University of California Davis
Davis, California

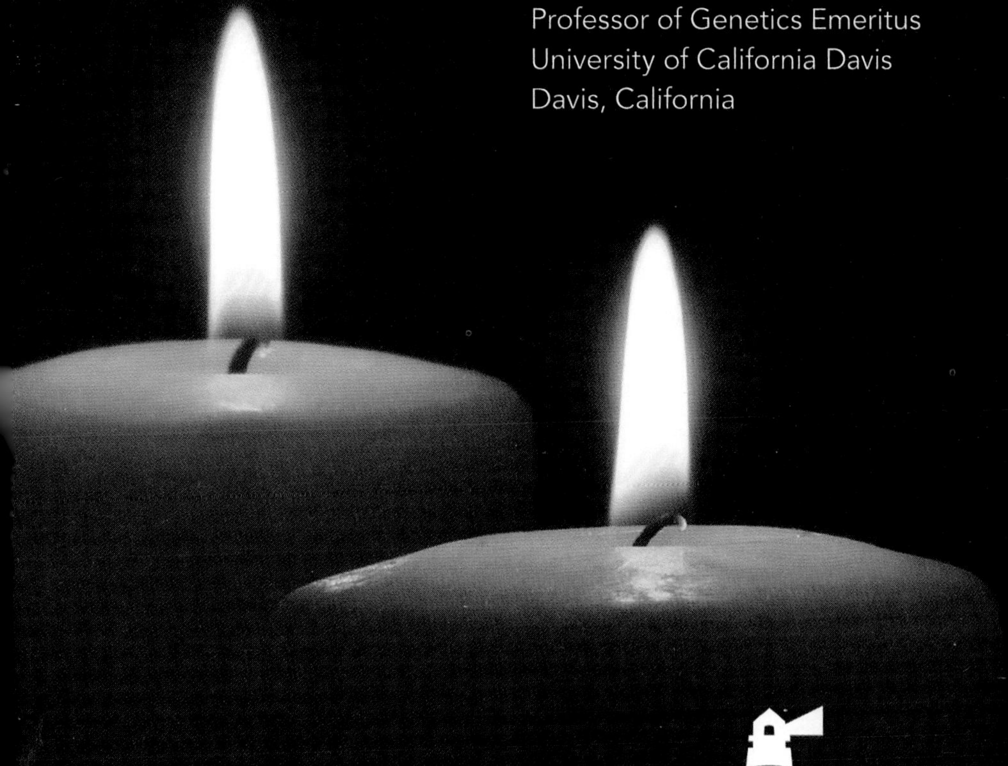

JONES & BARTLETT
LEARNING

*World Headquarters*
Jones & Bartlett Learning
40 Tall Pine Drive
Sudbury, MA 01776
978-443-5000
info@jblearning.com
www.jblearning.com

Jones & Bartlett Learning
Canada
6339 Ormindale Way
Mississauga, Ontario L5V 1J2
Canada

Jones & Bartlett Learning
International
Barb House, Barb Mews
London W6 7PA
United Kingdom

Jones & Bartlett Learning books and products are available through most bookstores and online booksellers. To contact Jones & Bartlett Learning directly, call 800-832-0034, fax 978-443-8000, or visit our website, www.jblearning.com.

Substantial discounts on bulk quantities of Jones & Bartlett Learning publications are available to corporations, professional associations, and other qualified organizations. For details and specific discount information, contact the special sales department at Jones & Bartlett Learning via the above contact information or send an email to specialsales@jblearning.com.



Production Credits
Chief Executive Officer: Ty Field
President: James Homer
SVP, Chief Operating Officer: Don Jones, Jr.
SVP, Chief Technology Officer: Dean Fossella
SVP, Chief Marketing Officer: Alison M. Pendergast
SVP, Chief Financial Officer: Ruth Siporin
SVP, Editor-in-Chief: Michael Johnson
Publisher, Higher Education: Cathleen Sether
Senior Acquisitions Editor: Shoshanna Goldberg
Senior Associate Editor: Amy L. Bloom
Editorial Assistant: Prima Bartlett
Production Manager: Julie Champagne Bolduc
Production Editor: Jessica Steele Newfell
Associate Marketing Manager: Jody Sullivan
VP, Manufacturing and Inventory Control: Therese Connell
Composition: Publishers' Design and Production Services, Inc.
Interior Design: Anne Spencer
Cover Design: Scott Moden
Associate Photo Researcher: Sarah Cebulski
Cover and Title Page Image: © Tischenko Irina/ShutterStock, Inc.
Printing and Binding: Courier Kendallville
Cover Printing: Courier Kendallville

Library of Congress Cataloging-in-Publication Data
Golanty, Eric.
Human sexuality : the basics / Eric Golanty, Gordon Edlin.
p. cm.
Includes bibliographical references and index.
ISBN-13: 978-0-7637-3652-1 (pbk. : alk. paper)
ISBN-10: 0-7637-3652-X (pbk. : alk. paper)
1. Sex—Textbooks. 2. Sex (Biology)—Textbooks. I. Edlin, Gordon, 1932– II. Title.
HQ21.G5995 2012
306.7—dc22

2010049181

6048
Printed in the United States of America
15 14 13 12 11 10 9 8 7 6 5 4 3 2 1

# Brief Contents

# Contents

# Preface

A study in human sexuality is among the most diverse of all academic college courses. Human sexuality courses must include discussions of sexual biology, psychology, and behavior as well as changes in sexuality that occur over one's lifetime. Courses must include information on sexual assault and unusual sexual behaviors; moral, ethical, and legal issues; and sexuality in different cultures and the media.

Most human sexuality textbooks attempt to address almost all of the numerous and diverse perspectives of sexuality. As a result, however, the typical college human sexuality text is overwhelming in size, content, and cost. Instructors cannot transmit all or even a significant part of the material, nor can students learn and understand all of the material in the limited time available.

Our goal in writing *Human Sexuality: The Basics* is to distill the most relevant information and research into "the basics" to provide instructors and students with the core knowledge underlying the vast subject of human sexuality. Our text also differs from others in that we include a chapter on genetics as it pertains to normal and abnormal sexual development. Modern genetics helps us to understand why people differ not only in sexual preferences but also in anatomy; not everyone is fortunate enough to be born with unambiguous male or female anatomy. As a society, we have learned to be tolerant of racial differences that are inherited. We still must learn to be tolerant of sexual differences and preferences that are due to genetic differences among people.

Our perspective in this text is based on the belief that sexual expression is as basic to human nature as eating and learning. Each of these activities has a biological basis but also is molded and modified by environmental influences throughout life. Furthermore, we believe that sexual expression refers not solely to sexual intercourse and its consequences but also to all forms of intimacy and human communication. Facial expressions, touches, words, and gestures can convey sexual meaning. Healthy sexual behaviors, successful relationships, and satisfying physical interactions must all be learned. We hope that *Human Sexuality: The Basics* provides students with the knowledge, skills, and confidence to enable them to understand and to express their sexuality in healthy and enjoyable ways at all stages of life.

# Additional Resources

## Student Resources

The companion website to accompany *Human Sexuality: The Basics* (http://health.jbpub.com/sexuality/basics) offers additional resources for students and instructors. Students can further explore and study topics in the text by accessing the following resources: interactive glossary, flashcards, crossword puzzles, web links, and practice quizzes.

## Instructor Resources

Resources for instructors include the following materials to assist and enrich the instruction of this text: Instructor's Manual, computerized TestBank, and PowerPoint presentations.

# Acknowledgments

We wish to thank our many students who have taken our courses in human development, human sexuality, human genetics, and health over the past three decades. We also want to thank colleagues—too many to mention—who have helped us improve our teaching and writing skills over the years. And, once again, we are grateful to the editorial and production teams at Jones & Bartlett Learning for the encouragement and enthusiasm that made this book possible.

Thank you also to Virginia Thomas for creating the ancillary materials that accompany this book. Lastly, thanks to the following reviewers, who provided valuable feedback on our manuscript:

- Stephan A. George, MA, Paradise Valley Community College, Phoenix, Arizona
- Mary Goodwin, MEd, Brigham Young University, Provo, Utah
- Gina Gray, MEd, Penn State Worthington Scranton, Dunmore, Pennsylvania
- Shelley Hamill, PhD, CHES, Winthrop University, Rock Hill, South Carolina
- Steven J. Hoekstra, PhD, Kansas Wesleyan University, Salina, Kansas
- Laura Jones, PhD, Southern Oregon University, Ashland, Oregon
- Pat Lefler, PhD, Bluegrass Community and Technical College, Lexington, Kentucky
- Peter Malo, PhD, JD, Richard J. Daley College, Chicago, Illinois
- Mikki Meadows, PhD, Eastern Illinois University, Charleston, Illinois
- Jane A. Petrillo, EdD, Kennesaw State University, Kennesaw, Georgia

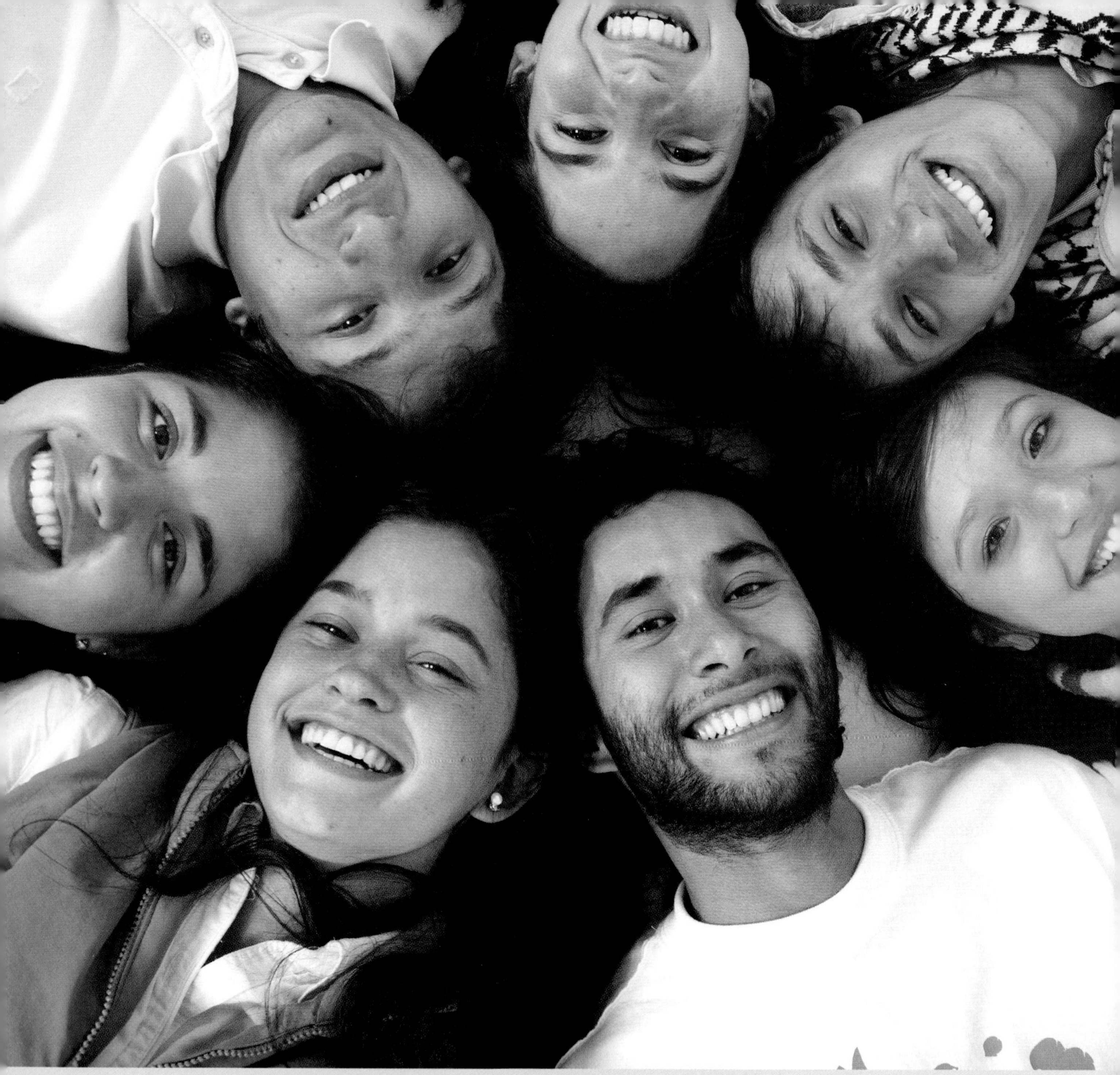

*"A loving heart is the beginning of all knowledge."*

— Thomas Carlyle

CHAPTER 1

# Introduction to the Study of Sex and Sexuality

## Student Learning Objectives

1 List eight reasons for studying human sexuality

2 Explain the three definitions of *sex*

3 List and describe the six dimensions of human sexuality

4 Explain the advantages and limitations of *sampling* in the scientific study of human sexuality

5 Compare the research methods of clinical case study, laboratory observation study, naturalistic observation study, and ethnographic study

6 Compare survey and experimental methods of sexuality research

7 Distinguish between the concepts of statistical average and socially normal

Nearly all human adults have innate needs for sexual activity and sexual expression with peers. However, people are not born knowing how to meet these needs. That's where learning about sex and sexuality come in. Beginning in early childhood and continuing throughout life, individuals learn their culture's beliefs, values, and rules of behavior for seeking and engaging in sexual experiences. In some cultures, values, attitudes, and rules regarding sexual behavior and expression are relatively stable over generations, and group members think and behave as their elders do and did. However, in modern, highly technological, mass-media–dominated cultures, sexual values and attitudes tend to change rapidly. For example, compared with today, sexual behaviors and values in the nineteenth and early twentieth centuries in much of Europe and North America were different. Guided by Victorian morality (referred to as such because Queen Victoria of England set the cultural standards of the time), sexual activity was to be restrained and sexual speech modest. Passionate behavior or expressions of intimacy were not tolerated in public. During the 1920s, however, Victorian sexual mores were rejected, particularly by women, as being puritanical, moralistic, and highly repressive. Sexual expression was expected to be more open and equal among the sexes. In the 1940s and 1950s, sexual conservatism was the norm, only to be replaced by the sexual openness of the 1960s, a trend that continues today.

Sex and love emerge from the rich and varied core of our humanity; they are essential to many aspects of our lives and overall health and well-being. Although it may be difficult to obtain healthful guidance and knowledge in our rapidly changing environment cluttered with mixed messages and self-serving advertisements, it is nevertheless possible to identify some basic goals for our sexual learning. These are:

1. To develop healthy, constructive, responsible, positive attitudes about sexuality and sexual expression
2. To accept oneself and others as sexual beings so that one can take pleasure in one's body and sexual interactions
3. To gain knowledge of sexual functions and responses
4. To develop skills for enhancing sexual relationships
5. To assess one's own sexuality education and to undertake the role of sex educator of one's children

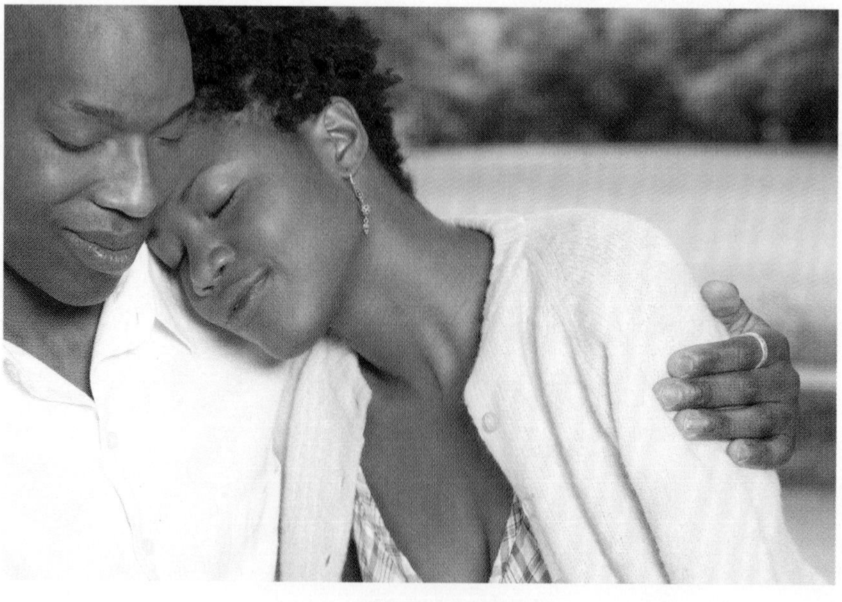

Sex and love emerge from the rich and varied core of our humanity; they are essential to many aspects of our lives and overall health and well-being.

6. To increase knowledge and acceptance of sexual values and practices different from one's own
7. To foster confidence in one's own values and capacity for making wise sexual decisions
8. To increase one's capacity for intimate relationships and communication

## The Definitions of Sex

### The Word *Sex*

To study a subject, one must first define it. According to the *Oxford English Dictionary*, the English word *sex* entered the language in the late fourteenth century. At that time, the word referred to "either of the two divisions of organic beings, the males and the females" (spelled in those days *maals* and *femaals*). The word was based on the phoneme 'sek,' which is derived from the Latin adverb *secus*, meaning "in another way, otherwise, differently," and its cognate, the Latin verb *secare*, meaning to cut, cleave, or divide, which is the root of the modern word *sect* and related words suggesting separating wholes into parts. Some ancient cultures and religions teach that the two sexes originated from dividing a unisex individual in two.

By 1600 the English word *sex* also came to denote aspects of an individual's personal characteristics that were thought to derive from her or his sexual biology.

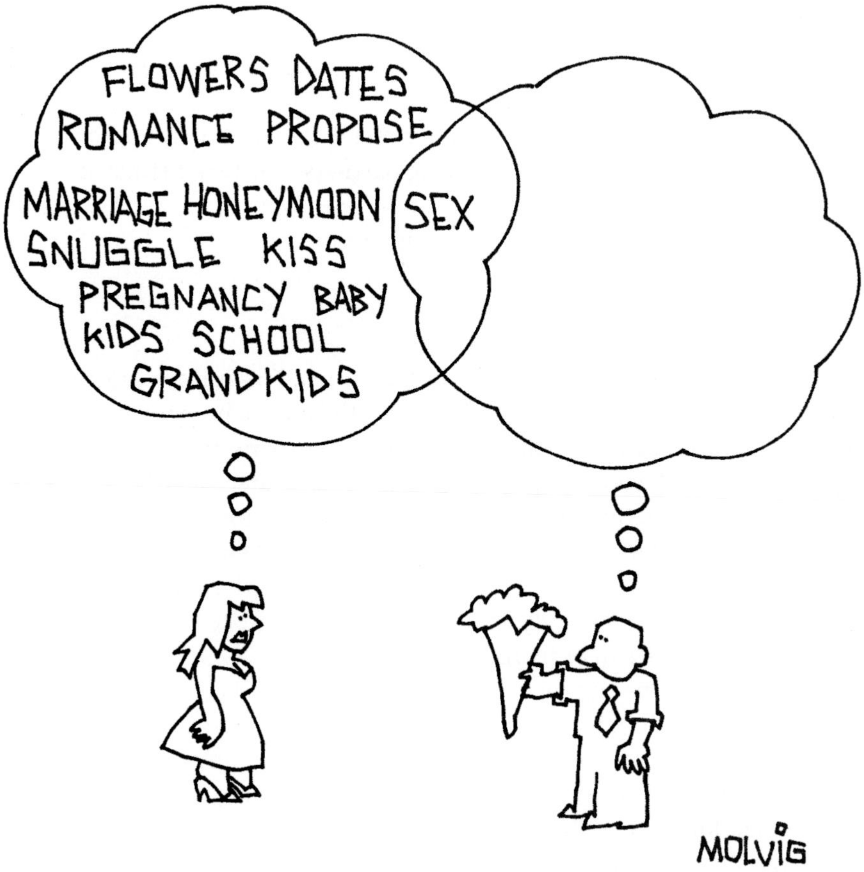

Thus, the biological property of "femaleness" became associated with the social quality of "femininity," and the biological property of "maleness" became associated with the social quality of "masculinity." Although most modern dictionaries still define *sex* as having to do with personal characteristics, this concept is more accurately referred to as *gender* to distinguish its origins primarily in culture rather than in biology.

The Latin *secus* implies not only "otherwise" but also "badly" or "wrongly." In English, the word *sex* came to refer to one's personal qualities, but it carried with it the notion that males were the "better, sterner" sex and females the "softer, weaker"—and possibly dangerous—sex, as illustrated by these words written in 1613: "Strong Sampson and wise Solomon are witnesses, that the strong men are slaine by this weaker sexe." Thus, imbedded in the origins of the definition of the word *sex* are the roots of our culture's history of discrimination against women.

In the early twentieth century, the word *sex* became associated not only with biological and social classification but also with activities associated with biological reproduction and any experiences having to do with those activities, such as sexual gratification or the urge for it.

## Sex-as-Classification

At the most fundamental biological level, *sex* refers to the manner in which humans (and most other multicelled organisms) reproduce. Generally, among animals (there are a few exceptions) sexual reproduction involves the mating of a sperm-producing individual (the male) with an egg-producing individual (the female). In humans, males deposit sperm inside the body of females, and fertilization and fetal development take place within specific organs inside the female body (see Chapters 3 and 4).

Besides reproduction, the genitals and other sex-specific anatomical characteristics (e.g., body size, body shape, pattern of body hair, appearance of breasts) can signal (depending on a society's values) which individuals are socially appropriate and individually desirable as sexual and mating partners. The two distinct sexual anatomies also provide a classification scheme to which a variety of social expectations are applied, called the *gender role* (see Chapter 9).

## Sex-as-Activity

Social groups define certain activities as *sex* or *having sex*. For example, some American young adults (and even a federal court in the impeachment proceedings of President Bill Clinton) consider oral stimulation of the penis or clitoris/vagina *not* to be actual sex because it is not penis-in-vagina intercourse.

Humans are sexually active a lot. A couple having sexual intercourse once or twice a week (the average for American married couples) will engage in more than 2000 acts of intercourse in a 50-year relationship. Even if they have 10 or more children, this degree of sexual activity indicates a strong desire to engage in sexual intercourse for reasons other than reproduction.

One reason that humans engage in frequent sexual activity is that they can. Unlike many other animals, which are physically capable of mating only during specific periods, adult humans are capable of sexual activity at any time. Furthermore, most people find sex pleasurable, which motivates them to do it often.

Another reason for frequent human sexual activity is that humans have the capacity for symbolic thought, which permits them to place a variety of meanings on sexual experience and activity—for example, proving attractiveness, enhancing social standing in a group (peer pressure), earning money, expressing love or other emotions, and developing and maintaining emotional attachment (Table 1.1).

## Sex-as-Experience

Besides biological and social classification and specific activities, the word *sex* can mean particular kinds of pleasurable experiences that have unique and identifiable qualities, often described as *erotic*, *lusty*, or *intimate*, which distinguish them from other kinds of pleasure, such as the satisfaction of hunger by food, the relief of pain, or winning the lottery. Sexual experiences can be described in terms of the following:

1. *Sexual gratification or pleasure.* This experience is commonly referred to as "getting off." It involves a powerful genital focus, high sexual excitement, sensations of sexual pleasure, and mental processes (e.g., sexual fantasies, focus on one's own experience) and behaviors intended to heighten sexual arousal and produce orgasm.
2. *Sexual intimacy.* This experience is often described as "making love." It generally involves a sense of mutuality and emotional sharing with the partner that is heightened in mutual sexual activity, the partner's personality

**Table 1.1** Reasons for Sexual Activity Given by American College Students

| Reason | Examples |
|---|---|
| Reproduction | To have children |
| Curiosity and Adventure | How will this feel? |
| | What's that person like? |
| | What would it be like to____ with _______? |
| Sexual Release | Feeling "horny" |
| | Relief of sexual tension |
| Love/Intimacy | Couple communication |
| | To express love |
| | To feel emotionally close |
| Other Reasons | To prove one's femininity/masculinity |
| | Relationship maintenance |
| | Duty |
| | To control another |
| | To abuse another |
| | To make money |
| | To relieve stress |
| | To relieve boredom |
| | To relieve loneliness |
| | To have fun |
| | To give/receive comfort |
| | To gain a sense of accomplishment |
| | To prove one's attractiveness |
| | To prove adult status |
| | To gain/maintain acceptance in a social group (peer pressure) |

mattering more than her or his physical qualities, and a sense of emotional closeness, affection, and personal investment in the partner.

Sexual intimacy is associated with *sexual self-disclosure*, which is making known to the partner aspects of one's sexuality that one considers private. During sexual activity, your body is generally unclothed; you allow yourself to be touched in "private" places to create intense feelings, urges, and responses; you may make noises and have or share unusual images; and you may experience powerful emotions. A partner's acceptance and appreciation of the private, innermost aspects of your sexuality creates a sense of trust and deepens the level of sexual and emotional intimacy.

3. *Sexual transcendence.* This experience is sometimes referred to as "sexual trance" or "tantric sex." It involves the shifting of mental awareness from everyday thoughts and concerns to deep, focused psychological involvement in the sexual experience, perhaps even to an altered state of consciousness characterized by a sense of timelessness, profound significance, dissolution of self-boundaries, and an oceanic feeling of oneness.

Defining sex as an experience helps account for the fact that some individuals may consider certain activities to be sexually pleasurable (oral stimulation of the penis or anal intercourse, for example) while other individuals may find those same activities unpleasant or repugnant. Furthermore, identical behaviors may in some instances be erotically pleasurable, whereas in others they may not be. Kissing a child or a grandparent can be quite a different experience than kissing a lover. The touching of the genitals in a medical examination is not the same as the touching of the genitals when expressing love and affection to a peer. Furthermore, any number of activities that are socially defined as sex may produce neither a sexual experience nor pleasure. And, a variety of activities that are not socially defined as sex may be used to create sexual experiences (**Table 1.2**).

**Table 1.2** Nontraditional Sexual Practices

| Sexual Practice | Description |
|---|---|
| Fetishism | Sexual arousal from (1) wearing or holding an article of clothing or inanimate object (e.g., shoes, boots, underwear, stockings, gloves, diapers, leather, rubber, lace, satin, spandex, skintight suits); (2) bodily functions (e.g., urination, defecation, lactation; or (3) physical disability (e.g., amputation, anatomical abnormality) |
| Partialism | Sexual arousal from observing or touching a specific body part (e.g., foot, hand, navel, ear) |
| Transvestic Fetishism | A heterosexual male deriving sexual arousal from wearing women's clothes ("cross dressing") |
| Exhibitionism | Exposing the genitals to an unsuspecting stranger |
| Frotteurism | Touching or rubbing against nonconsenting persons |
| Voyeurism | Sexual arousal from observing an unsuspecting person |
| Sexual Masochism | Sexual arousal from the act (not simulated) of being humiliated, tied up, beaten, or made to suffer |
| Sexual Sadism | Sexual arousal from acts (not simulated) that cause others to suffer |
| Pedophilia | Sexual arousal from fantasies or behaviors involving sex with prepubescent children |

Nontraditional sexual practices (medically called paraphilias, "para" meaning along the side and "philia" meaning "love" or emotional involvement in) generally involve fantasizing about or using objects, activities, or situations not considered sexually arousing by most others. Sometimes referred to as "deviant," "kinky," or "perverted," some of these practices may be harmless, whereas others may have serious social and legal consequences. Also, the practitioner's behavior may seriously affect nonconsenting others.

Notice that defining sex in terms of the experience makes no reference to any particular goal or outcome other than what is experienced. Sex is *not* defined by certain genital changes, such as erection of the penis, vaginal lubrication, or orgasm. Also, defining sex in terms of experience makes no reference to interaction with any particular person. Sexual experience can be brought about through self-stimulation (masturbation) and/or fantasy with someone of the same or the other sex. Sexual experiences may take place in a variety of social and emotional contexts (e.g., marriage, friendship, with strangers, with or without love).

Defining sex as an experience rather than a set of activities allows sexual partners to create a wide variety of experiences that they find erotically pleasing and allows them to define for themselves what they consider satisfying sex to be. This can lessen worries about whether they are "doing it right" and permits them simply to enjoy themselves.

## Definitions of Sexuality

**Sexuality** consists of aspects of one's personhood that are involved with sexual classification, sexual activity, and creating erotic experiences. Human sexuality has six dimensions.

**sexuality** aspects of one's personhood that are involved with sexual classification, sexual activity, and creating erotic experiences

1. *The physical dimension* consists of any regions of the body that contribute to sexual classification, sexual activities, and sexual experiences. These include the sexual organs, brain, nervous system, skin, body hair, body shape, and facial features that are considered attractive (or unattractive). The physical dimension also includes general physical health and well-being.
2. *The psychosocial dimension* includes one's sexually related values, beliefs, attitudes, and emotions; one's sexual identity, the sense of oneself as a sexual being; the gender identity, the sense of oneself as male or a female; the gender role, the personal and behavioral expectations of individuals of either sex set forth by their cultural group; and sexual orientation, the propensity to be sexually attracted to and feel most comfortable being emotionally close with someone of a particular biological sex.
3. *The reproductive dimension* consists of physiological and social processes that contribute to the conception and birth of children and their nurturance until they are capable of an independent life. This dimension also consists of efforts to alter and control by various means one's reproductive capacity.
4. *The developmental dimension* consists of one's personal sexual history, the physical, psychological, and social experiences (and self-interpretations of them) that change as one navigates the life course. Throughout life the physical sexual self changes, especially during fetal life when the body develops, and again at puberty when the child's body changes to that of an adult. One's beliefs about sex and sexuality also change throughout life, particularly with regard to the personal meanings of sexual activity and sexual experience.
5. *The erotic dimension* consists of feelings, images, and behaviors intended to create erotic experience, including sexual interest and desire, attracting a sexual partner, knowing how to satisfy sexually oneself and one's sexual partner, being intimate, and maintaining a sexual relationship. This dimension also consists of physical and psychological difficulties related to creating erotic experiences.

6. *The relationship dimension* consists of various kinds of interpersonal relationships in which sexual activity and experience occur. Such relationships might be between virtual strangers, friends, or marital partners. In most cultures, sexual activity and experience are considered rights and responsibilities of marital partners. In some cultures, sexual activity and experience are integral to interpersonal relationships characterized by feelings of love, intimacy, and emotional closeness.

## The Scientific Study of Sex and Sexuality

How does the world we live in work? This is an important question, for knowing the answer can help individuals and communities live harmoniously within their physical and social environments. Also, *believing* one knows the answer can make one feel secure in a world that otherwise might seem overwhelmingly chaotic, incomprehensible, or threatening.

For most of human history, people have relied on religion, philosophy, myth, intuition, and their personal experiences to understand how the world works. Whereas these ways of knowing might make people feel secure, because they lack precision and predictability, they have caused debate and violence as often as they have created workable guidelines for living harmoniously.

**scientific method** a way to gain knowledge of the world utilizing observations, measurements, and experiments

Contrary to religion and philosophy, the **scientific method** is a way to gain knowledge of the world utilizing observations, measurements, and experiments. The scientific method can be applied to both animate (living) and inanimate (nonliving) things. It can be applied to the largest things (the universe) as well as the smallest (the subatomic particles of matter). The scientific method was first applied effectively to the study of the planets, the properties of physical matter, and the biological world. In the past 100 years, the scientific method has been applied to the study of human thought and behavior, including sex and sexuality. The scientific method incorporates the following elements:

1. *Unbiased observations.* Descriptions of how the world works are based on what is actually observed and not the observer's preconceived ideas, assumptions, and prejudices. Most important, the scientific method prohibits discarding valid observations because they are deemed inappropriate or undesirable. Observations can be made with the naked eye or with instruments that make visible small or distant objects. Observations can also be responses to questions posed to individuals about their beliefs, attitudes, and behaviors. One observation is called a *datum* (Latin meaning "what is given"); many observations are *data* (the plural of datum).
2. *Reproducibility.* Once a measurement or experiment has been described, anyone who repeats the experiment the same way should get the same result.
3. *Falsification of hypotheses.* An observer may propose a hypothesis to explain observations or the outcome of an experiment, and similar observations may support it. Additional findings suggest that the hypothesis accurately describes the real world. However, a hypothesis gains the most support from efforts to *disprove* it. Repeated attempts that fail to falsify a hypothesis make it more and more acceptable and, if it survives many kinds of challenges, it may become a scientific theory or law, such as Newton's Laws of Motion. Here's how an observation or hypothesis can be falsified: Suppose someone observes that all the roses in a garden are red. This leads to the

## Dear Penelope . . .

***Sex can be confusing, especially when it gets mixed up in personal relationships. What is a healthy sexual relationship?***
***— Wants It to Be Good***

*Dear Wants,*

Yes, sex can be confusing. That's because it touches so many parts of a person's life and also because there are many influences on sexual attitudes and behavior (e.g., peers, media, religion), the messages of which often conflict. Rather than offer my definition of a healthy sexual relationship, I asked some American college students to offer theirs. They said a healthy sexual relationship consists of openness, trust, honesty, understanding, attraction, good sex, spontaneity, communication, mutual interest, responsibility, enjoyment, not fearing any aspect of sex, interest, respect, willingness to change, creativity, fun, loyalty, being disease-free, willingness to compromise, fidelity, caring, love, unselfishness, and knowing how to please the partner.

The students described an unhealthy sexual relationship in terms of lacking communication, sexual/relationship experience, cooperation, and trust, and consisting of guilt, physical dominance, one-sided gratification, dishonesty, spreading diseases to partner, cheating, jealousy (of friends and time alone/apart from partner), criticism, totally different interests, boredom, faking orgasm, too high/too low expectations, harmful practices, poor hygiene, and using the partner for sex.

Courtesy of the UC Davis *Aggie*

hypothesis that all roses in the world are red. When some white roses are discovered in a different garden, however, the original hypothesis about the universality of red roses must be discarded.

4. *Cause-and-effect relationships.* The ultimate goal of the scientific method is to explain an observation by identifying the reasons it occurred (causes). Furthermore, the relationships between causes and their effects must be predictable. Mathematical formulas are often used to describe cause-and-effect relationships. Because sexuality is so complex, a single cause of any observation is often not possible to discern. The best that can be achieved is to identify several possible causes and to try to determine how strongly each contributes to the observed effect.

**cause-and-effect relationships** predictable patterns and outcomes in scientific investigations

## Sampling

When a scientific question calls for such an enormous number of observations that it is not feasible to make them all, a smaller, more manageable number of observations are made and it is *assumed* that the smaller number, called a sample, is an accurate representation of the total number of possible observations had they been made. For example, suppose you wanted to know the percentage of American college students who have sexual fantasies. You could try to ask all 16 million American college students, but that would be an enormous task. Instead, you could ask a few hundred students at several colleges (a "sample") and assume that they represent reasonably accurately the entire college population. This method is called sampling.

**sample** a small number of observations assumed to represent accurately all possible similar observations
**sampling** making a small number of observations from a large group

A variety of sophisticated techniques enable researchers to gather reliable data for very large numbers of people by studying relatively small samples. However, it is always possible that observations made on a sample do not accu-

**sampling bias** drawing conclusions from samples that do not accurately represent the larger group from which they are draw

rately represent the entire group from which it is drawn. This error is called **sampling bias**. For example, in the determination of the extent of sexual fantasizing among all American college students, sampling bias might occur if only 19-year-old Asian American male students were queried. Obviously, a group of 19-year-old Asian American males does not represent younger or older Asian American males, males of other ethnic backgrounds, and women.

Human sex research is highly prone to sampling bias because many people will not divulge aspects of their sexuality to researchers. Thus, observations are made only on willing participants, and these observations may not be representative of everyone. Furthermore, much sexuality research is carried out on college students because many researchers are college professors, and students are readily available and generally willing (especially if extra course credit is offered) to participate in a study. However, college students may not represent people who do not go to college.

Before you accept as valid a report of any sex or sexuality research, find out how the observations were made and critically evaluate if those observations justify conclusions offered by the researchers. Be especially mindful of potential sampling bias with regard to age, gender, ethnicity and cultural influences, and sexual orientation.

## Methods of Sex and Sexuality Research

### Case Study

**case study** drawing scientific conclusions from the study of one or more individuals

In a **case study**, one or more individuals are observed and conclusions are drawn about them. Sometimes conclusions about "the case" are extended to the group which the "case" is a part of, even though others in the group are not observed.

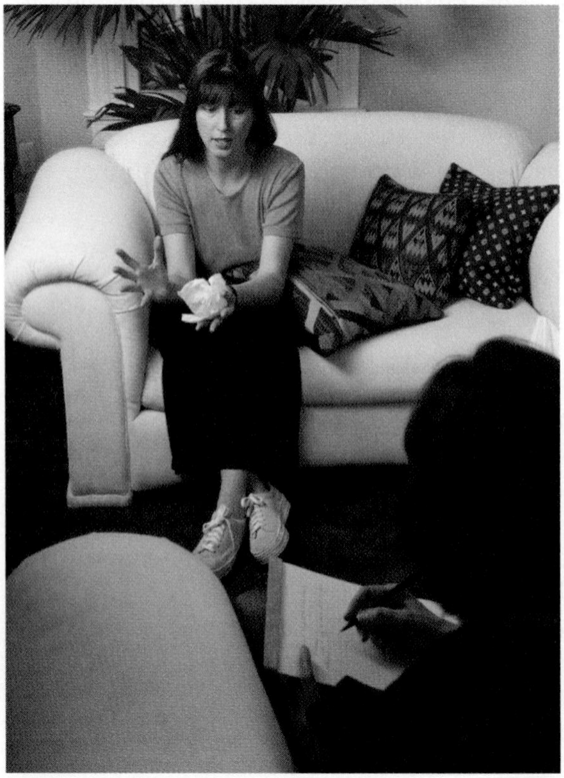

The clinical case study is a method of sex research in which a health practitioner reports observations based on clinical encounters with clients.

**Table 1.3** Sigmund Freud's Basic Concepts

| Concept | Description |
|---|---|
| Unconscious Mind | Thought processes that take place out of conscious awareness |
| Defense Mechanisms | Mental processes used to cope with perceptions, misperceptions, and interpretations of reality and presumed dire consequences |
| Basic Psychic Structures: Id, Ego, and Superego | *Id:* Instinctual drives and impulses, including sex, aggression, and immediate satisfaction |
| | *Ego:* Conscious awareness, reasoning, harmony-seeking |
| | *Superego:* Parental and social rules designed to mold, direct, and contain the id |
| Libido | Instinctual sexual drive that can become fixed on various persons or objects for its release |
| Oedipus and Electra Complexes | *Oedipus:* fixation of a male child on the mother as a sexual object |
| | *Electra:* fixation of a female child on the father as a sexual object |
| Stages of Sexual Development | *Oral:* Libidinal pleasure from nursing (infant) |
| | *Anal:* Libidinal pleasure from bowel function (toddler) |
| | *Phallic:* Libidinal pleasure from manipulation of the genitals (child–adult) |
| Penis Envy | The realization of young girls that they do not have a penis, thus establishing development of female gender identity |
| Castration Anxiety | The realization of young boys that girls do not have a penis and the consequent fear of losing the penis for some misbehavior |

Friends carry out case studies with each other all the time, although they don't call them that. They observe what a friend does ("she's seeing him again") or what a friend says ("I can't let him go") and draw conclusions ("she's dependent"). If they notice similar behaviors among similar individuals, they might draw a conclusion about the group ("most women are dependent").

## Clinical Case Study

In a clinical case study, health practitioners report observations made of people who seek their help. Nearly all of Sigmund Freud's research was derived from clinical case studies. Freud listened to patients recount their experiences (sometimes the patients were hypnotized so they could recall memories that were otherwise blocked from consciousness) and drew conclusions about basic aspects of human psychology (**Table 1.3**). A problem with clinical case studies, of course, is that the observations are derived from people who are seeking help, and the observer often is their professional helper, so the observations and conclusions may be biased and also may not pertain to everyone.

clinical case study drawing scientific conclusions from observations made of one or more individuals who seek help for medical problems

laboratory observation study observations derived in laboratory settings rather than clinical or real-life ones

## Laboratory Observation Study

In a laboratory observation study, observations are made in a laboratory setting rather than a real-life or clinical one. For example, to study the effects of alcohol consumption on sexual arousal, subjects' physiological reactions (e.g., heart and breathing rates, blood pressure, changes in pelvic blood flow) to watching sexually explicit films before and after consuming alcohol could be measured in a laboratory with a variety of scientific instruments. A major bias in this kind of study, of course, is the assumption that the people who are studied are capable of authentic sexual responses (intoxicated or not) while in a laboratory setting and are willing to be observed by others after having imbibed alcohol and become sexually aroused.

**naturalistic observation** studying many people at one time in their natural setting
**epidemiological study** comparing two or more groups in their natural setting
**ethnographic study** observations of an entire community in which the observer lives for a period of time

## Naturalistic Observation Study

Naturalistic observation is a case study approach in which many people are observed in a natural setting as opposed to a laboratory or clinical setting. For example, a graduate student in psychology might go to a party not to participate in the festivities but to observe and report on the effects of alcohol on the interactions of the guests.

## Epidemiological Study

Epidemiological studies are naturalistic studies in which observations of people in different groups are compared, generally using sophisticated statistical methods. For example, the effects of taking a daily vitamin on the frequency of sexual activity could be studied by comparing the frequency of sexual activity of a group of vitamin takers with that of a matched group of non-vitamin takers.

## Ethnographic Study

Ethnographic studies are naturalistic studies of an entire community in which the observer lives for an extended period of time. Between 1850 and 1930, ethnographic studies were carried out on hundreds of what were then referred to as "primitive" or "preliterate" cultures in every part of the world. Comparisons of the sexual behaviors and attitudes of these cultures were used to provide a

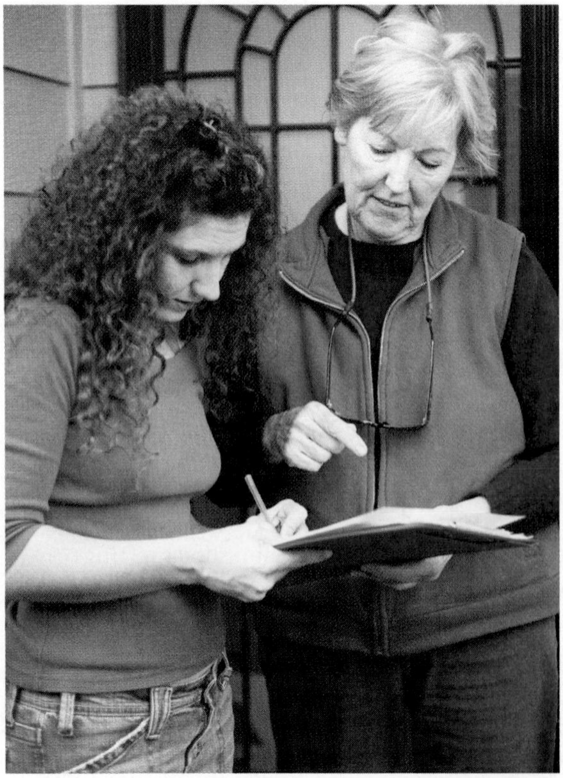

deeper understanding of sexuality than studies of American society alone could provide.

## Survey Methods

In **survey methods**, the scientist is not the observer. Instead, the scientist asks others to report *their* observations, generally of their own thoughts, feelings, and experiences. Most often, surveys involve a standard set of questions to which people ("subjects") respond. The questions can be administered in a face-to-face or telephone interview, or by a self-administered hard copy or online questionnaire. Observations obtained by survey methods can be unreliable. For example, some people might exaggerate or otherwise distort their observations. They may tell the researcher what they think the researcher wants to hear. An observation may be remembered inaccurately. Furthermore, many sex surveys conducted by television programs, Internet polls, and consumer magazines suffer from sampling bias because the observations are derived from the viewers and readers of those media, who are unlikely to be representative of everyone.

**survey methods** asking people to report their observations, generally of their own thoughts, feelings, attitudes, and behavior

**experimental study** scientific results derived from comparing a test or experimental group with a matched control group

## Experimental Studies

In an **experimental study**, the results from at least two similar groups are compared: (1) the *experimental group*, which receives some kind of test, intervention, or treatment, and (2) the *control group*, which is similar to the experimental group but does not receive the test, intervention, or treatment. Observed differences between the two groups are assumed to be *only* from the test, intervention, or treatment. Experimental studies are the only valid way in which the safety and efficacy of medications are determined. An experimental group (or groups) receives a test drug, and a control group receives a placebo ("sugar pill"). In the 1990s, a large experimental study exposed some risk of taking hormonal drugs during and after menopause.

# Interpreting Sexuality Research

To do their jobs well, professional educators, counselors, health practitioners, and researchers must be able to assess critically the findings and interpretations reported in sexuality research. They must judge the risk of sampling and other kinds of bias. They must carefully examine both the data that are reported and the statistical or other analytical tools that are used to interpret them. Finally, they must carefully and critically assess the interpretations and conclusions drawn by the researchers about their research, taking into account any source of funding for the research that might bias their conclusions.

Compared with professional educators, counselors, health professionals, and researchers, most individuals lack the specialized training to assess critically the findings from scientific sexuality research and the conclusions drawn from studies. In the best case, nonprofessionals can receive unbiased explanations of research from professionals they trust and whose goal is to enhance others' health and well-being. Accurate and unbiased accounts of sexuality research can sometimes be found in the mass media (e.g., newspapers, magazines, television, Internet). However, because the primary goal of mass media is profit and not necessarily accurate and unbiased reporting, the media may skew presentations about sexuality research to capture interest (and to sell products and services) rather than to enlighten and educate. With regard to information derived from sexuality research, keep in mind the following:

- What organization or individual is providing the information? What is the provider's stated or implied intention? Assessing the motives for providing information on the Internet is especially important because a Web site can be made to appear educational when, in fact, its goal is to influence attitudes and behaviors, including purchases.
- What is the information provider's training and expertise? Popular magazine articles often quote psychologists or sex counselors to support the article's thesis. Can you really be sure that the person being quoted is a reliable authority?
- What is the source of the data in the research? Is the information based on an observer's experience (a case study), a survey, or a study comparing a "treatment" group with a group of "matched controls" (epidemiological or experimental study)?
- Who benefits? What benefits might the source of the information be receiving for communicating it?

You want to avoid being manipulated by bias presented in the guise of scientific truth.

Occasionally, a study's results are described as *statistically significant*, which means that an observation, or a comparison of observations, is highly likely not to be the result of mistakes made by researchers or to have occurred by chance. For example, suppose researchers report the statistically significant finding that the number of sexual partners among unmarried members of a particular group is two per year. It might be that the actual annual number of sexual partners in this group is zero, one, two, three, or more. Findings are statistically significant if a mathematical analysis of the data show a very small—or *insignificant*—chance that the actual number of partners is *not* two. However, this does not mean that the actual number of partners is always two. It means only that there is a small chance that the findings from this analysis are wrong. Scientists are generally willing to accept a finding if the chance it is wrong is less than 1 in 20 (reported as $p < 0.05$).

In some situations, a result is statistically significant but otherwise not very meaningful. For example, one research study might show that the risk of unintended pregnancy for a new birth control method is 3.0 per 100 female users per year, and another study might show it to be 2.9 per 100 female users per year. Even if the difference in efficacy is statistically significant, it is not very meaningful because the difference is negligible.

## Comparing Yourself with Research Findings

Because people are concerned about their sexual desirability and/or sexual abilities, many compare themselves with results of scientific sexuality research, thinking that the results measure what is normal, good, and desirable. This is a mistake because normal, good, and desirable are socially, not scientifically, defined. Remember that scientific research reports *what is* and not what should be, although research can report what people *think* should be, and in that sense set a norm for people in a particular group.

Two common errors in interpreting scientific research are to equate (1) "average" with "good/normal" and (2) "infrequent" (sometimes referred to as *atypical*)

## HEALTHY SEXUALITY

### Tips for Enhancing Sexual Experience

- Create pleasure by stimulating the whole body, not just the genitals.
- Vary the manner and intensity of stimulation. Allow sensations to build and wane.
- Try not to make sex = work.
- Set aside time that is free of intrusions and distractions. Disconnect the phone; lock the door to ensure privacy.
- Make yourself an open, effective channel for sexual arousal before sexual activity begins. Satisfying sex is not a mechanical activity involving only bodies, but a blending of mind–body energies. Remove sex-negative energies such as hunger, fatigue, and anger, and focus your energy on sex through deep breathing or other relaxing activity.
- Be aware of differences between you and your partner in the state of readiness for sexual activity. Try to synchronize both partners' states of sexual arousal through talking, light touching, dance, massage, and so on, before sexual activity begins.
- Address concerns about birth control and sexually transmitted diseases prior to sexual experience.
- Take your time. Go slowly.
- Communicate likes and dislikes to your partner either verbally or nonverbally.
- Do not focus just on orgasms. Learn to appreciate the many sexual sensations from touching all parts of the body.
- Either partner may reach orgasm through manual, oral, or other means of stimulation before or after intercourse.
- Sexual activity need not stop after one partner reaches orgasm. If a couple chooses, lovemaking can continue until both wish to stop.
- It is possible that neither individual may desire an orgasm during a particular sexual episode. Physically expressing love and caring does not require orgasm.

with "bad/deviant." In each case, a scientific term (e.g., average, infrequent) is mistakenly used as a social term (e.g., normal, deviant). For example, the average height of American men is 5 feet 8 inches. Obviously, we do not consider men who are 5 feet 8 inches tall normal and men of different heights abnormal or socially deviant.

Although averages are generally reported in sexuality research, it is a mistake for individuals to use them as standards of normal for their own thoughts, feelings, and behaviors. Such standards reflect the values and norms of social groups, and they vary from group to group and from time to time in the same group. Also, it is vital to realize that human sexual behaviors vary enormously, and some individuals' sexual attitudes and behaviors may fall outside of their group's definition of "normal." Unless these behaviors are harmful to the participant(s) or others, as in instances of sexual assault or child sexual abuse, to label them as "abnormal" is often more a matter of opinion than scientific fact.

## SEXUALITY IN REVIEW

- Human sexuality is studied to develop healthy, constructive, responsible, and positive attitudes about ourselves and others as sexual beings; to undertake the role of sex educators of our children; and to increase our capacity for creating and experiencing sexual pleasure and sexual intimacy.
- *Sex* is defined as one's classification as a biological male or female, as activities personally or socially defined as sex, and as specific experiences, such as erotic pleasure and sexual intimacy.
- Sexuality has six dimensions: physical, psychological, reproductive, developmental, erotic, and relationship.
- Sexuality is studied scientifically using observational, survey, and experimental methods.
- Human sexual behaviors vary enormously from person to person and from group to group.

## CRITICAL THINKING ABOUT SEXUALITY

1. This chapter has presented three definitions of *sex*. What is your personal definition of sex? In what ways has your definition of sex changed as you've become older?
2. List five criteria for a healthy sexual relationship and explain the reasons for your choices.
3. Sexual images are prevalent in consumer advertisements. Find three examples of advertisements that used sexual imagery to sell a product or an idea. For each example:
   - Identify the source.
   - Identify the intended audience.
   - Describe the sex-related imagery and its relationship to the advertiser's intention. Is the ad effective?
   - Describe the sex-related messages and values that are communicated in the ad.
   - Offer your opinion of the ad.
4. A reputable news source reports that scientists at a leading university have discovered a brain chemical that is responsible for creating feelings of sexual pleasure. The report also states that a pharmaceutical company is interested in developing a drug based on the scientists' discovery. Using criteria presented in this chapter regarding evaluating media reports of sexuality research, what information would you require to evaluate the validity of this scientific finding?

## REFERENCES AND RECOMMENDED RESOURCES

### References

Cott, N. F. (Winter 1978). Passionlessness: An interpretation of Victorian sexual ideology, 1790–1850. *Signs, 4*, 219–236.

Fernández-Villaverde, J., et al. (2010). From shame to game in one hundred years: An economic model of the rise in premarital sex and its de-stigmatisation. *Vox*. Available at: http://www.voxeu.org/index.php?q=node/4649. Accessed July 13, 2010.

Freud, S. (1905). *Three essays on the theory of sexuality.* New York: Basic Books.

Mosher, W. D., et al. (2005). Sexual behavior and selected health measures: Men and women 15–44 years of age, United States, 2002. Advance data from vital and health statistics; no. 362. Hyattsville, MD: National Center for Health Statistics.

Reiss, I. L. (1986). *Journey into sexuality.* Englewood Cliffs, NJ: Prentice Hall. Available at: http://www2.hu-berlin.de/sexology/Reiss3/index.htm. Accessed June 5, 2006.

Smith, T. W. (2006, March). American sexual behavior: Trends, socio-demographic differences, and risk behaviors. General Social Survey Topical Report No. 25, Version 6. Available at: http://www.norc.org/NR/rdonlyres/2663F09F-2E74-436E-AC81-6FFBF288E183/0/AmericanSexualBehavior2006.pdf. Accessed November 1, 2009.

### Recommended Resources

Ford, C. S., & Beach, F. A. (1952). *Patterns of sexual behavior.* New York: Harper. This text is a classic reference based on ethnographic research comparing sexual attitudes and behaviors among 192 human cultures.

Go Ask Alice. http://www.goaskalice.columbia.edu. This health—including sexual and relationship health—question-and-answer Internet resource is produced at Columbia University.

Haavio-Mannila, E., et al. (2002). *Sexual lifestyles in the twentieth century.* London: Palgrave Macmillan. This text is an exploration of the evolution of sexual behavior and relationships during the twentieth century.

Mayo Clinic. http://www.mayoclinic.com. The authoritative medical institution offers information on a variety of sexuality topics (use the search tool).

MedlinePlus. Female reproductive system. http://www.nlm.nih.gov/medlineplus/femalereproductivesystem.html. Information for females.

MedlinePlus. Male reproductive system. http://www.nlm.nih.gov/medlineplus/malereproductivesystem.html. Information for males.

Stearns, P. N. (2009). *Sexuality in world history.* London: Routledge. This book examines sexuality in the past and explores how it helps explain sexuality in the present. The subject of sexuality is often a controversial one, and exploring it through a world history perspective emphasizes the extent to which societies, including our own, are still reacting to historical change through contemporary sexual behaviors, values, and debates.

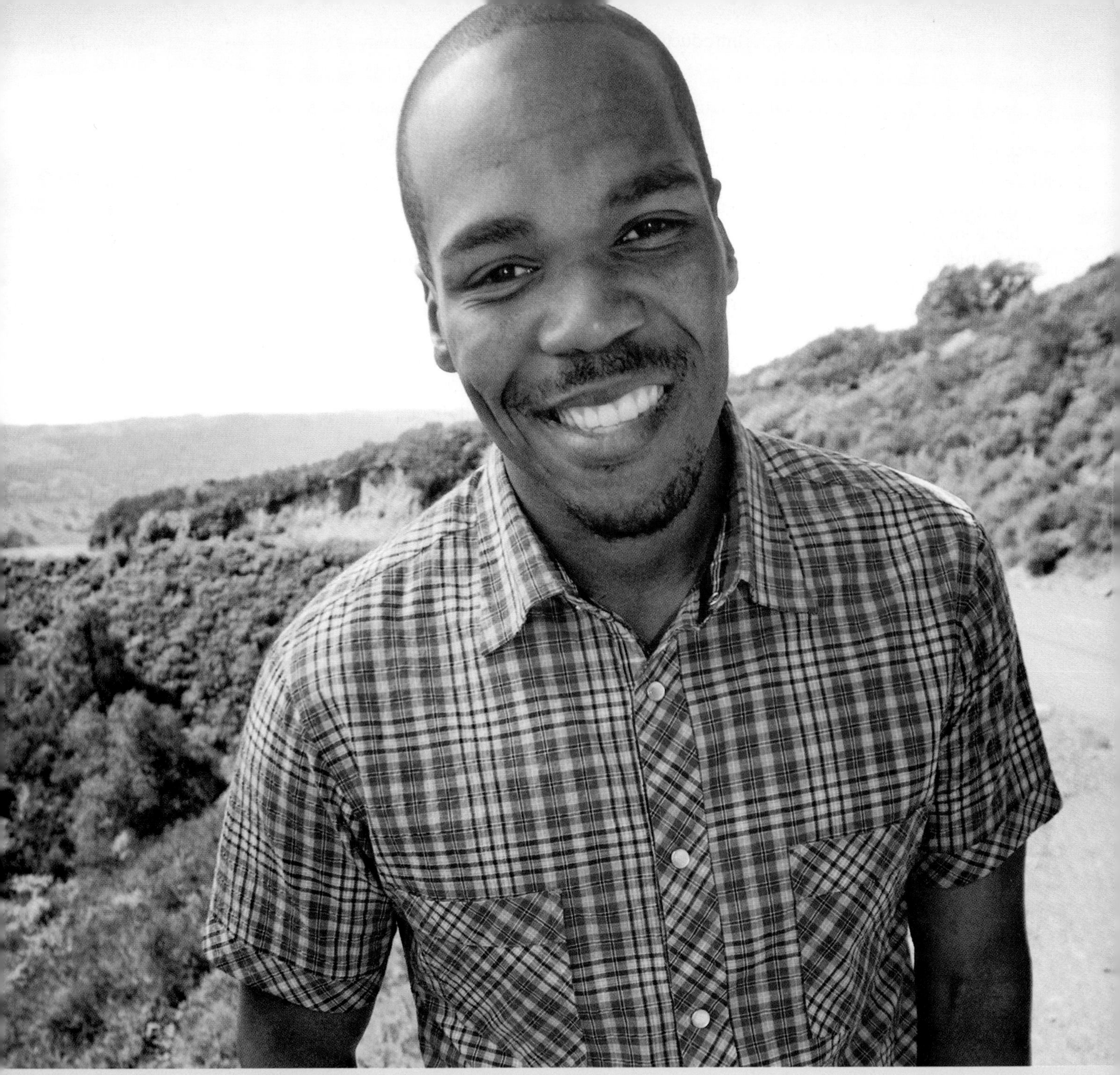

*"A healthy body is the guest-chamber of the soul."*

— Francis Bacon

CHAPTER 2

# Male Sexual Biology

## Student Learning Objectives

1. Describe how the testes produce sperm and androgenic sex hormones
2. Describe the four parts of the genital (sperm) duct system
3. Name the glands that contribute to formation and release of seminal fluid
4. Describe the two phases of ejaculation
5. Explain the physiological mechanisms that produce penile erection
6. List at least three functions of androgenic sex hormones
7. Name and describe male secondary sex characteristics

Human sexual biology consists of specific anatomical structures and physiological functions called *sex characteristics*, which contribute to a person's ability to participate in sexual activities, to reproduce, to attract sexual and/or romantic partners, and to be classified as male or female. Primary sex characteristics are directly involved in the production and delivery of sperm or eggs, fertilization, and pregnancy. Human male primary sex characteristics consist of the pair of testes in which sperm and sex hormones are produced, the genital duct system through which sperm are transported from their site of production in the testes to the outside, the glands that produce seminal fluid, and the penis (FIGURE 2.1).

**primary sex characteristics** body structures directly involved in the production and delivery of sperm or eggs, fertilization, and pregnancy
**penis** the male organ of copulation and urination
**secondary sex characteristics** body structures associated with each sex that are not involved in the manufacture and delivery of sperm or eggs, fertilization, or pregnancy

Secondary sex characteristics are anatomical and physiological features not primarily involved in the manufacture and delivery of sperm or eggs or the maintenance of pregnancy, but they are nevertheless specific to members of a particular sex. For example, compared with women, men tend to be larger and stronger, have broader shoulders and slimmer hips, and have prominent facial hair (FIGURE 2.2). Also, compared with women, men tend to be aggressive, dominant, and adept at certain spatial–cognitive tasks. Secondary sex characteristics are generally the result of the actions of androgenic ("male-producing") hormones on androgen-

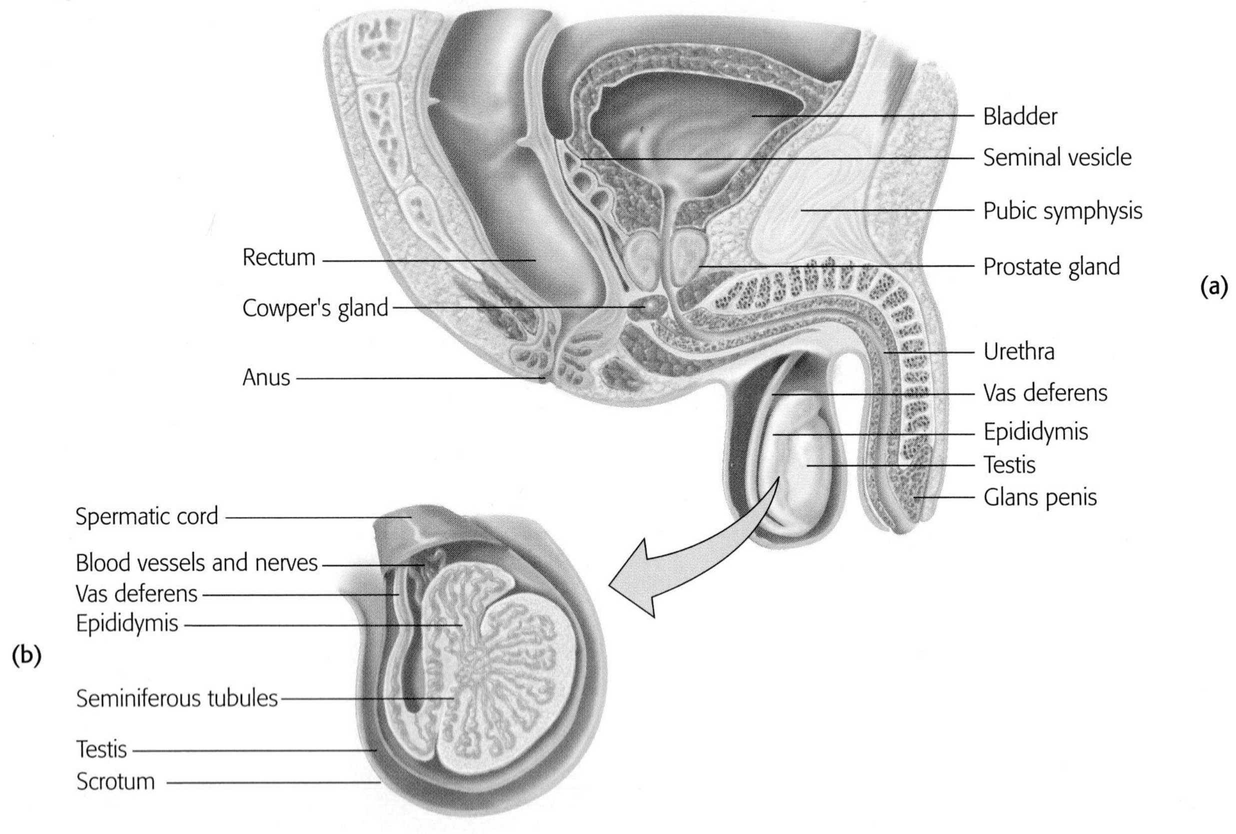


FIGURE 2.1 **Male Primary Sex Characteristics.** (a) The male primary sex characteristics consist of the testes, the genital duct system, the glands that produce seminal fluid, and the penis. (b) Each testis is suspended at the end of a fibrous sheath called the spermatic cord, which contains a vas deferens, blood vessels, nerves, and the cremaster muscle. Sperm and androgenic sex hormones are manufactured in the testes. Sperm are produced in seminiferous tubules. Sperm move from the testes to the outside through a series of connected tubes (epididymis, vas deferens, ejaculatory duct, and urethra). As they prepare to exit the body, sperm become mixed with fluids produced by the seminal vesicles and prostate; the Cowper's glands produce fluid that lubricates the urethra, the tube that courses through the penis. Androgens enter the bloodstream through blood vessels that course from the testes through the spermatic cord.

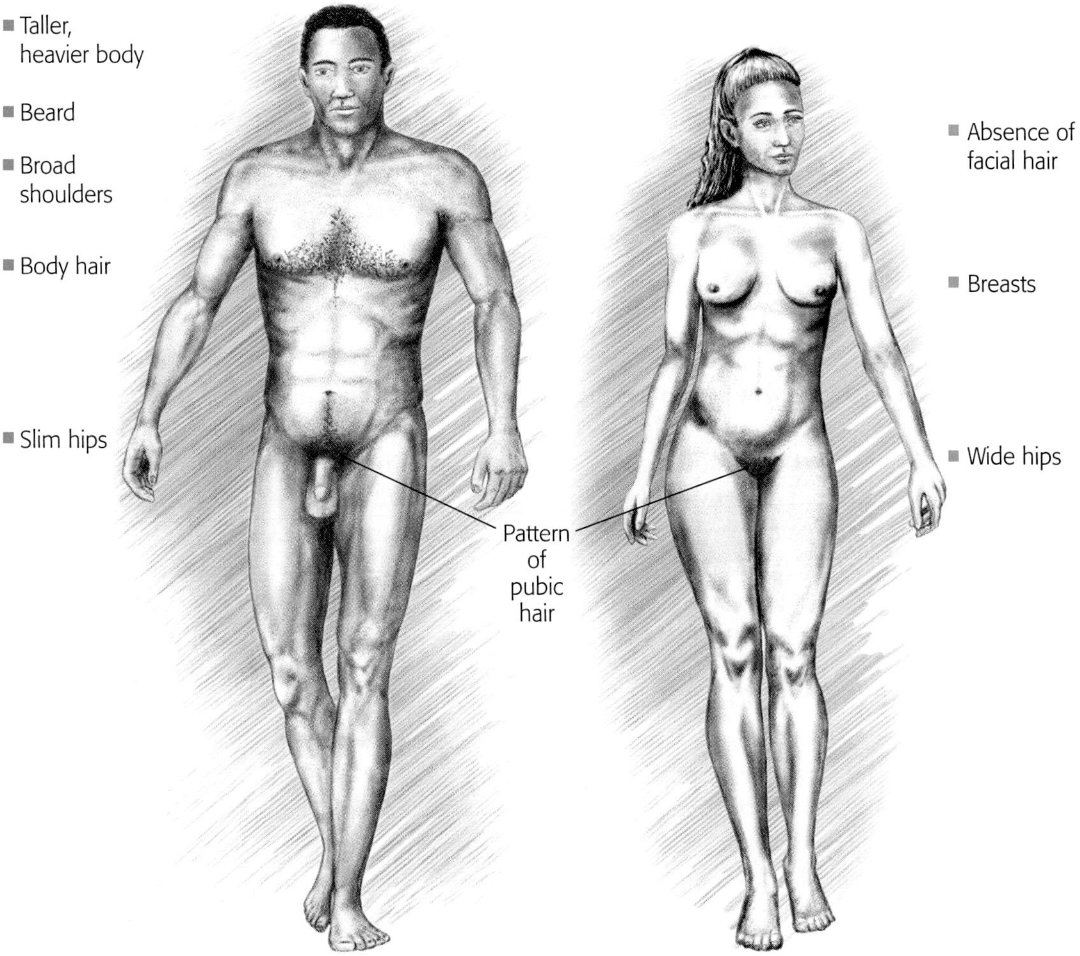


FIGURE 2.2 **Male Secondary Sex Characteristics.** Compared with females, men tend to have broader shoulders, slimmer hips, a larger proportion of muscle to body fat, lower voice, and facial and more body hair. These differences are the result of the androgenic ("male-producing") steroid hormones acting on androgen-sensitive body structures.

sensitive body structures. Knowing about one's own and a partner's sexual biology can foster healthy sexuality in the following ways:

1. Increasing understanding and appreciation of one's own and a partner's sexual functions
2. Increasing one's ability to attend to, and communicate about, sexual needs, matters of reproductive and sexual health, and pregnancy
3. Developing ways to use physical sexual experiences to foster intimacy, mutuality, and enjoyment in emotionally close relationships
4. Avoiding unintended pregnancy and the transmission of sexual infections
5. Assessing critically messages about your body and erotic experience portrayed in media, advertising, fashion, and social trends
6. Being a knowledgeable sex educator of children

As you read this chapter, keep in mind that sexual biology affects nonbodily dimensions of sexuality. For example, individuals are often socially classified as males or females by the presence of specific primary and secondary sex characteristics. Sexual biology can influence the ability to attract sexual and/or romantic partners, which, in turn, affects attitudes about oneself as attractive and desirable. Sexual biology also can affect intimacy and trust because the skin is both a psychological and a physical boundary of the self. Letting someone see the "outer you" partially or completely unclothed is a way of trusting that person to accept and value the "inner you," even if you judge some aspects of your "outer you" as unattractive (e.g., stretch marks, blemished skin, thinning scalp hair). It also requires a degree of trust to let someone touch you in "private," sensitive places or to join your body with someone else's to produce intense sensual/emotional experiences.

## The Testes

**testes** the pair of male reproductive organs that produce sperm cells and steroid sex hormones
**scrotum** the sac of skin that contains the testes
**cremaster** a thin muscle that raises and lowers the scrotum relative to the body
**seminiferous tubules** small tubules in the testes in which sperm are produced

The testes are a pair of oval-shaped organs about 3 centimeters long and 2 centimeters wide. They produce sperm and sex hormones, principally testosterone and related substances. The word *testis* is derived from the Latin word meaning "witness" or "spectator" and, as such, is the root of the words *testify, testament,* and *testimony.* The reasons for this association are not clear. One hypothesis is that in Roman society, only males could bear witness, so the act of testifying became associated with the male organs themselves. Holding one's own scrotum, or another's, came to signify telling the truth.

The testes are located in the scrotum, a sac-like structure that is attached to the front of the pelvis. Each testis is suspended in the scrotum at the end of a fibrous structure (*spermatic cord*) that contains nerves, blood vessels, a sperm duct called the vas deferens, and a thin muscle called the cremaster (see Figure 2.1B). The cremaster surrounds a testis and raises and lowers it inside the scrotum. The cremaster raises the testis in response to cold, fear, anger, and sexual stimulation. Normally, one testis is a bit higher than the other.

During fetal life both testes develop inside the body, but shortly before birth they descend into the scrotum where they remain for life. Inside the scrotum the testes are kept about 5°F cooler than internal body temperature, which is necessary for sperm viability. Prolonged exposure to heat from wearing tight-fitting underwear or sitting in spas or hot tubs can diminish viable sperm production.

Each testis is subdivided into several hundred small segments containing one or more coiled seminiferous tubules, where, in a healthy adult male, about 150 million sperm are produced daily. Each seminiferous tubule is about 0.1 millimeter in diameter and between 30 and 70 centimeters (between 10 and 25 inches) long. Their combined length in both testes is almost a kilometer (about 1 mile). Interspersed among the seminiferous tubules are interstitial cells, which synthesize and release testosterone and other androgens.

## The Genital (Sperm) Duct System

**genital duct system** a four-segment biological tube for transporting sperm and seminal fluid
**epididymis** a coiled tube connected to the testis that stores and matures sperm

The genital duct system is a long, Y-shaped tube divided into four parts through which sperm move from the testes to the outside (see Figure 2.1).

### Epididymis

Sperm manufactured in the seminiferous tubules leave the testis through a small number of tubes (*rete testis*) and enter an adjacent structure called the epididymis, which lies on the back of the testis. Each epididymis is composed of about 6 meters of tubule, which is densely coiled into a structure about 4 centimeters long. In the epididymis, damaged sperm are removed, and those that remain are concentrated into a dense mass and become capable of fertilizing an egg. Periodic

HEALTHY SEXUALITY

### Penis Enlargement Scams

Want to make a fortune? Then market a pill, pump, salve, lotion, stretching device, or exercises (e.g., "jelqing") that promise to enlarge the penis. That's what Steve Warshak did when he promoted Enzyte, a combination of vitamins, minerals, and the amino acid arginine, as a penis enlargement product. Enzyte grossed hundreds of millions of dollars before Warshak and his business partner (his mother) were sent to jail for fraud. Nothing other than risky surgery can alter the anatomy of the penis.

Many men believe that their masculinity and sexual desirability are reflected in the size of their penis. Believing their masculinity is at stake, it is no wonder that many men seek penile enlargement to bolster their self-image and, they imagine, increase their esteem in the eyes of sex partners. Whereas some people are turned on by the fantasy of a large penis, in reality, most men and women concede that what is important is that a penis function normally.

The length of nonerect penises ranges from 8 to 10 centimeters (3–4 inches), whereas erect penises are between 12 and 18 centimeters (5–7 inches). Penis size, like the size of the feet, brain, or liver, is determined by one's genes and biology. All medical experts agree that no drug, vitamin, exercise, or device can alter the anatomy of the penis. Penis enlargement scammers know this, too, and their advertising often confuses penis size and erectile capability in order to dupe potential customers. Erections are the result of increased blood flow to the penis, not alterations in penile anatomy. An erect penis is, indeed, larger than a nonerect one, but the change in size is determined by penile anatomy, which cannot be altered other than surgically. Certain drugs (e.g., Viagra, Cialis, Levitra), called PDE5 inhibitors, and possibly some plant extracts, can alter penile blood flow to create and prolong erections, and these substances are sometimes added secretly (since it is illegal to add a prescription drug to an herbal medicine) to a penis enlargement product. So, don't be fooled. Men, your sexual anatomy is OK just as it is.

contractions of smooth muscle in the epididymis move sperm through it. Because an epididymis is coiled, it is firmer than its associated testis, and its ridges can be felt in the back of the scrotum.

### Vas Deferens

Each epididymis is connected to a **vas deferens**, a relatively straight tube about 35 centimeters long. Each vas deferens courses upward in the spermatic cord from the scrotum into the body's pelvic cavity. Each vas deferens is lined with smooth muscle, the contractions of which force sperm through it. The fertility control method called *vasectomy* involves blocking movement of sperm into the penis, usually by surgically removing a portion of the vas (see Chapter 5).

**vas deferens** a tube that transports sperm from the scrotum into the body

**ejaculatory duct** a straight tube that connects a vas deferens to the urethra

**urethra** the tube that courses through the penis and through which urine and semen pass

### Ejaculatory Duct

Each vas deferens connects to an inch-long, straight tube called an **ejaculatory duct**, which opens into a single tube, the **urethra**. The urethra courses through the penis to the outside.

### Urethra

The urethra is the exit tube for both sperm and urine. It courses through the penis from the bladder to outside the body. A small band of smooth muscle surrounds the urethra near the bladder. When that muscle contracts, that portion of the tube is closed off. This prevents ejaculate from entering the bladder (called *retrograde ejaculation*). Contraction of this band of muscle makes it difficult for a man to urinate when the penis is erect.

## Fluid-Producing Glands

As they move through the genital duct system on their way out of the body, sperm become mixed with secretions from several fluid-producing glands (see Figure 2.1).

When a man ejaculates, the fluid-producing glands empty their contents into tubes that connect to the genital ducts. The fluid-producing glands are the following:

1. A pair of seminal vesicles. These are located near the junction of each vas deferens and ejaculatory duct.
2. The prostate gland. This is a chestnut-sized organ surrounding the urethra near its origin at the bladder.
3. Cowper's (bulbourethral) glands. These are a pair of pea-sized organs located along the urethra near the prostate.

**seminal vesicles** a pair of glands near the bladder that manufacture part of seminal fluid
**prostate gland** an organ at the base of the bladder that produces part of seminal fluid
**Cowper's (bulbourethral) glands** a pair of glands that produce lubricating fluid
**seminal fluid** fluids produced by the seminal vesicles and prostate
**semen** the mixture of seminal fluid and sperm that is ejaculated

The seminal vesicles and prostate produce a white, semiviscous seminal fluid, made up of water, fructose as an energy source for sperm movement, vitamins, minerals, and a variety of proteins. Seminal fluid nurtures sperm, protects sperm from attack by the female immune system, and neutralizes the acidity of the vagina. The mixture of sperm and seminal fluid is called semen. By volume, semen is about 95% seminal fluid and 5% sperm.

The Cowper's glands produce small amounts of a lubricating fluid ("pre-ejaculate" or "precum") that enters the urethra soon after a man becomes sexually aroused and before ejaculation. Sometimes drops of this fluid can be seen at the tip of the erect penis. It was once incorrectly thought that pre-ejaculate contained sufficient sperm to effect fertilization and thus contributed to the ineffectiveness of penile withdrawal as a fertility control method (see Chapter 5). In truth, pre-ejaculate contains few if any sperm and thus is highly unlikely to contribute to a pregnancy. However, this fluid can carry human immunodeficiency virus (HIV), the virus that causes acquired immune deficiency syndrome (AIDS).

## Ejaculation

**ejaculation** the release of semen
**emission phase** the movement of semen to the back part of the urethra
**expulsion phase** the release of semen from the penis

Ejaculation is the release of semen (seminal fluid plus sperm) from the penis. When a man ejaculates, nerve signals from the brain (where the ejaculation center is located) travel down the spinal cord to the smooth muscle tissue that surrounds the tubes of the genital ducts and the fluid-producing glands.

In the emission phase of ejaculation, contraction of this smooth muscle forces seminal fluid into the genital duct system and propels seminal fluid plus sperm (semen) to the prostate. The semen's journey is blocked temporarily by stricture of the portion of the urethra that courses through the prostate (*prostatic urethra*), and a man feels a sensation that ejaculation is about to occur. Learning to recognize this sensation and those that precede it is the key to developing ejaculatory control (see Chapter 10).

In the expulsion phase of ejaculation, semen that has collected in the prostatic urethra is forcefully propelled from the body by strong, rhythmic contractions of pelvic muscles and the coat of smooth muscle that surrounds the urethra. The rhythmic contractions force the semen out of the body in spurts. The amount of semen of a man who has not recently ejaculated is about a teaspoon. The volume of ejaculate increases the longer ejaculation is prolonged during a sexual episode. So-called wet dreams are spontaneous ejaculations during sleep, usually occurring during adolescence.

## The Penis

The surface of the penis has two distinct regions, the *glans* (or head) and the *shaft* (FIGURE 2.3). A rim or crown of tissue, called the *corona*, marks the junction of the

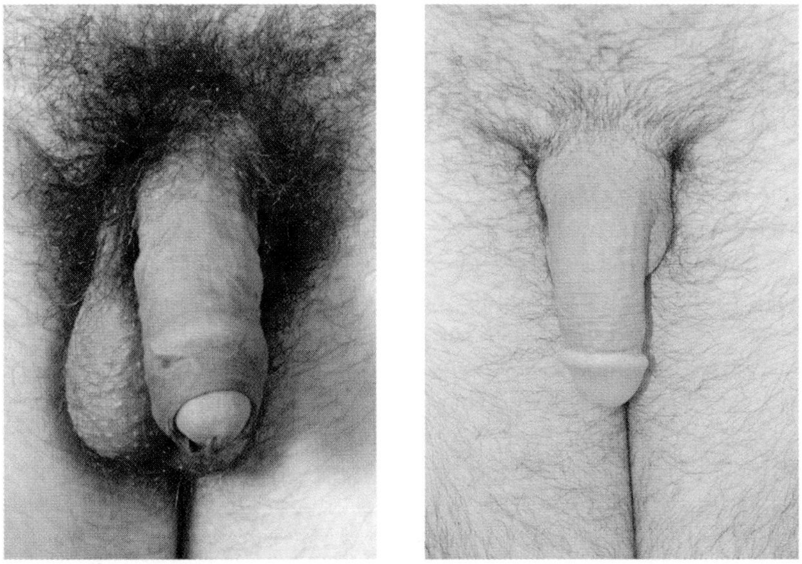

(a) (b)

FIGURE 2.3 **The Penis.** (a) Uncircumcised penis. (b) Circumcised penis.

glans and shaft. The glans and regions of the shaft can be quite sensitive to tactile stimulation. There is no particular technique or site of penile sexual stimulation that is preferred by all men. Individuals have preferences with regard to penile sexual stimulation.

The shaft of the penis is composed of three sponge-like, cylindrical structures, the two *corpora cavernosa* and the single *corpus spongiosum* (FIGURE 2.4). The two

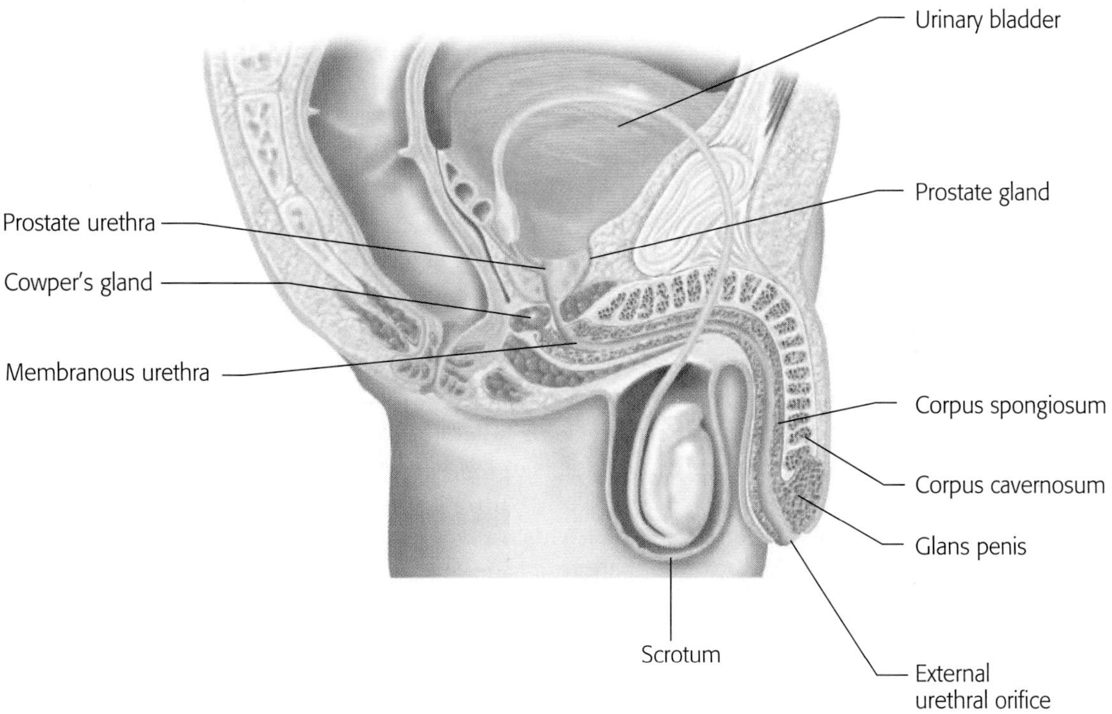


FIGURE 2.4 **Spongy Tissues of the Penis.** The penis is composed of three cylinders of spongy tissue arranged in a triangle: a *corpus cavernosum* on each side of the top of the penis and a *corpus spongiosum* on the bottom. The urethra courses through the *corpus spongiosum*. Erection occurs when blood flowing into the penis fills the spongy tissues.

corpora cavernosa lie next to each other and make up the top side of the penis. The corpus spongiosum lies underneath the corpora cavernosa; it contains the urethra. The penis is not a muscle and, unlike in many other animals, it does not have a bone. The back portion of the penis extends inside the body, where it is attached to the bony pelvis.

Normally the penis is soft (*flaccid*). However, it can become hard and enlarge when arteries that carry blood into the penis expand (*dilate*), which increases the amount of blood flowing into the penis and decreases the amount flowing out. The extra blood goes into the cylindrical spongy tissues, especially the two uppermost ones (*corpora cavernosae*), and this causes the penis to swell and become erect. When the arteries bringing blood to the penis go back to their normal size, the penis returns to its nonerect state. Drugs that promote erectile capability (e.g., Viagra, Cialis, Levitra) act by slowing the rate by which the penile arteries return to their normal diameter. Whereas there may be considerable variation among men in the size of the penis when flaccid, there is less variation in penis size when erect; smaller flaccid penises tend to enlarge relatively more than larger flaccid penises do. Contrary to advertisements and folklore, it is not possible to permanently enlarge a penis with drugs, devices, or manipulation.

Erections can occur when a man is sexually excited (*psychogenic erection*), when the penis is touched, from the pressure of a full bladder or an enlarged prostate (*spinal erection*), and during sleep (*REM erection*). Erections resulting from sexual excitement involve the brain, which interprets thoughts, memories, and sensory stimuli (e.g., what is seen, felt, smelled, heard) as erotic, decides that a sexual response is personally and socially permissible, and then sends nerve signals down the spinal cord to the nerves that control blood flow into the penis (**FIGURE 2.5**). This is the excitement phase of the male sexual response cycle.

Some erections, known as spinal erections, do not involve the brain; nerves in the spinal cord that control blood flow to the penis are stimulated by nerves in various parts of the pelvis—for example, the skin of the penis, the bladder, and the prostate. Spinal erections also can occur spontaneously without any apparent stimulus. Spontaneous erections can occur in children (even infants), but they are most common in the early and late teens (often accompanied by great embarrassment); they tend to diminish in frequency in adulthood.

REM erections (also called *nocturnal penile tumescence* [*NPT*]) occur several times a night during episodes of rapid eye movement (REM) sleep. Typically, a person dreams during REM; however, REM erections do not necessarily mean that a man is having sexy dreams. No one knows why REM erections occur. A man awakening right after a period of REM sleep may have an erection. He may not feel sexually aroused at first, but noticing the erection may suggest to him (or his partner) that he is.

**foreskin** a fold of skin that covers the glans penis
**circumcision** surgical removal of the foreskin
**smegma** a white, cheesy substance that can accumulate under the foreskin

Males are born with a fold of skin called the **foreskin** or *prepuce* covering the end of the penis. In the United States today, parents of male infants can elect to have the foreskin removed surgically within hours after a child's birth. Removal of the foreskin is called **circumcision**. Muslim and Jewish traditions call for the circumcision of all males. Although circumcision is associated with several health benefits, including protection against penile cancer, HIV/AIDS, and the transmission of human papillomavirus (HPV) to female sex partners, the American Academy of Pediatrics does not recommend routine neonatal circumcision. The removal of the foreskin does eliminate the buildup of **smegma**, a white, cheesy substance that can accumulate under the foreskin. Careful hygiene, however, also is a way to handle the buildup of smegma. The belief that circumcision, by exposing the head of the

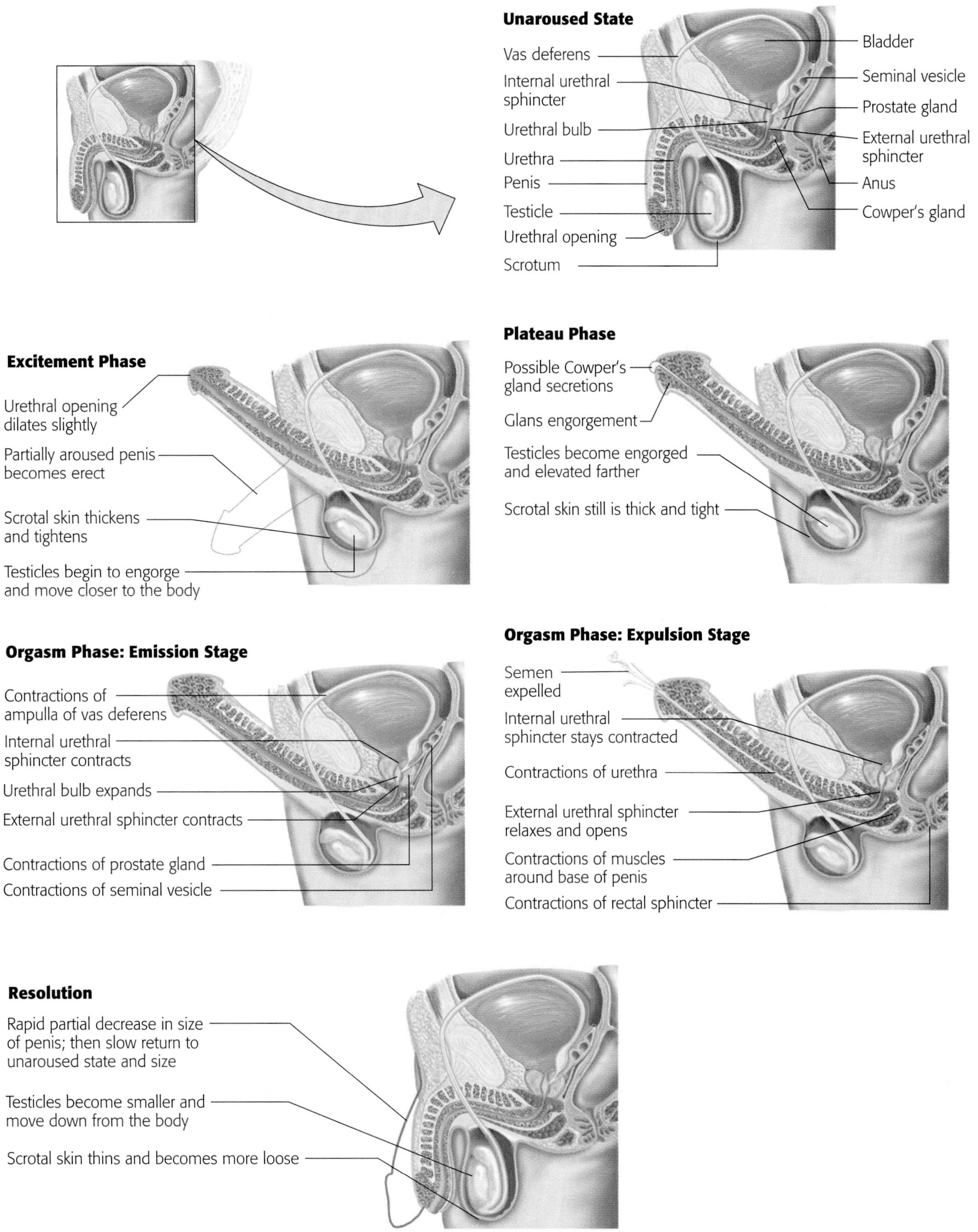
Unaroused State
Vas deferens
Internal urethral sphincter
Urethral bulb
Urethra
Penis
Testicle
Urethral opening
Scrotum
Bladder
Seminal vesicle
Prostate gland
External urethral sphincter
Anus
Cowper's gland
Excitement Phase
Urethral opening dilates slightly
Partially aroused penis becomes erect
Scrotal skin thickens and tightens
Testicles begin to engorge and move closer to the body
Plateau Phase
Possible Cowper's gland secretions
Glans engorgement
Testicles become engorged and elevated farther
Scrotal skin still is thick and tight
Orgasm Phase: Emission Stage
Contractions of ampulla of vas deferens
Internal urethral sphincter contracts
Urethral bulb expands
External urethral sphincter contracts
Contractions of prostate gland
Contractions of seminal vesicle
Orgasm Phase: Expulsion Stage
Semen expelled
Internal urethral sphincter stays contracted
Contractions of urethra
External urethral sphincter relaxes and opens
Contractions of muscles around base of penis
Contractions of rectal sphincter
Resolution
Rapid partial decrease in size of penis; then slow return to unaroused state and size
Testicles become smaller and move down from the body
Scrotal skin thins and becomes more loose

FIGURE 2.5 **Male Sexual Response Cycle.**

penis, makes men more easily aroused sexually and, therefore, unable to control ejaculation is untrue. The belief that the presence of a foreskin blocks sexual pleasure is also untrue. When a man becomes aroused, the glans protrudes beyond the foreskin.

Penis size often is mistakenly considered a measure of masculinity and sexual prowess. This belief tends to occur in societies in which the penis is a symbol of male strength and fertility. One must not confuse a symbol, and the expectations and fantasies that it generates, with reality. Although there is variation among men in the size of the penis, just as there is variation in body height, the size of the penis has no bearing on an individual's personality characteristics, and only at the extreme limits of anatomical variation does it have any functional significance.

## Androgenic Steroid Hormones

Hormones are chemicals produced in one part of the body, generally a specific hormone-producing tissue or organ, that bring about changes in other parts of the body. During fetal life and at puberty, *sex steroid hormones* produced by the testes or ovaries bring about the development of reproductive and sexual anatomy (see Chapter 8), and in adulthood, they maintain and influence the functions of these structures.

**androgens** hormones that promote the development and maintenance of male and some female sex characteristics
**testosterone** the principal male sex steroid hormone

Androgens (*andros* is from the Greek, meaning "male") are a group of sex steroid hormones that are responsible for the growth and development in the male fetus of the penis, genital ducts, fluid-producing glands, and some parts of the brain; during puberty for the growth, development, and functioning of those organs, and the formation of secondary sex characteristics associated with maleness; and during adulthood for the maintenance and function of male primary and secondary sex characteristics (Table 2.1).

There are several types of androgenic hormones (Table 2.2). The principal androgen is testosterone, which is produced by special (*interstitial* or *Leydig*) cells in the testes and then transported within the testes to testosterone-sensitive structures or carried throughout the bloodstream to testosterone-sensitive cells and organs. Cells capable of responding to testosterone and other androgens have receptors that specifically bind the hormone. The interaction of hormone and receptor is similar to the way a key (the hormone) fits into a lock (the receptor). In some instances, an androgen–receptor interaction triggers an almost immediate response; in other instances the response may occur after several hours. In some cells, testosterone is converted inside the cell to a different hormone that brings about biological changes.

**Table 2.1** Functions of Androgens in Males

| |
|---|
| Develop the sperm ducts, semen-producing glands, and the penis in the fetus |
| Maintain function of the sperm ducts, semen-producing glands, and the penis during adult life |
| Support sperm development |
| Support semen production |
| Initiate development of male secondary sex characteristics: male pattern of body hair, deep voice, muscle mass and tone |
| Cause interest in engaging in sexual activity |

The manufacture and release of testosterone from the testes is governed by the male hypothalamo-pituitary-gonadal (HPG) system (FIGURE 2.6), which is composed of the following:

- *Hypothalamo* refers to certain nerve cells in the brain's hypothalamus that manufacture and secrete into the bloodstream a hormone called gonadotrophin releasing factor (GnRF).

**hypothalamo-pituitary-gonadal (HPG) system** a "team" of hormone-producing structures responsible for sperm and androgen production
**gonadotrophin releasing factor (GnRf)** stimulates follicle-stimulating hormone (FSH) and luteinizing hormone (LH) production

**Table 2.2** Types of Androgens

| Type of Androgen | Source |
|---|---|
| Testosterone | Testes, ovaries |
| Dehydroepiandrosterone (DHEA) | Adrenal glands |
| Androstenedione (Andro) | Testes, adrenal glands, ovaries |
| Androstenediol | Testes, adrenal glands |
| Androsterone | Liver (from testosterone) |
| Dihydrotestosterone (DHT) | Testes |

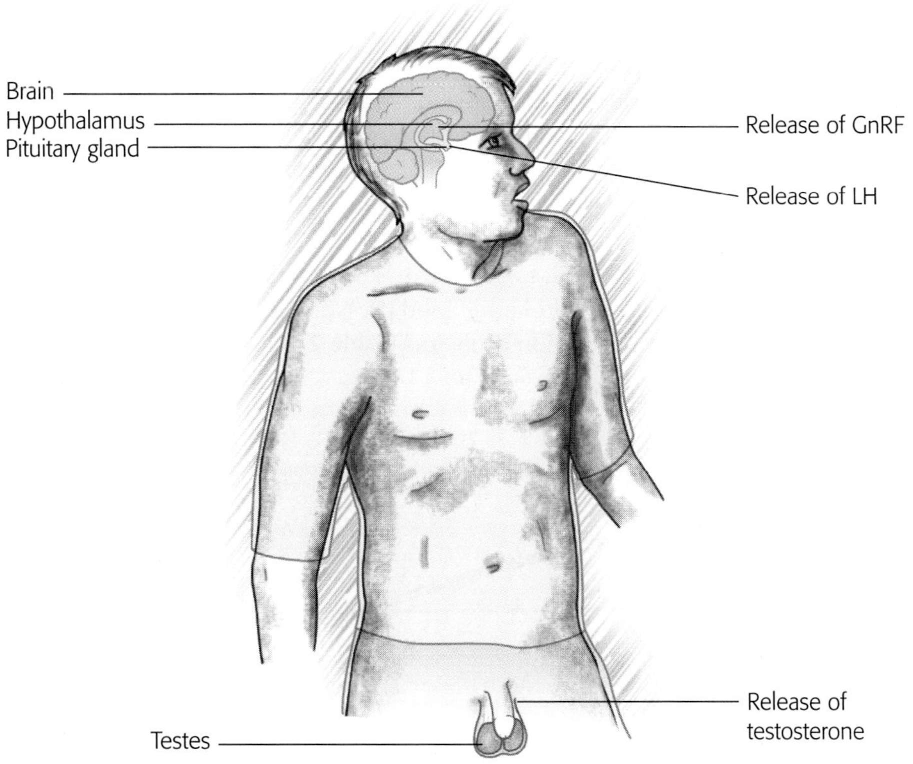


FIGURE 2.6 **The Male Hypothalamo-Pituitary-Gonadal (HPG) System.** Gonadotrophin releasing factor (GnRF) is manufactured by specific cells in the hypothalamus of the brain and released into the bloodstream. GnRF stimulates certain cells in the pituitary gland, located at the base of the brain, to manufacture and release luteinizing hormone (LH) into the bloodstream. In the testes, LH stimulates the interstitial cells to manufacture and release testosterone in the bloodstream. Testosterone circulates throughout the body and brings about biological responses in specific target cells. It also regulates the amount of GnRF manufactured by the hypothalamus.

**luteinizing hormone (LH)** a hormone produced by the pituitary gland that is responsible for releasing the egg from the ovary and stimulating the production of progesterone

**anabolic steriods** testosterone-like substances

- *Pituitary* refers to the pituitary gland, which is located at the base of the brain. It responds to GnRF by releasing into the bloodstream a substance called **luteinizing hormone (LH)**, which circulates throughout the body.
- *Gonadal* refers to cells in the testes that respond to LH by manufacturing and releasing testosterone into the bloodstream.

The amount of testosterone in the bloodstream controls the activity of the HPG system. When blood levels of testosterone rise, the hypothalamus slows the production of GnRF, which slows the pituitary's production of LH, which ultimately results in a slowdown of testosterone production by the testes. As blood levels of testosterone fall, GnRF and LH levels rise, resulting in a rise in testosterone secretion.

The amount of testosterone in a male's body varies across the life span (**FIGURE 2.7**). During fetal life and at puberty, testosterone levels are relatively high. In childhood, testosterone levels are the lowest in a male's lifetime. During adulthood, testosterone levels vary on daily, monthly, and possibly seasonal cycles.

Besides their effects on male reproduction and sexuality, androgens are responsible for the growth of genital and underarm hair in both sexes, and to some degree the maintenance of interest in erotic experience and feelings of aggression in both sexes (discussed later). Androgens contribute to acne in both males and females by stimulating the growth of *sebaceous glands* in hair follicles in the skin and the production of a waxy substance called *sebum*. Acne occurs when sebum and cell debris become trapped in the opening of a hair follicle. Androgens also contribute to *male pattern baldness*.

Testosterone and a variety of related androgens are used illegally (generally by athletes) as **anabolic steroids** (*anabolic* means "growth promoting") to increase muscle mass and bone density. In an untrained individual, anabolic steroids have little effect on muscle growth. In trained athletes, however, anabolic steroids accelerate the healing of muscle tissue that has been damaged during intense strength training. With less rest required between workouts, an athlete can become stronger, faster. Anabolic steroids are associated with a variety of unintended effects, including elevated blood cholesterol and blood pressure, liver and heart damage, acne, infertility, cancer, and erection problems (**Table 2.3**).

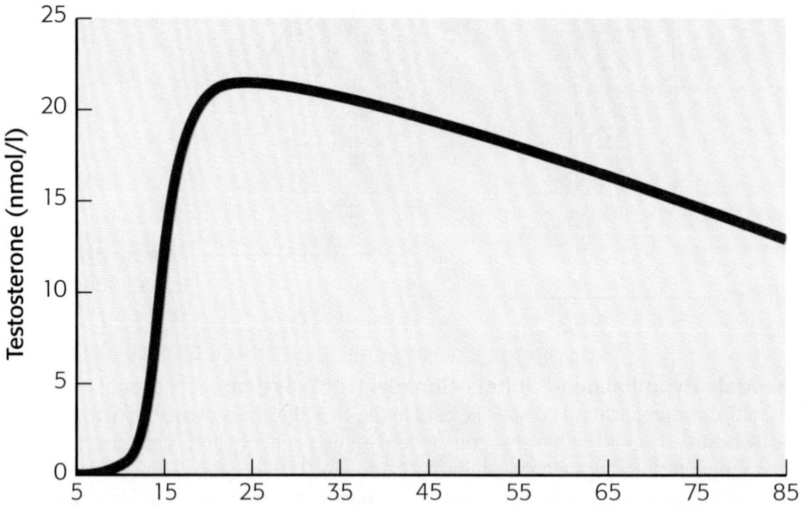


FIGURE 2.7 **Amounts of Androgens in the Male Body Across the Lifespan.**

Adapted from Vermeulen, A. (1996) Declining androgens with age: An overview. In: Vermeulen, A. & Oddens, B. B. (eds.). *Androgens and the aging male.* New York: Pantheon.

**Table 2.3** Health Effects of Anabolic Steroids

| Men and Women | Men | Women |
|---|---|---|
| Liver tumors and cancer | Erection problems | Growth of facial hair |
| Jaundice (yellowish pigmentation of skin, tissues, and body fluids) | Shrinking of the testicles | Loss of head hair |
| Fluid retention | Reduced sperm count | Changes in or cessation of the menstrual cycle |
| High blood pressure | Infertility | Enlargement of the clitoris |
| Increases in LDL (bad cholesterol) | Baldness | Deepened voice |
| Decreases in HDL (good cholesterol) | Development of breasts | |
| Kidney tumors | Increased risk for prostate cancer | |
| Severe acne | | |
| Trembling | | |
| Premature halting of growth and premature onset of puberty (in adolescents) | | |

## Androgens and Behavior

Laboratory experiments with a variety of nonhuman animals show that androgens can influence certain behaviors. For example, in male laboratory rats, testosterone stimulates mating behavior and aggression. In humans, androgens affect several aspects of behavior, including sensation seeking and risk taking, sexual interest, aggression, the tendency to want to dominate others, and some cognitive abilities.

### Sensation Seeking and Risky Behavior

Levels of testosterone are related to the tendency to become bored easily and seek novel, varied, complex, and intense sensations. Testosterone levels are also related to the willingness to take risks for the sake of such experiences, with an increased risk of smoking cigarettes and using other drugs, reckless driving, and risky sexual behaviors (e.g., not using condoms).

### Sexual Interest

At puberty, a dramatic increase in testosterone levels in both sexes correlates with a large increase in interest in sex. Medically, low levels of androgen in adults are associated with loss of interest in sex, and in many cases sexual interest can be restored when androgen levels are increased (see Chapter 10). Not only can androgens stimulate sexual interest, but sexual interest also can stimulate androgen production. A unique example involves a man who spent periods of several weeks in isolation on a remote island who carefully collected and weighed his daily beard shavings. Beard growth, which is stimulated by androgens, increased in anticipation of going to the mainland and reuniting with his sex partner, and it fell after he returned to the island.

## Dear Penelope . . .

***How do you know what a man likes sexually?***
***— New To Lovemaking***

*Dear New To Lovemaking,*

Despite what you may read in a popular magazine about male sexuality, male sexual needs, desires, and responses vary widely, and even the same man may prefer different sexual sensations from one sexual episode to the next. For example, magazine articles often report that men prefer stimulation of the end (or glans) of the penis because it possesses many nerve endings. However, some men find stimulation of the end of the penis irritating. Indeed, pressure or light touching on the underside of the penile shaft, or even a passionate kiss on the mouth, might be more stimulating.

It isn't helpful or fun if attempts to stimulate a man's penis are experienced by him as unpleasant. It's also a shame if a man thinks there's something wrong with him because he isn't that turned on by something that a magazine or book says he should be.

One way to know what a man likes is to ask him. You can do this by asking him to guide you either verbally or with his hand and to indicate to you with words, movements, or gestures how things are going. You also can ask directly with an open question, such as: "I want to make you feel good. What's the best way to do that?"

Courtesy of the UC Davis *Aggie*

## Competition

Prior to and during sports competition, testosterone levels rise in both male and female athletes. After the competition, testosterone levels in victorious male competitors remain high, whereas they return to normal in women and in losing male competitors. This same pattern holds for male observers of sports; fans who identify strongly with winning or losing teams also show elevated androgen levels.

## Aggression and Dominance

Aggression can be physical (hitting), verbal (shouting, swearing), angry, and hostile (resentful, suspicious). Elevated testosterone level is associated with aggres-

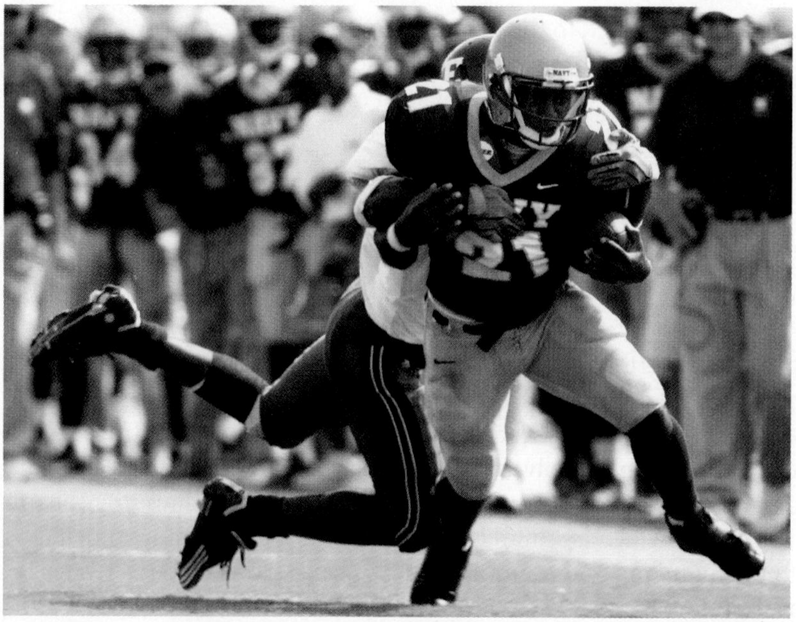

sion in both sexes. In males, aggression tends to be offensive; the goal is to dominate another person or group. In females, aggression tends to be defensive; the goals are to protect oneself and one's group (e.g., family, children).

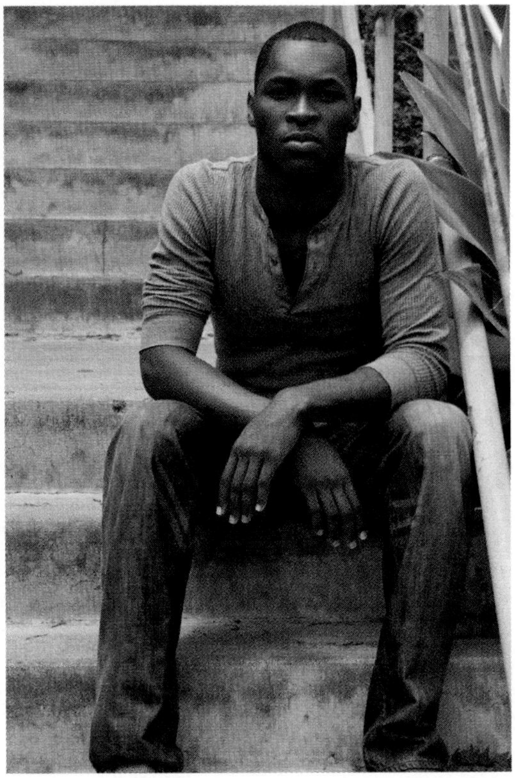

## Cognitive Abilities

Androgen levels are related to mathematical reasoning (problem solving with numbers) and performance of certain visual–spatial tasks, such as mentally rotating or manipulating an object, navigating a maze or map, and target-directed motor skills like throwing a ball.

Androgens can affect behavior by direct activation of brain cells that possess androgen receptors (*activating function*). Androgens can also alter brain structure (*organizing function*). For example, during fetal life, the fetal testes, adrenal glands, and/or the mother's body (either her own hormones or from hormone-like environmental pollutants she has ingested), produce androgens that circulate to the developing fetal brain and organize certain brain cells into functional units that, when activated or "switched on" later in life by a thought, environmental cue, or hormones, automatically bring about a specific, pre-programmed behavior.

To ascertain the effects of androgens on human brain development, scientists have studied females with a condition called *congenital adrenal hyperplasia* (CAH), the result of which is production of large amounts of androgen by the adrenal glands in fetal life. Even though they are genetic females and have ovaries, because of prenatal exposure to large amounts of androgen, at birth the genitalia of these individuals appear male-like. Often, these children undergo surgery to establish female-appearing genitalia, and they are raised as females. Although they think of themselves as female, as children these girls tend to prefer playing with trains, trucks, and other vehicles rather than dolls; rough-and-tumble play; and playing outdoor games with boys. Although not overly aggressive, they tend to be competitive and dominant compared with other girls, including non-CAH sisters.

The effects of androgens in a particular individual can affect *others'* behavior. For example, androgens in males produce a large jaw and prominent brow, which others generally regard as characteristics of a dominant individual. Depending on their outlook, other males may respond to the perception of dominance in another man by being aggressive in order to dominate him or being submissive or distant to avoid his anticipated aggressive behavior. Females may respond by being attracted to or repulsed by facial features suggesting dominance.

Human evolutionary psychologists hypothesize that androgen-stimulated behaviors exist because over the thousands of years of human evolution they have contributed to *reproductive fitness*—that is, the ability to outcompete others for sexual/reproductive mates and to foster the raising of offspring who themselves are likely to reproduce more successfully. For example, the real purpose of the changes in testosterone in men prior to, during, and shortly after athletic competition represents a biologically based capacity that supports reproduction, not athletics. The pre- and during competition rise in testosterone represents the activation of brain centers that govern aggression. The continued post-competition rise in testosterone among winners represents the need to remain aggressive to defend that which is won, whereas the drop in testosterone in losers represents acknowledgment of the loser's status in the competition for mates. In a woman, testosterone rises in response to being provoked by another's aggression, which is biologically advantageous to protect herself and her children.

## SEXUALITY IN REVIEW

- Primary male biological sex characteristics (those that contribute directly to reproduction) are the testes, sperm ducts, semen-producing glands, and penis.
- Secondary male sex characteristics include a large body size, small waist-to-hip ratio, greater proportion of muscle to fat, deep voice, and facial and body hair.
- The testes produce androgenic sex steroid hormones.
- Ejaculation is a two-phase process controlled by the brain.
- The penis is normally flaccid but enlarges and becomes erect due to sexual psychological arousal, touching, and during REM (dream) sleep.
- Androgenic sex hormones (principally testosterone) bring about a variety of characteristically male biological and behavioral features.

## CRITICAL THINKING ABOUT SEXUALITY

1. A large and increasing number of men believe they are not sufficiently muscular despite the fact that their bodies appear normal. In many instances, men who believe themselves to be insufficiently muscular feel less masculine, and freely admit that they wish to be bigger. Some men become so focused on pursuing greater muscularity that they consume dietary supplements and nutritional aids, lift weights almost obsessively, and in some cases take dangerous and illegal anabolic steroids. Researchers suggest that concerns over muscularity are due to the influence of media images of super-muscular men, such as professional athletes, film actors, and models in advertising. What is your assessment of this hypothesis?
2. Beer and cars top the list of products advertised on television sports programs. But ads for drugs for erectile dysfunction (ED) get plenty of television time, too. Why is that? Erectile dysfunction is most prevalent in men over 70 years old, a small portion of the population of adult men. Advertising ED drugs to this group on national television seems not worth the financial costs. Also, the actors in television ads for ED drugs appear to be in their 40s, not their 70s. Furthermore, sales of ED drugs are quite brisk among young men without erection problems. Critics argue that while the ads directly address ED, they cleverly suggest that all men can use these drugs as "sex enhancers." Find some ads on television, in magazines, or on the Internet that describe drugs for ED. In your view, do any of the ads encourage male fears about sexual performance or their masculinity? Are such ads appropriate in mass media? Do they really encourage men to "talk to their doctors about ED," as the advertisers claim?
3. Depending on geographic region, in the United States between 40% and 80% of newborn males are circumcised. Since circumcision is of little or no benefit, what are the reasons for the large degree of elective circumcision? What is your personal opinion of circumcision of newborn males?
4. What is your personal definition of masculinity?

## REFERENCES AND RECOMMENDED RESOURCES

### References

American Academy of Pediatrics. (1999). Circumcision policy statement. *Pediatrics, 103*, 686–693. Available at: http://aappolicy.aappublications.org/cgi/content/full/pediatrics.

Arnold, A. P. (2009). The organizational-activational hypothesis as the foundation for a unified theory of sexual differentiation of all mammalian tissues. *Hormones and Behavior, 55*, 570–578.

Basaria, S. (2010). Androgen abuse in athletes: Detection and consequences. *Journal of Clinical Endocrinology and Metabolism, 95*, 1533–1543.

Chiras, D. G. (2008). *Human biology.* Sudbury, MA: Jones & Bartlett Learning.

Frisén, L., et al. (2009). Gender role behavior, sexuality, and psychosocial adaptation in women with congenital adrenal hyperplasia due to CYP21A2 deficiency. *Journal of Clinical Endocrinology and Metabolism, 94*, 3432–3439.

Jones, R. E. (2006). *Human reproductive biology, 3rd ed.* San Diego: Academic Press.

Kerr, J. D. (2010). *Functional histology, 2nd ed.* New York: Mosby.

### Recommended Resources

Jones, R. E. (2006). *Human reproductive biology, 3rd ed.* San Diego: Academic Press. A most-readable undergraduate text.

Mayo Clinic. (2009). Penis enlargement scams: You're more normal than you think. Available at: http://www.mayoclinic.com/health/penis/MC00026. Information on penis enlargement scams.

MedlinePlus. (2010). Male reproductive system. Available at: http://www.nlm.nih.gov/medlineplus/malereproductivesystem.html. Information on the male reproductive system.

Nieschlag, E., et al. (2009). *Andrology: Male reproductive health and dysfunction.* London: Springer. An authoritative medical text.

Zilbergeld, B. (1999). *The new male sexuality.* New York: Bantam. An authoritative guide to all aspects of male sexuality.

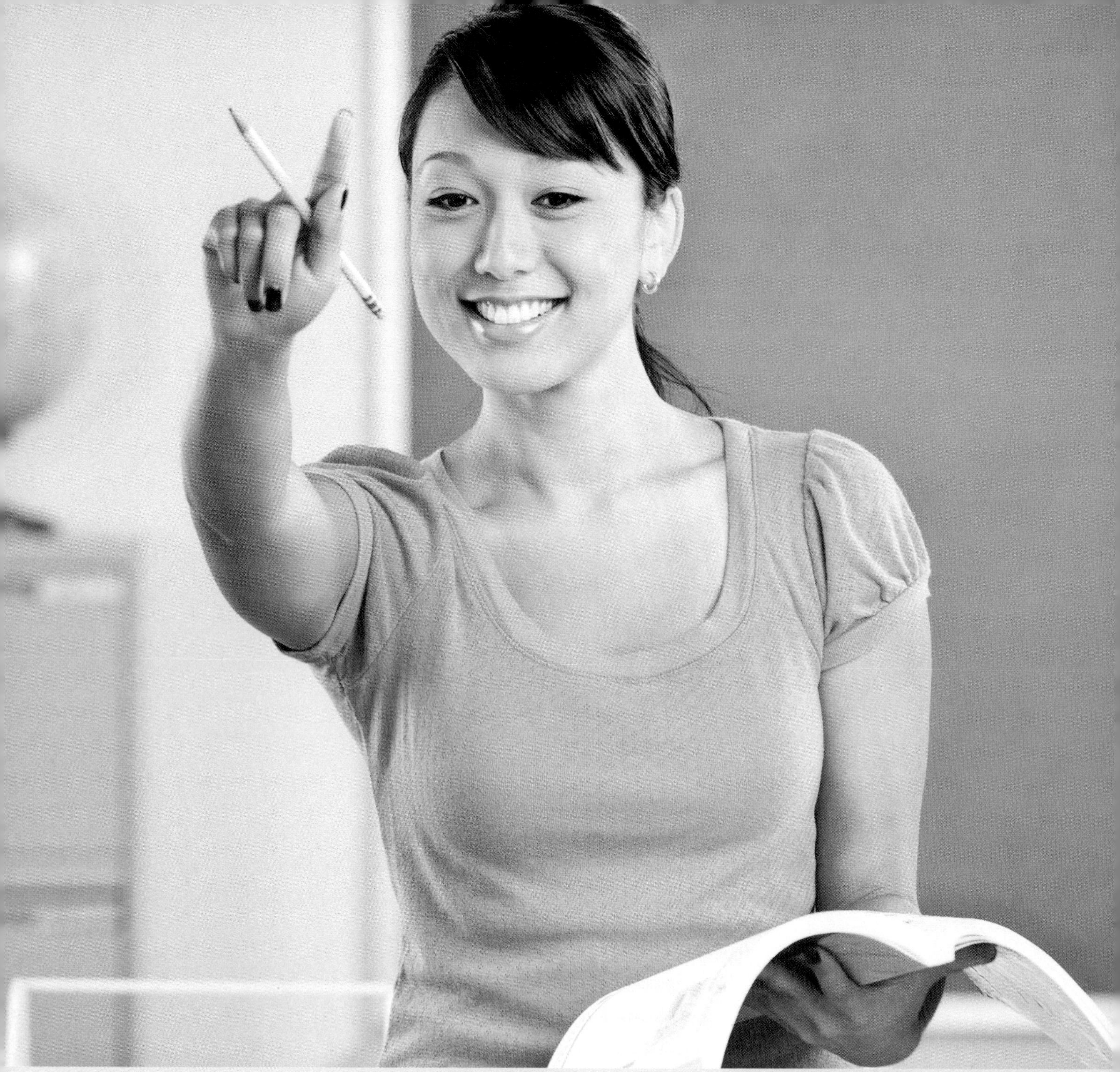

*"The kind of beauty I want most is the hard-to-get kind that comes from within—strength, courage, dignity."*

— Ruby Dee

CHAPTER 3

# Female Sexual Biology

## Student Learning Objectives

1. List and describe the female primary sex characteristics
2. List and describe the female secondary sex characteristics
3. Identify the functions of the ovaries
4. Describe the structure and function of the fallopian (uterine) tubes
5. Describe the structure and function of the uterus and cervix
6. Identify the two principal female sex hormones and list their functions
7. Describe the structure and function of the breasts
8. List and describe the stages of the menstrual cycle

From its origins about 3 or 4 billion years ago, life on Earth has maintained itself through the production of new individuals from existing ones. In some animal species, individuals produce many, many new offspring to ensure that at least some will survive disease, environmental hazards, and predation so that they too can reproduce. In other animal species, including humans, only a few offspring are usually produced by each female, but offspring are protected during development to increase their chances of surviving to reproductive age. The basic human female reproductive processes are the following:

1. *Internal ovulation.* In many species, ova are released into the environment where they are at high risk for predation and destruction. However, human ova remain inside the female body, which offers considerable protection from environmental hazards.
2. *Insemination.* Through sexual intercourse, sperm are deposited into the female vagina leading to fertilization within the female body.
3. *Internal fertilization.* Ova are fertilized inside a fallopian tube.
4. *Intrauterine development.* Embryonic and fetal development take place inside a female's uterus; the female's body provides nutrients for fetal development and protection from predators, disease, and environmental hazards.
5. *Postnatal care.* Infants are fed milk produced by the female breasts.

## Female Primary and Secondary Sex Characteristics

**primary sex characteristics** body structures that contribute to reproduction and sexual activity
**internal female primary sex characteristics** ovaries, fallopian tubes, uterus, vagina
**external female primary sex characteristics** mons veneris, labia minora, labia majora, clitoris
**female secondary sex characteristics** female-specific body structures not involved in the production or delivery of eggs or maintenance of pregnancy
**ovaries** a pair of organs in the pelvic cavity in which eggs and sex hormones are produced
**estrogen** a sex steroid hormone that is predominant in females
**progesterone** a sex steroid hormone involved in the maintenance of pregnancy
**ovarian (graffian) follicle** an egg and its surrounding nutrient and hormone-producing cells

Female primary sex characteristics consist of the organs that contribute to reproduction and sexual activity (FIGURE 3.1). Some structures are located inside the body and others are outside. Internal female primary sex characteristics include the ovaries, fallopian tubes, uterus, and vagina. External female primary sex characteristics include the vaginal labia and the clitoris. Besides producing fertilized eggs and fostering pregnancy, female primary sex characteristics often mark a newborn *socially* as a female, meaning that her social group will expect her to demonstrate certain personality characteristics (*gender stereotyping*) and to behave in accordance with her social group's rules for appropriate female behavior (*gender role*) (see Chapter 8).

Female secondary sex characteristics consist of the breasts, and in comparison to males, wider hips; a greater proportion of body fat; less hair on arms, legs, and torso; and smaller stature. Secondary sex characteristics appear at puberty when hormones change specific body structures from child to adult form.

### The Ovaries

Each female has two ovaries. These slightly flattened, oval-shaped organs are each about the size of an almond. Located in the pelvic cavity, they are separated from one another by the uterus and fallopian tubes. Each ovary is attached by ligaments to the body wall and the uterus. The ovaries produce ova and sex hormones, principally estrogen and progesterone (discussed later). The ova lie near the surface of the ovary and are surrounded by clusters of nutrient and hormone-producing cells. Each ovum and its contingent of encircling cells are called an ovarian (or graffian) follicle.

The ovaries develop in a fetus about the fifth week after fertilization, and soon thereafter immature, nonfertilizable ova begin to develop in them. By the fifth month after fertilization, the ovaries contain a combined total of about 7 million

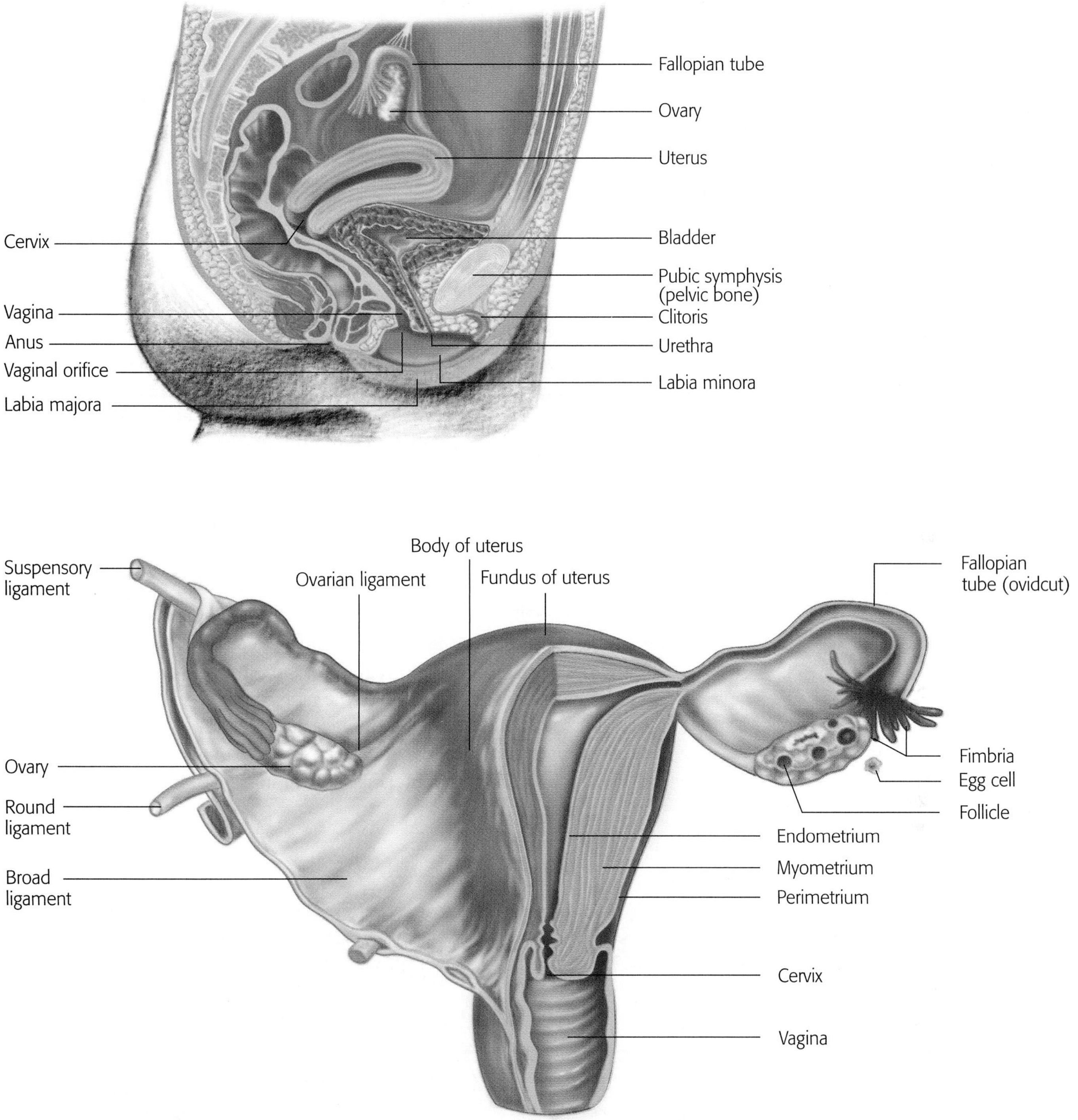


FIGURE 3.1 **Female Primary Sex Characteristics.** Eggs (ova) are produced in the ovaries. When an egg is released from the ovary, it is taken up by an adjacent fallopian tube and transported toward the uterus. Sperm deposited in the vagina travel through the uterus to the fallopian tubes. If an egg is present in a tube, fertilization may take place. The fertilized ovum travels to the uterus, where pregnancy takes place.

immature ova, all that a woman will ever have in her lifetime. From that point on, the immature ova continually die (a process called *follicular atresia*), such that at birth the total in both ovaries is about 2 million, and by age 50 no viable ova are left. The cessation of ovum production is associated with the cessation of menstrual periods, called the **menopause**.

**menopause** the cessation of menstrual periods

## The Fallopian (Uterine) Tubes

**fallopian (uterine) tubes** a pair of structures responsible for transporting eggs from the ovaries to the uterus
**uterus** an organ in the pelvic cavity in which the fetus develops
**endometrium** the inner lining of the uterus responsible for nurturing the fetus

There are two fallopian tubes, one on each side of the pelvic cavity. Each fallopian tube is about 10 centimeters long and lies adjacent to an ovary. One end of a fallopian tube is connected to the uterus. The other end is open to the pelvic cavity—that is, the ovary and the fallopian tube are not connected. The open end has fingerlike projections called *fimbriae* that sweep over the surface of the adjacent ovary. When an ovum is released from the ovary, it rises off the surface of its ovary, and the fimbriae of the adjacent fallopian tube capture it; fertilization may occur inside the tube if sperm are present. Occasionally, an ovum enters the fallopian tube on the other side of the uterus instead of the adjacent tube.

## The Uterus

The uterus is a hollow, pear-shaped organ about the size of a woman's closed fist and is situated in the pelvic cavity behind the bladder. Sperm travel from the vagina through the uterus to the fallopian tubes to fertilize an egg. The fertilized egg then travels down the fallopian tube and into the uterus, where *implantation* (see Chapter 4) and subsequent development take place. The uterus is composed of these three layers:

1. *Outer:* Made up of fibrous connective tissue that helps support the uterus in the pelvic cavity.
2. *Middle:* Muscle fibers that provide the strong contractile forces necessary to expel a baby at birth.
3. *Inner:* A soft, glandular tissue called the endometrium, which nurtures a fetus during the first three months of pregnancy. During each menstrual cycle, the endometrium thickens to prepare the uterus for pregnancy. If fertilization does not occur, the thickened tissue and some of the tiny blood vessels of the endometrium are sloughed off, resulting in a menstrual period. Occasionally, dense masses of uterine smooth muscle tissue called *fibroids*

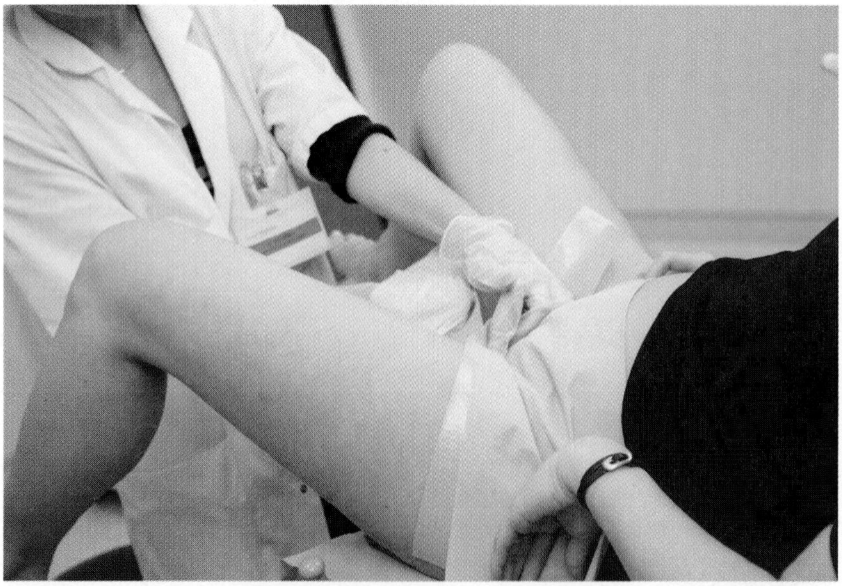

The gynecological exam is a medical examination of a woman's sexual and reproductive system can form and cause irregular menstrual bleeding and interfere with fertility. Fibroids can be removed from a uterus by surgical techniques.

The lower part of the uterus, the cervix, is connected to the vagina. The cervix is composed of fibrous tissue and has many mucus-secreting glands. The fibrous tissue resists stretching and thus helps to retain the fetus, amniotic fluid, and placenta (which collectively weigh about 10 pounds by the time the baby is born) during pregnancy. The glands secrete cervical mucus, which changes in composition and consistency during the menstrual cycle. Examining the cervical mucus is a fertility awareness method of contraception (see Chapter 5). The Pap smear is a medical test to examine the cervix for the presence of cancer or precancerous cells, which usually is caused by infection of the cervix by certain viruses. An effective vaccine is now available that protects women from cervical cancer. It is recommended that all young women receive this vaccine before becoming sexually active.

**cervix** the lower part of the uterus
**Pap smear** a diagnostic test for cancer of the cervix
**vagina** a tube extending from the uterus to the outside of the body
**vaginitis** yeast or bacterial infection of the vagina
**hymen** tissue that partially covers the opening of the vagina

## The Vagina

The vagina is a hollow tube extending from the cervix to the outside of the body. Normally the vaginal canal is a relatively narrow space, like the sleeve of a shirt. However, the vagina can widen to accommodate a tampon during menstruation, a penis during intercourse, or the passage of a baby during childbirth.

When a woman becomes sexually excited, the flow of blood to the pelvic region increases. This causes drops of lubricating fluid to appear on the vaginal walls. With continued sexual stimulation, more drops of fluid appear and eventually the walls of the vagina become wet. The function of this fluid is to reduce friction from penile thrusting during sexual intercourse.

Some women have a region in the vagina called the *G-spot* (*Graffenberg-spot*). When present, the G-spot is about the size of a dime and is located about one-third to one-half of the way from the vaginal opening. Some women find stimulation of their G-spot sexually arousing.

The vagina possesses a unique physiology that is maintained by secretions that continuously emanate from the vaginal walls. These secretions help control the growth of microorganisms that normally inhabit the vagina, and they also help to cleanse the vagina. It is usually unnecessary to employ extraordinary vaginal cleansing measures such as douching because they often upset the natural chemical and biological balance of the vagina and increase the risk of developing vaginal infections, called vaginitis. Symptoms of vaginitis include irritation or itching of the vagina and vulva, unusual vaginal discharge, and sometimes a disagreeable vaginal odor.

Vaginitis is commonly referred to as a *yeast infection.* Whereas yeast (typically *Candida albicans*) can cause vaginitis, other microorganisms, such as the protozoan *Trichomonas vaginalis,* bacteria, and viruses, also cause it. Even irritation from vaginal sprays, spermicidal products, and other chemicals can produce symptoms of vaginitis. Anyone with symptoms of vaginitis should see a health practitioner to obtain an accurate diagnosis and treatment.

The hymen is a thin piece of connective tissue at the entrance of the vagina, the purpose of which is unknown. Hymens vary in shape and size; they may cover a larger or smaller portion of the vaginal opening. Normally, hymens do not block the opening of the vagina, so menstrual discharge can pass, tampons can be used, and a pelvic exam can be performed. However, the hymen is likely to be torn or disrupted by a penis during intercourse. As hymens can tear for a variety of reasons, including athletic activity, the absence of a hymen is not a sign of a woman's

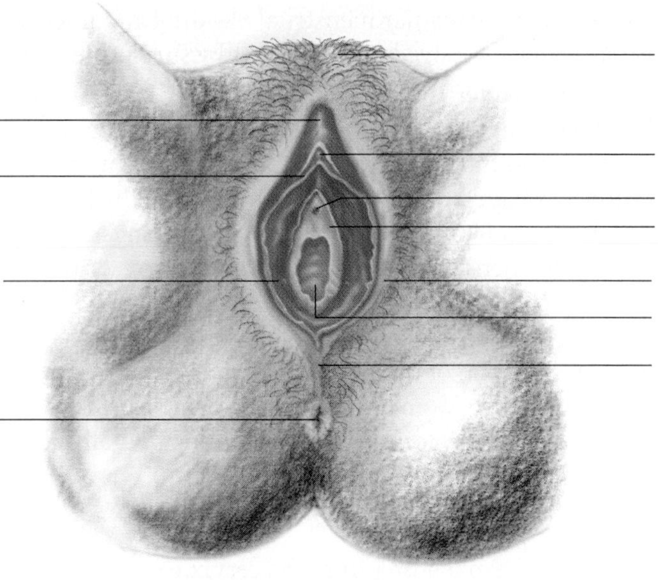


FIGURE 3.2 **Female External Genitalia.**

sexual experience. At first intercourse, tearing of the hymen may result in a small bit of bleeding. However, the tear is usually not painful. A painful first intercourse is generally the result of insufficient vaginal lubrication and tightening of the muscles surrounding the vagina brought about by anxiety and inexperience.

## External Genitalia

**vulva** the lower part of the pelvis and between the legs where the external genitalia are located
**mons veneris** a mound of fatty tissue covering the vulva
**perineum** the region between the lower part of the vagina and the anus
**labia minora** the inner fleshy folds that cover the vagina
**labia majora** the outer fleshy folds that cover the vagina
**clitoris** a sexually sensitive organ located near the urethra
**urethra** the exit tube for urine

A woman's external genitalia are located in the **vulva**, the region in the lower part of the pelvis and between the legs (FIGURE 3.2). The vulva is covered by a small mound of fatty tissue called the **mons veneris** ("Mountain of Venus"), sometimes referred to simply as the *mons*. The mons is covered by pubic hair. The pattern (generally either triangular or rhomboid), extent, and thickness of pubic hair varies among women. The region between the lower part of the vagina and anus is the **perineum**. Many women (and men) find this region to be sexually sensitive.

Two pairs of fleshy folds surround the opening of the vagina. The **labia minora** are a smaller, inner pair of folds. The **labia majora** are a larger, outer pair. When a woman becomes sexually excited, both pairs of labia become engorged with blood, swell, and, in some women, darken in color.

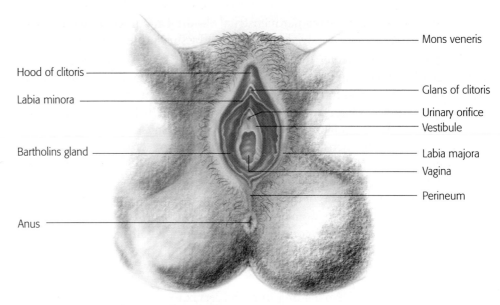

The **clitoris** is an erotically sensitive organ, the tip of which is located just above the urethra where the inner vaginal lips converge to form a fold of tissue called the *clitoral hood*. The clitoris is composed of a glans and a shaft. The shaft is made up of two cylindrical spongy bodies that extend along the sides of the vagina. When a woman becomes sexually excited the spongy bodies become engorged with blood, which causes the clitoris to swell and become firm and also causes a sensation of fullness in the pelvic region (see Chapter 10).

## The Urethra

The **urethra** is the exit tube for urine. It connects the bladder, where urine is stored before it is excreted, to the outside. The opening of the urethra is located in the vaginal region just below the clitoris. Because the female urethra is about one-half inch long and situated close to the vagina, bacteria (principally the rectal bacterium, *E. coli*) can be introduced inadvertently into the urethra, causing an infection (**urethritis**). Moreover, the bacterial cells can migrate to the bladder, also causing an infection (**cystitis**). The occurrence of urethritis and/or cystitis is referred to medically as a **urinary tract infection (UTI)**.

**urethritis** infection of the urethra
**cystitis** infection of the bladder
**urinary tract infection (UTI)** urethritis and/or cystitis

A frequent cause of UTIs is irritation of the opening of the urethra from frequent sexual intercourse and/or the introduction of bacteria from the anal region into the vaginal region and into the urethra. To prevent UTIs:

- Urinate immediately after intercourse
- Wipe from front to back after urinating
- After anal stimulation, cleanse fingers or penis before vaginal entry

The symptoms of a UTI are a frequent urge to urinate and/or a burning sensation upon urination. UTIs can be successfully treated with medications. A mild case of cystitis often can be helped by drinking a lot of fluids to flush bacteria from the body and by acidifying the urine by taking vitamin C or by drinking cranberry juice. One should not ingest alcohol, caffeine, or spices, as they may irritate an already inflamed urinary tract. A physician should be consulted in cases of severe pain or blood in the urine.

As many as 25% of women will experience difficulty controlling urination (called *urinary incontinence*) at some time in their lives. Loss of control tends to manifest as involuntary leakage of urine, which may be preceded by an urgent need to urinate. In some persons, urinary incontinence may occur only in certain situations—for example, when lifting, sneezing, coughing, or laughing. Surgery, medications, and pelvic muscle strengthening exercises can help restore and maintain normal bladder function.

## Female Sex Steroid Hormones

Ovaries produce several kinds of estrogenic hormones, progesterone, and testosterone. The female adrenal glands produce the androgen *dehydroepiandrosterone* (DHEA).

Estrogens are responsible for the growth and development in the female fetus of the female sexual and reproductive organs, and at puberty, the development of breasts, the female pattern of body hair, and the female pattern of body fat deposition. Estrogen is responsible for maintaining the health of the vagina and the ability to produce lubrication during sexual arousal. Estrogen also helps maintain the elasticity of the skin.

Progesterone is primarily responsible for preparing the female body for pregnancy and for maintaining pregnancy. The function of progesterone in males is not known.

Androgen production in females, although produced in smaller amounts than is typical for males, is responsible for the growth of genital and underarm hair and to some degree the maintenance of interest in erotic experience and feelings of aggression. Androgens contribute to the development of acne by stimulating the growth of *sebaceous glands* in hair follicles in the skin and the production of a waxy substance called *sebum*. Acne is the result of the trapping of sebum and cell debris in the opening of a hair follicle.

A large number of agricultural (generally pesticides) and industrial chemicals are able to enter the human body and affect normal estrogen activities. Such chemicals are called *xenoestrogens* ('xeno' meaning foreign); some inhibit and others stimulate an estrogen-dependent process. For example, phthalates (used in the manufacture of thousands of plastic products) have been associated with premature breast development. Several xenoestrogenic pesticides (aldrin, lindane) are associated with higher risk of breast cancer.

## Breasts

**breasts** milk-producing organs that also can be sexually sensitive

The **breasts** are made up of glandular (milk-producing) tissue, fat, connective tissue, blood vessels, and nerves (FIGURE 3.3). Glandular tissue accounts for less than 20% of the breast volume; fat cells account for nearly all the rest. Regardless of the size of their breasts, nearly all women have sufficient glandular tissue to provide milk for their infants.

The glandular tissue in the breast is divided into 15–20 segments called *lobules*, which converge on the nipple like spokes to a wheel's hub. Every lobule contains clusters of individual milk-producing units called *alveoli*. When a woman

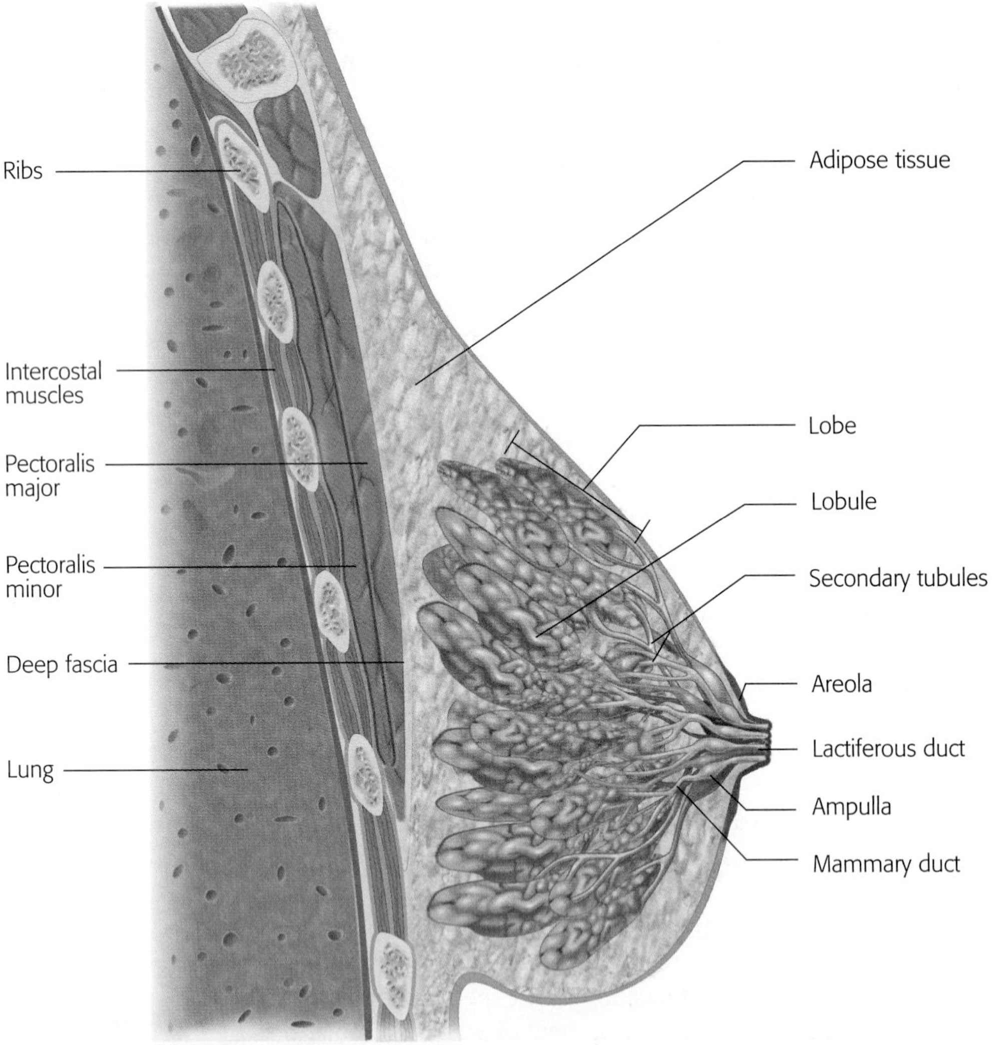


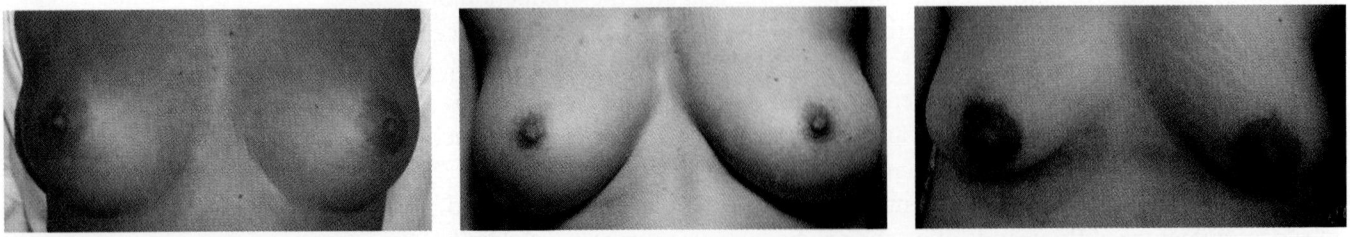

FIGURE 3.3 **The Breasts.** The breast is a modified sweat gland. It is composed of several compartments, each of which has milk-producing lobules. Ducts carry milk from the lobules to the nipple. The breast is attached to the body wall by ligaments, which tend to stretch over time, causing breasts to become distended. With aging, a woman's breasts lose tissue and fat to become smaller and less full.

HEALTHY SEXUALITY

### Elective Breast Augmentation Surgery

About 300,000 American women undergo elective breast augmentation surgery annually, making it the most common plastic surgery procedure in the United States. Most women who undergo elective breast augmentation surgery say they want to look and feel better and to fit into their clothes. And, they say, the decision to change their bodies is personal rather than an accommodation to males in their lives.

That women undergo 90% of the 11 million cosmetic surgeries in the United States each year is not surprising, given the relentless bombardment of media messages telling them that their bodies are flawed because they do not match the ideal set forth by models, actresses, celebrities, and even professional athletes, such as volleyball player Holly McPeak, who had breast augmentation surgery to increase her appeal to fans and her income.

Suggesting a flaw (not only physically, but *personally*) and selling something to remove it is a time-honored sales strategy. The current female ideal, consisting of slim hips, muscularity, and disproportionately large breasts, is a financial winner because most women cannot achieve that body shape naturally. With the help of extensive advertising by cosmetic surgeons, implant manufacturers, and television shows such as *The Swan* and *Dr. 90210* that glorify cosmetic surgery and its supposed benefits, it is no wonder that business is booming.

Proponents of breast augmentation surgery emphasize the personal rewards and minimize the risks, which include complications from anesthesia, infection, bleeding, changes in nipple sensitivity, and interference with diagnostic mammography. Breast implants also need to be checked every three years with magnetic resonance imaging or ultrasound scans to look for leaks or ruptures; these tests usually are not covered by health insurance. It also is likely that implants will need to be replaced within 15–20 years. Finally, there is an association between breast implants and an increased risk of cancer or other forms of systemic disease. Whereas most recipients of implants are initially satisfied, within a year of two of the surgery some women become disappointed because their new bust line did not improve their relationships, job prospects, or self-esteem.

Most of us want to feel good about ourselves and have others appreciate us. Breast augmentation surgery is largely motivated by social pressures that encourage women to define their self-worth and attractiveness in terms of their body shape. To a large extent, it represents exploitative economic forces that prey upon women's desires to feel attractive and accepted.

*Source:* Walden, J. L., Panagopoulous, G., & Shrader, S. W. (2010). Contemporary decision making and perception in patients undergoing cosmetic breast augmentation. *Aesthetic Surgery Journal, 30*, 395–403.

produces milk, the cells in each alveolus manufacture milk products including proteins, sugars, fats, salts, and antibodies, and secrete them into a duct that courses to the nipple. Breast cancer is most often the result of uncontrolled, often estrogen-stimulated, reproduction of cells that line the milk ducts. Eventually the cancer cells form a dense mass, or tumor, that hopefully can be detected with a special x-ray test (mammography), a medical exam, a breast self-exam, or an aware sex partner before the cells spread to other parts of the body.

**areola** the pigmented region of the breast surrounding the nipple

The **areola** is the circular, pigmented region around the nipple. The pigment-producing cells in the areola often become activated during pregnancy, causing the areola to darken. The areola contain numerous sebaceous glands that provide a protective lubricant for the areola and nipple, especially during nursing. The nipple and areola contain muscle fibers that contract in response to suckling, cold, and erotic arousal. Contraction of these muscle fibers produces nipple erection.

The skin of the breast tends to be soft and thin. It contains sebaceous and apocrine glands and may produce hair, except on the nipple. Because body hair is considered "unfeminine" in our culture, women often are embarrassed by hair on the chest or breasts. It can be removed without harm if desired.

The size and shape of breasts tend to be inherited, probably by genes from both parents. The amount of fat in the breasts can be affected by factors that influence the overall fat content of the body, such as diet and exercise. The size and shape of the breasts may change during a woman's lifetime. In adolescence, the breasts are likely to be dome shaped or conical. In mature women who have not had children, the breasts often are hemispheric. After pregnancy and in later life, the breasts may become pendulous as the ligaments that attach a breast to the body wall weaken and stretch.

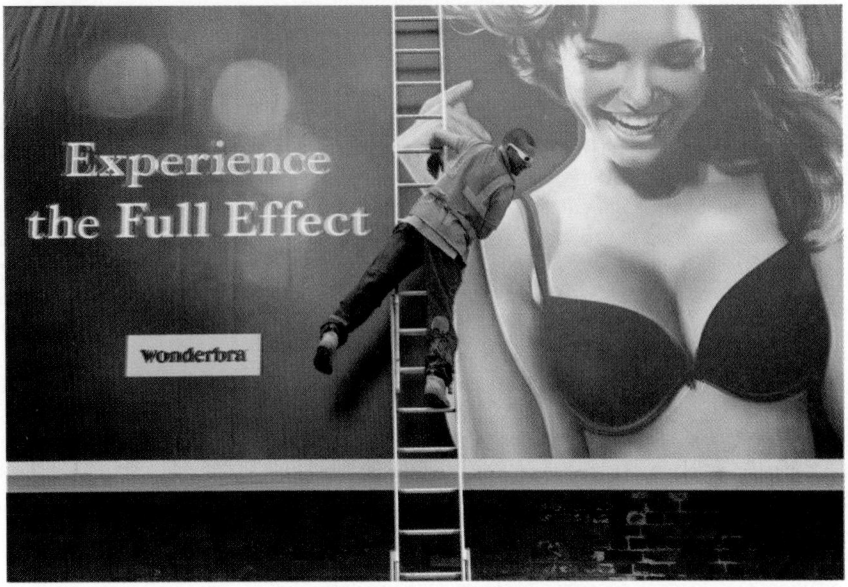


In some cultures, female breasts are symbols of femininity and sexual attractiveness. Commercial idealization of the size and shape of female breasts reinforces the value that how one looks is less important than who one is.

In North America and Europe, female breasts are symbols of femininity and sexual attractiveness. Men tend to be interested in, and aroused by, the sight of breasts, as evidenced by the widespread use of partially exposed breasts and breast symbolism in advertising and other media. Clothes that display and emphasize the bust also are popular. In American culture, what is considered ideal breast size varies largely because of changes in fashion and media trends, which thrive economically on change. There are periods when a large bust is a standard of feminine beauty, and other times when the ideal feminine body is curveless. Nowadays, fashion calls for women to have ample breasts and slim hips.

Males also have glandular breast tissue that can produce milk if hormonally activated. Indeed, newborns of both sexes occasionally express milk (so-called witch's milk) because breast glandular tissue has been activated by the mother's hormones. Male breasts can be sensitive to touch, and some men enjoy manual or oral nipple stimulation during sexual activity.

## The Menstrual (Fertility) Cycle

Beginning at puberty, the time of life when individuals become biologically capable of reproducing, females produce usually one (although sometimes two or more) fertilizable ovum approximately every month. The near-monthly production of ova is the basis of a woman's **menstrual (fertility) cycle**.

**menstrual (fertility) cycle** the period of time from one menstruation to another
**menstruation** the near-monthly discharge of uterine tissue debris and blood from the vagina

During each cycle of ovum production, a woman's body undergoes several hormonally induced changes to prepare her body for pregnancy. One of these changes is the thickening of the lining of the uterus (the *endometrium*) to support the first stages of pregnancy. Another change is the growth of special blood vessels in the endometrium. Should conception occur, these blood vessels bring nutrients from the mother to the embryo and carry away waste products. If conception does not occur, the endometrium and the special blood vessels are sloughed off and leave the body via the vagina. This process is **menstruation**.

Menstruation generally spans three to six days, during which between 35 and 85 milliliters (about 1–3 teaspoons) of material are discharged. Women taking hormonal contraceptives may experience minimal blood loss; women using a contraceptive IUD may lose more blood than usual. A one-time, later-than-usual loss of considerable blood may be due to the early loss of a pregnancy (*miscarriage*). Repeated heavy menstrual flow may lessen the amount of iron in the blood (*iron-deficiency anemia*) and thus reduce the efficiency with which oxygen is transported throughout the body. Consuming dark-green leafy vegetables or taking iron-containing dietary supplements can restore iron lost to the body via menstruation. Some brands of combination oral contraceptives contain iron.

For most adult women the length of a menstrual cycle is between 24 and 35 days. The most common cycle lengths are 28 or 29 days. Some cycles occur at regular intervals; others recur irregularly. Irregular cycles are common when women first begin to menstruate (*menarche*; see Chapter 8) and as menopause approaches. Some women take hormonal contraceptives to regulate their menstrual cycles, to extend the time between periods (often for special events), or to suppress menstruation altogether—for example, in cases of heavy menstrual flow, severe menstrual discomfort, and endometriosis (discussed later).

The menstrual cycle is controlled by the female version of the **hypothalamo-pituitary-gonadal (HPG) system** (FIGURE 3.4), which is composed of the following:

- *Hypothalamo* refers to certain nerve cells in the brain's hypothalamus that manufacture and secrete into the bloodstream a hormone called **gonadotrophin releasing factor (GnRF)**. During the menstrual cycle, levels of GnRF rise

**hypothalamo-pituitary-gonadal (HPG) system** a "team" of hormone-producing structures responsible for ovum and sex hormone production

**gonadotrophin releasing factor (GnRf)** stimulates follicle-stimulating hormone (FSH) and luteinizing hormone (LH) production

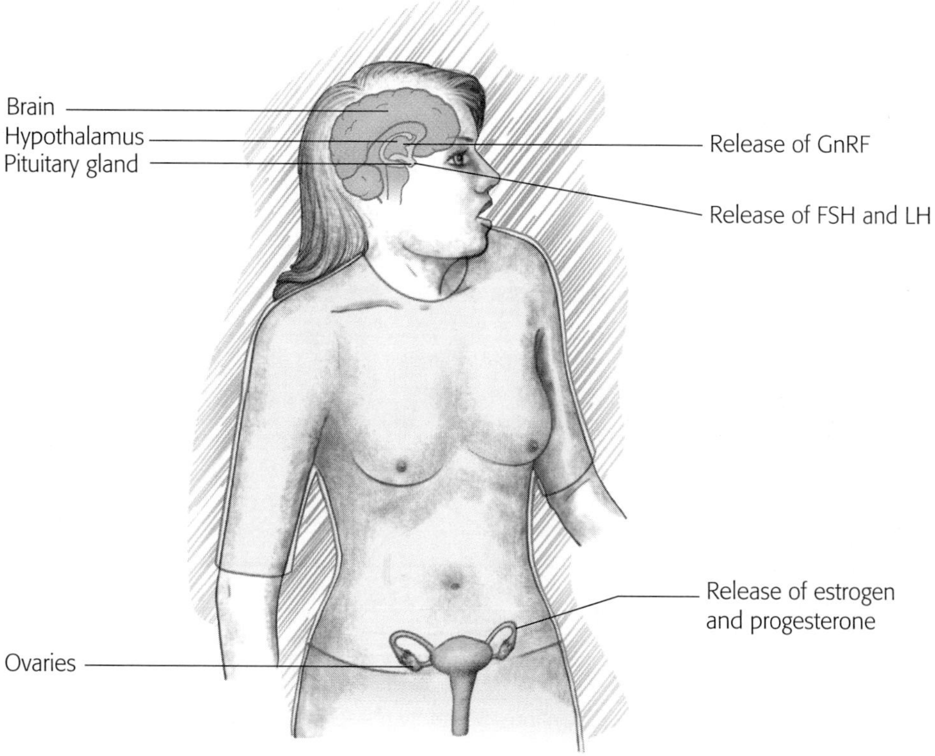


FIGURE 3.4 **Female Hypothalamo-Pituitary-Gonadal System.** Gonadotrophin releasing factor (GnRF) is manufactured by specific cells in the hypothalamus of the brain and released into the bloodstream. GnRF stimulates certain cells in the pituitary gland, located at the base of the brain, to manufacture and release follicle-stimulating hormone (FSH) and luteinizing hormone (LH) into the bloodstream. In the ovaries, FSH stimulates the development of premature ova and hormone-manufacturing cells to make estrogen. LH induces release of a fertilizable ovum from the ovary and the production of progesterone. Estrogen and progesterone regulate the amount of GnRF manufactured by the hypothalamus.

and fall in a specified manner, which gives rise to the cyclic nature of the menstrual cycle.

- *Pituitary* refers to certain cells in the pituitary gland, located at the base of the brain, that respond to GnRF by releasing into the bloodstream the hormones follicle-stimulating hormone (FSH) and luteinizing hormone (LH).
- *Gonadal* refers to estrogen and progesterone production by the ovaries. Estrogen production is controlled by FSH; progesterone production is controlled principally by LH. Estrogen and progesterone circulate through the bloodstream and bring about specific biological changes, including regulation of the HPG system. When blood levels of estrogen rise, FSH production falls. As levels of progesterone rise, LH production falls.

**follicle-stimulating hormone (FSH)** facilitates maturation of ova
**luteinizing hormone (LH)** a hormone produced by the pituitary gland that is responsible for releasing the egg from the ovary and stimulating the production of progesterone

### Phases of the Menstrual Cycle

The menstrual cycle occurs in phases (FIGURE 3.5). The beginning phases are dedicated to preparing an ovum and the woman's body for fertilization. The latter

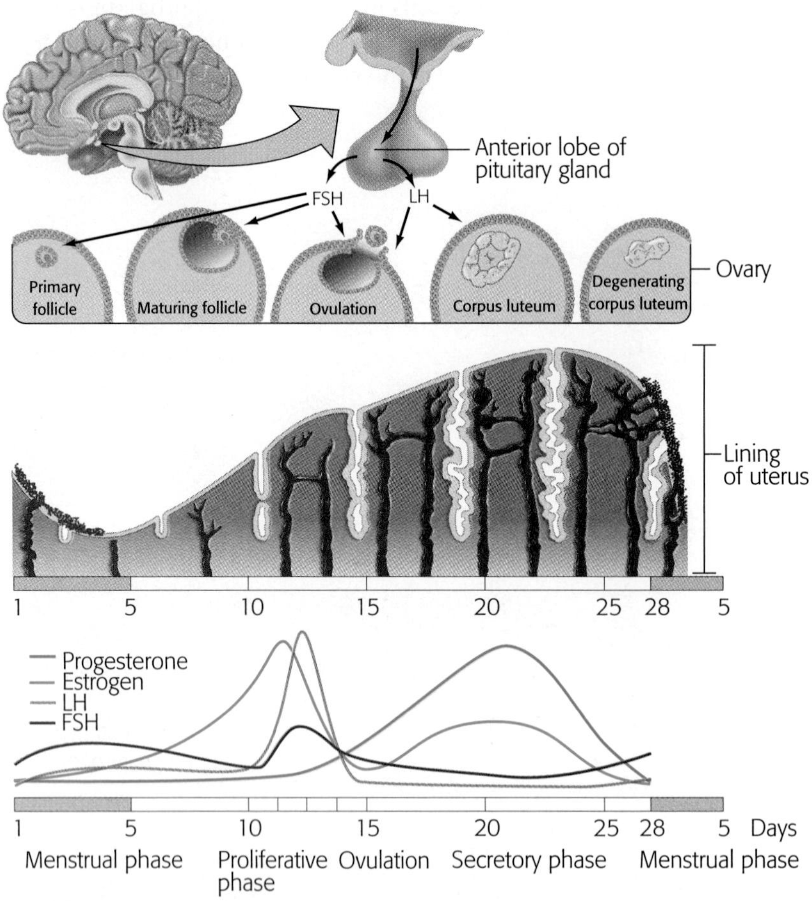


FIGURE 3.5 **The Menstrual Cycle.** This figure represents of a 28-day menstrual cycle during which ovulation takes place on day 14 (note the egg being released from the ovary, caused by a surge in the pituitary hormone (yellow line). In the days prior to ovulation (days 5–13), FSH (purple line) from the pituitary gland stimulates egg maturation and estrogen production (blue line) in the ovary. Estrogen causes the lining of the uterus to thicken. In the 14 days after ovulation (days 15–28), FSH and LH stimulate the manufacture of estrogen and progesterone (green line), which cause nutrient-producing glands and blood vessels in the lining of the uterus to develop. If pregnancy does not occur, hormone levels drop and menstruation ensues.

phases are dedicated to preparing the woman's body for pregnancy. All of these activities are coordinated by hormones. The phases of the menstrual cycle are as follows:

- *Menstrual phase* (days 1–5): The first day of menstrual bleeding marks the beginning of a cycle. During this time estrogen and progesterone levels are low, although several ova and their surrounding support and hormone-producing cells begin to develop.
- *Proliferative phase* (days 6–14): Low amounts of estrogen production during the menstrual phase stimulate the production of GnRH and FSH, which cause an ovum to mature and the ovaries to produce estrogen. Estrogen, in turn, stimulates proliferation of the lining of the uterus and uterine blood vessels.
- *Ovulation phase* (days 14–15): Rising levels of estrogen cause a surge in LH production, which triggers the release of a mature ovum from an ovary.
- *Secretory phase* (days 16–28): After an ovum is released from its ovary, FSH and LH stimulate the production of estrogen and progesterone from a structure in the ovary called the *corpus luteum*. Progesterone stimulates the development of nutrient-producing glands in the lining of the uterus.
- *Next menstrual phase:* If pregnancy does not occur, the corpus luteum disintegrates, hormone levels drop, and menstruation ensues.

## Menstrual Difficulties

For some women, menstruation may be accompanied by unpleasant symptoms, the most common of which include the following.

### Dysmenorrhea

About half of menstruating women experience some abdominal pain, commonly referred to as "cramps" and medically referred to as **dysmenorrhea**, usually during the first day or so of menstruation. Although psychological, anatomical, and hormonal factors can contribute to menstrual cramps, in most cases they are

**dysmenorrhea** abdominal pain during menstruation ("menstrual cramps")

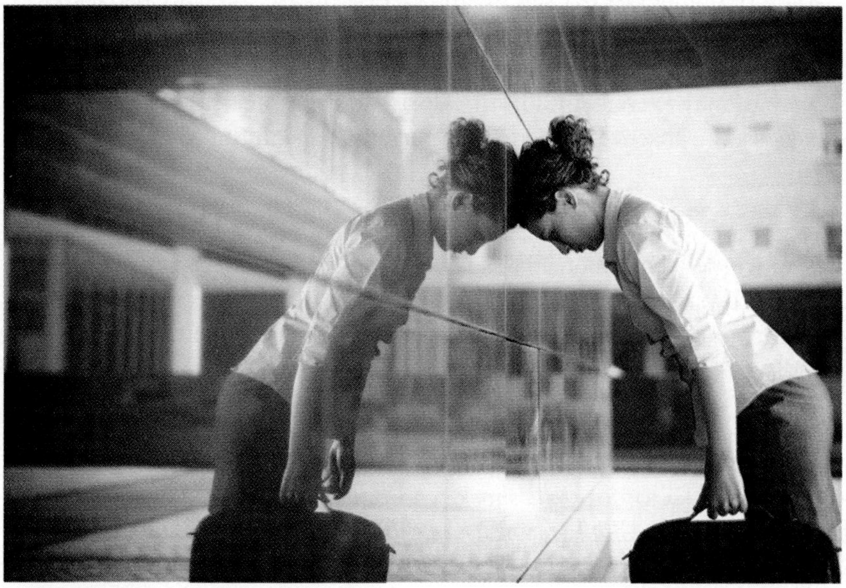

caused by naturally occurring substances called *prostaglandins*, which induce strong contractions of the uterine muscle tissue. The prostaglandins are formed when the uterine lining breaks down; their likely function is to promote removal of menstrual tissue from the body. In some instances dysmenorrhea is the result of medical problems such as endometriosis, pelvic inflammatory disease (PID), uterine fibroids, or tumors in the pelvic cavity.

In many instances, the severity of cramps is lessened or eliminated if no ovum is released, which is why women who take combination oral contraceptives ("the pill") often experience relief of cramps. Other ways to lessen menstrual cramps include having a flexible body, practicing meditation or other mental relaxation exercises, or taking medications that reduce levels of prostaglandins.

### Premenstrual Syndrome

At some time in their lives, 75% of women report experiencing changes in feelings and disposition as the time of menstruation approaches and during the first day or two of menstrual flow. These symptoms, known as premenstrual syndrome (PMS), may include headache, backache, fatigue, feeling bloated, breast tenderness, depression, irritability, unusual aggressive feelings, and social withdrawal. With the onset of menstruation, the symptoms virtually vanish. In about 5% of women, premenstrual symptoms are severe enough to cause a disorder called **premenstrual dysphoric disorder (PMDD)**, which is characterized by a combination of marked mood swings, depression, irritability, and anxiety.

**premenstrual dysphoric disorder (PMDD)** premenstrual symptoms severe enough to impair personal functioning
**amenorrhea** cessation of menstruation

Reducing the intake of caffeine, sugar, and salt around the time of menstruation, increasing exercise, increasing the intake of vitamin B-6, and having an adequate intake of calcium can provide relief from premenstrual symptoms.

### Amenorrhea

**Amenorrhea** is the interruption or cessation of regular menstrual periods. The most common reason periods stop is pregnancy, but the list of factors that can interfere with normal menstruation is quite long. Some factors are psychological stress, depression, marital or sexual problems, fatigue, ingestion of opiate drugs, depression medications, anxiety, hormonal imbalances, nutritional abnormalities such as severe calorie restriction diets, and anorexia nervosa.

Extreme physical activity and concomitant reduction in body fat (often from the combination of high levels of exercise and calorie restriction) can also lead to amenorrhea. Body fat is stored energy. When body fat is very low, some functions, including the menstrual cycle, temporarily shut down to conserve energy. Thus, although a woman may exercise and limit calories to promote health, self-esteem, and attractiveness, the absence of menstrual periods is a sign that she is overdoing it.

### Endometriosis

In about 10% of women, endometrial tissue occasionally detaches from the uterus and lodges in nearby structures (e.g., ovaries, fallopian tubes). This tissue remains responsive to hormones, so during regular menstrual cycles, it grows, degenerates, and bleeds, causing severe pain. Endometriosis is treated surgically or with medications.

### Toxic Shock Syndrome

Menstruation is a risk factor for *toxic shock syndrome* (TSS), caused by a toxin produced by the bacterium *Staphylococcus aureus*, which can colonize menstrual fluids. TSS is characterized by the sudden onset of fever, chills, vomiting, diarrhea,

## *Dear Penelope . . .*

***I've read that it's OK to have sex during a woman's menstrual period, but I'm wondering if that's really true. My girlfriend and I have tried it a few times, and, although she hasn't said anything, I notice that she doesn't seem to be quite as turned on because she doesn't get as lubricated. I'm concerned that she may not be interested in sex and is doing it just to please me.***

***— Concerned***

*Dear Concerned,*

The amount of vaginal lubrication depends on the level of certain hormones, particularly estrogen. What you notice may be due to the normal decrease in hormone levels at menstruation. Low estrogen level in hormonal contraceptives is also a reason that some women who use one of those methods lubricate less.

You're right to speculate, however, they she may not be as turned on. Although there's no particular physiological or psychological reason not to have sex during menstruation, your partner may nevertheless be uncomfortable with it. Perhaps she's feeling shy about sharing this personal body event with you. She may be having some menstrual discomfort.

Have you discussed this with her? Certainly you should.

Courtesy of the UC Davis *Aggie*

muscle aches, and rash. The condition can progress rapidly, causing a severe drop in blood pressure and malfunction of many body organs. TSS is fatal in about 5% of cases. The risk of menstrual TSS is reduced by frequently changing tampons, using less-absorbent tampons, and not using super-absorbent tampons.

## SEXUALITY IN REVIEW

- Female primary sex characteristics (those that contribute directly to fertilization) are the ovaries, fallopian tubes, uterus, and vagina.
- Female secondary sex characteristics include (as compared with males) a smaller body size, a smaller waist-to-hip ratio, a larger proportion of body fat, high voice, and minimal body hair.
- The ovaries produce eggs (ova) and steroid sex hormones, principally estrogens and progesterone.
- Ovulation produces an ovum that enters an adjacent fallopian tube, where it can be fertilized.
- Fetal development takes place in the uterus over a period of about nine months.
- Generally, one egg is produced during the near-monthly menstrual cycle. Production of ova cease at menopause.
- Breasts manufacture and deliver milk used to feed newborns.

## CRITICAL THINKING ABOUT SEXUALITY

1. A study revealed that the incidence of urinary tract infections (UTIs) among sexually active college women who were in steady relationships was highest after winter break and after final exams. What is the likely reason

that these women were susceptible to UTIs at these times of year? Design a study (see Chapter 1) that would test your hypothesis.

2. Several of the thousands of industrial and agricultural chemicals humans are exposed to each year are classified as *xenoestrogens* because they mimic the actions of sex hormones in the body. Scientists are concerned that some xenoestrogens may disrupt estrogen functioning and increase the risk of breast cancer in susceptible women. One of the most prevalent xenoestrogens is called bisphenol-A, or BPA. It is used to manufacture polycarbonate plastic food and beverage containers and the resin linings for canned foods. BPA can leach into food from these containers and thereby enter the body, where it can affect hormone function. To limit exposure to BPA, the FDA recommends choosing glass or BPA-free plastic bottles; using glass, porcelain, or stainless steel containers for hot foods and liquids; avoiding plastic containers with the No. 7 recycling symbol; not microwaving polycarbonate plastic food containers (use glass containers designed for microwaving instead); and limiting use of canned foods lined with BPA-containing resin. On a scale of 1 to 5 (1 = not at all; 5 = a lot), how concerned are you about exposure to BPA and other xenoestrogens? Can you identify *one* thing you could do to limit your exposure to BPA and other xenoestrogens?
3. Anorexia nervosa and bulimia were once common only in North America and Europe, but now they occur worldwide. Experts say that the growing prevalence of eating disorders is caused by young women trying to emulate models and actors, who often are unrealistically slim or trying to get that way. For example, prior to 1995, the island of Fiji had no television and very few cases of eating disorders among young women. However, after the introduction of television in 1995, with broadcasts of shows from Australia, the United States, and the United Kingdom, the incidence of eating disorders rose to 15%. To what extent, and in what ways, do you think media images affect women's susceptibility to eating disorders?

## REFERENCES AND RECOMMENDED RESOURCES

### References

Chiras, D. G. (2008). *Human biology*. Sudbury, MA: Jones & Bartlett Learning.

Jones, R. E. (2006). *Human reproductive biology, 3rd ed.* San Diego: Academic Press.

Kerr, J. D. (2010). *Functional histology, 2nd ed.* New York: Mosby.

Mannix, L. K. (2008). Menstrual-related pain conditions: Dysmenorrhea and migraine. *Journal of Women's Health, 17,* 879–891.

Pearlstein, T., & Steiner, M. (2008). Premenstrual dysphoric disorder: Burden of illness and treatment update. *Psychiatry and Neuroscience, 33,* 291–301. Available at: http://www.ncbi.nlm.nih.gov/pmc/articles/PMC2440788/?tool=pubmed. Accessed September 22, 2010.

### Recommended Resources

Boston Women's Health Book Collective. (2005). *Our bodies, ourselves, 4th ed.* New York: Touchstone. Considered the best all-around health reference for women.

Jones, R. E. (2006). *Human reproductive biology, 3rd ed.* San Diego: Academic Press. A most readable undergraduate text.

Mayo Clinic. Available at: http://www.mayoclinic.com/health/womens-health/MY00379/DSECTION=breast%2Dhealth. Information on breast health.

MedlinePlus. Available at: http://www.nlm.nih.gov/medlineplus/femalereproductivesystem.html. Information on the female reproductive system.

Merck Manual Online. Available at: http://www.merck.com/mmhe/sec22/ch241/ch241a.html. The biology of the female reproductive system.

Schuiling, K. D., & Likis, F. E. (2006). *Women's gynecologic health*. Sudbury, MA: Jones & Bartlett Learning. An authoritative text for students in the health sciences.

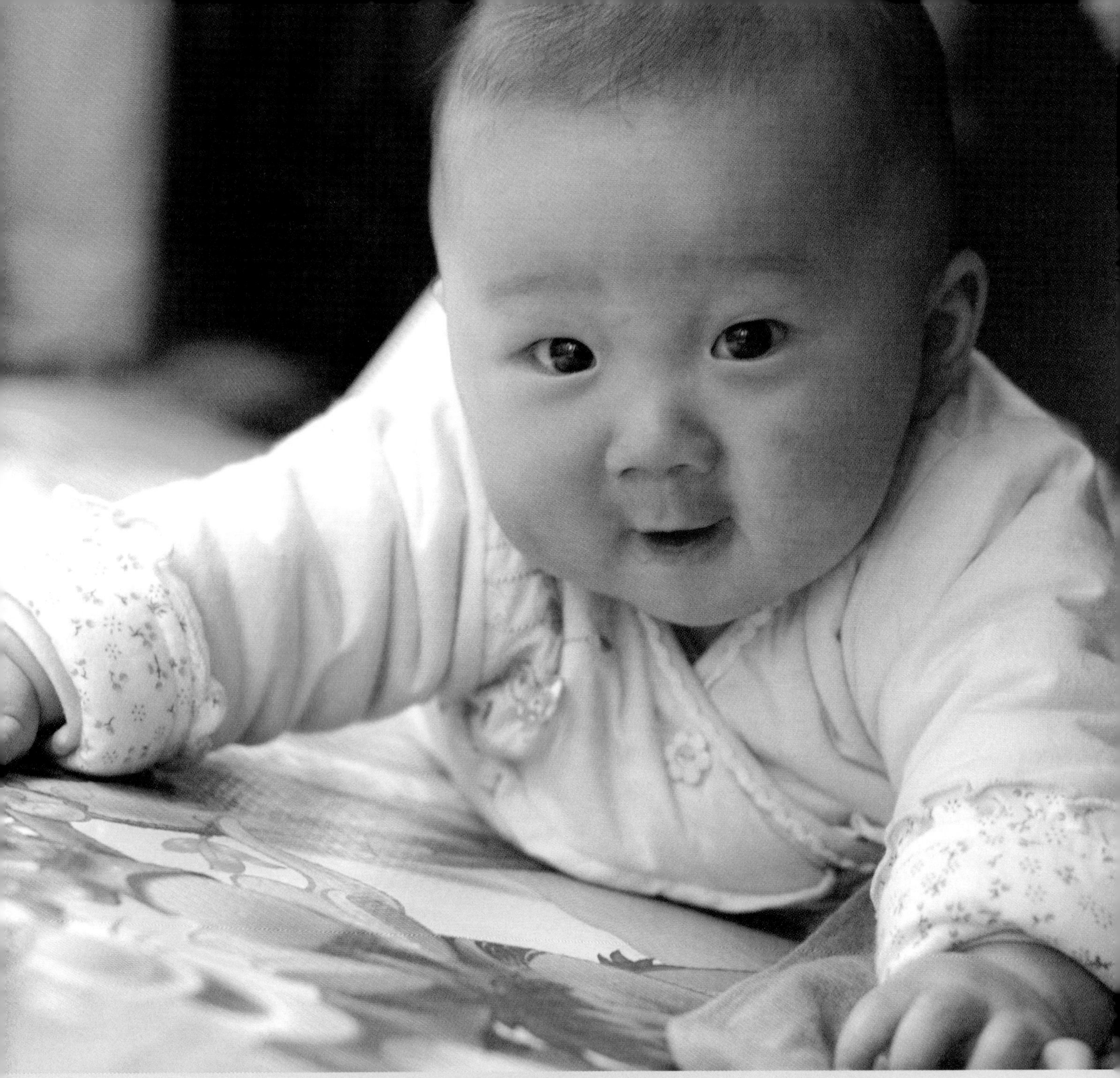

*"Recommend to your children virtue; that alone can make them happy, not gold."*

— Ludwig van Beethoven

CHAPTER 4

# Pregnancy and Childbirth

## Student Learning Objectives

1 Describe how sperm and eggs (ova) become capable of fertilization

2 Describe the process of ovum maturation and ovulation

3 Explain the process of implantation of the embryo in the uterus

4 List and describe the major health habits to practice during pregnancy

5 Describe the three stages of childbirth (labor)

6 List the major benefits of breastfeeding to the newborn and mother

7 Explain infertility and options for overcoming it

People become parents to (1) to create a family unit to which one can belong and share fun, love, and companionship; (2) to manifest a couple's sense of love and emotional attachment; (3) to leave a legacy to the world and carry on the family name; (4) to accede to social and family pressures to have children; and (5) to feel important, needed, loved, proud, and grown-up. Because human children are dependent on adult support, guidance, and protection for as many as 20 years, many parents and parents-to-be are awed by the tremendous responsibility for being the best parent possible in nurturing and raising a child to maturity.

Giving birth to and raising a child require major adjustments in the parents' lives. The career plans of one or both parents and the distribution of family resources—time, energy, physical space, and money—may change. Furthermore, the demands of parenting are often physically and psychologically intense. In virtually no other endeavor is there such responsibility, hard work, and intimacy as in creating and raising another human being.

About 5% of fertile American married couples choose not to become parents. Some see parenthood as infringing on their career goals or as an unnecessary or unwanted addition to their intimate partnership. Some may have doubts about their psychological or economic abilities to nurture and support children, or they may know or suspect that their children might inherit a genetic disease. Still others may feel that they do not want to contribute more children to an already overpopulated world.

Children do not ask to be born. Parents make that decision. Therefore, potential parents are wise to be as certain as they can be that their decision to have children is appropriate for their life goals and personal resources.

## Fertilization

**fertilization** the union of a sperm and egg (ovum) to form a zygote

Fertilization is the union of a sperm from a male and an ovum from a female. To become capable of fertilization, sperm and ova must undergo a maturation pro-

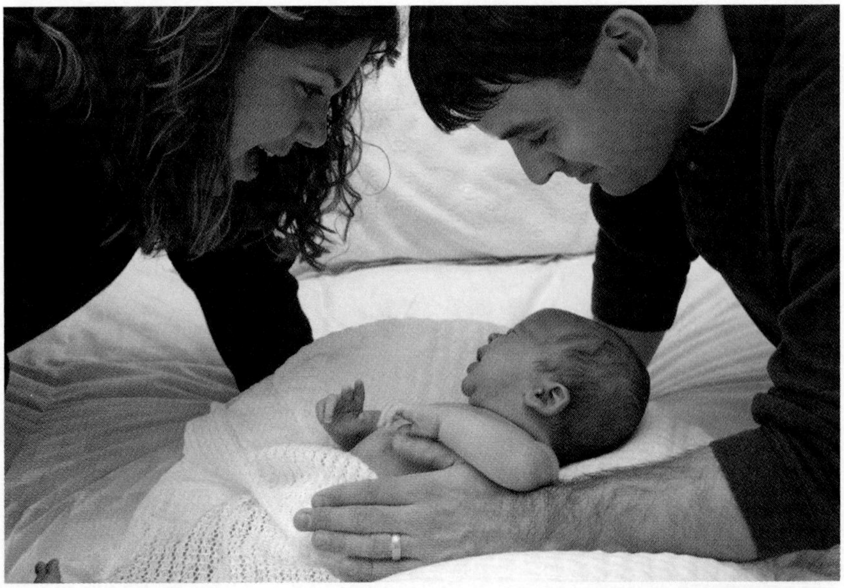

cess. Moreover, sperm must be transferred from the male into the female and transported within the female to a fallopian tube, where fertilization most often takes place (FIGURE 4.1).

## Maturation of Sperm

Sperm are produced in the seminiferous tubules of the testes (see Chapter 2), arising from round cells that are incapable of fertilization. Under the influence of hormones, and supported by neighboring nutrient-providing cells, immature sperm undergo a two-phase maturation process, called spermatogenesis.

**spermatogenesis** the process by which sperm cells mature

1. Phase 1: The number of chromosomes is reduced from 46 to 23 by a process called *meiosis*.
2. Phase 2: Round sperm cells containing 23 chromosomes develop the tadpole-like anatomy of mature sperm (FIGURE 4.2). Production of mature sperm in the testes takes about 70 days.

After developing in a testis, sperm move to an adjacent epididymis, where they are stored for up to several days and become capable of fertilization. At ejaculation, sperm move through the genital ducts and become mixed with fluids from the pair of seminal vesicles and the prostate gland (see Chapter 2). Fluid from the seminal vesicles nourishes sperm with fructose and other substances. Fluid from the prostate gland neutralizes the slightly acidic vaginal fluids, thereby making the vagina more hospitable to sperm survival.

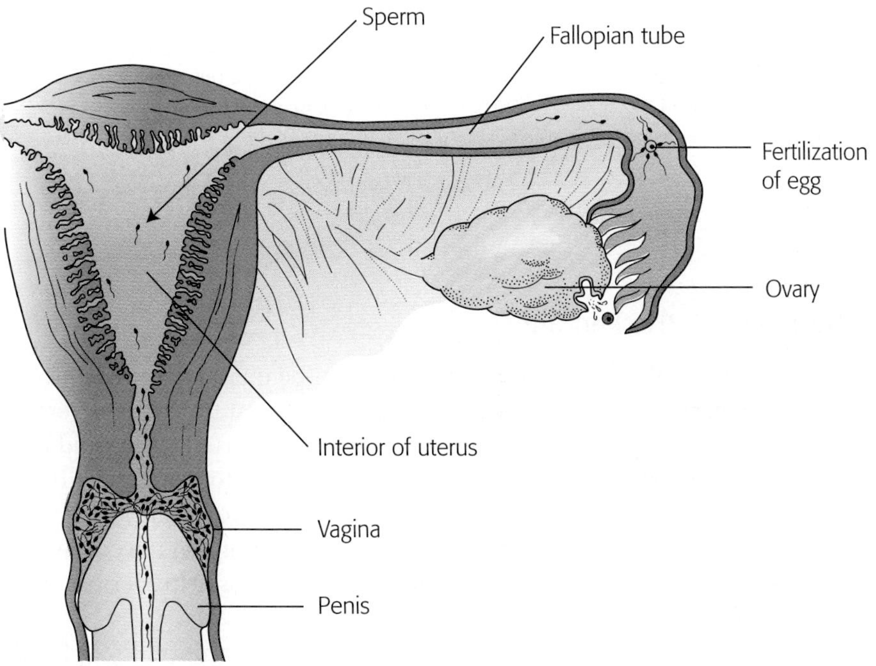


FIGURE 4.1 **Fertilization.** For fertilization to take place, an egg (ovum) must be released from an ovary and captured by a nearby fallopian tube, and sperm must be transferred from the male's body to the female's, where they travel through the uterus to the site of fertilization in a fallopian tube.

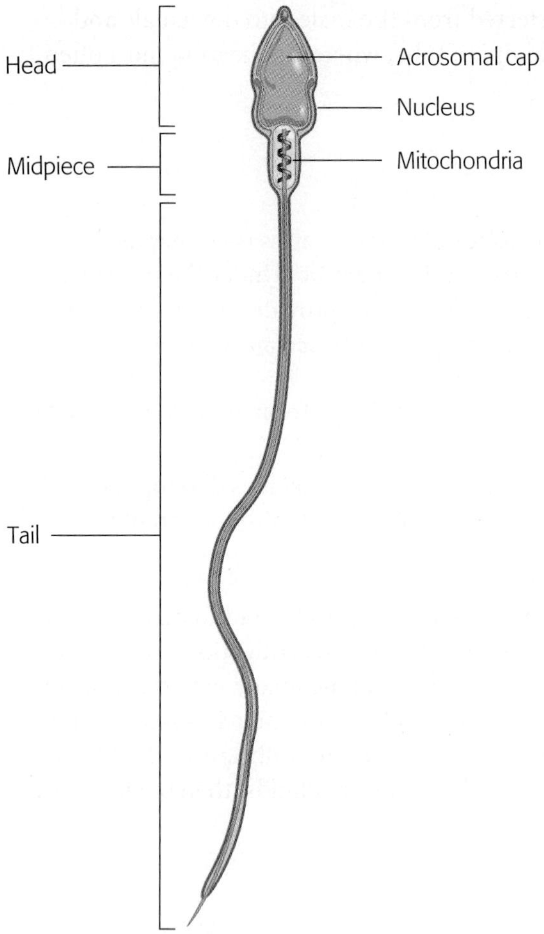


FIGURE 4.2 **Anatomy of a Mature Human Sperm Cell.** Mature sperm cells consist of three major parts: 1. *Head:* contains the sperm cell's nucleus and the 23 paternal chromosomes. The upper part of the nucleus is covered by a caplike structure (the *acrosome*), which contains enzymes that dissolve the outer membranes of the ovum, thus allowing the sperm to penetrate the egg. 2. *Midpiece:* contains many thousands of subcellular structures (*mitochondria*), which produce energy for sperm motility. 3. *Tail:* made up of filaments that provide the undulating motion that propels the sperm.

## Sperm Transport in the Female

After sperm enter the vagina, they must travel through the uterus to the site of fertilization in one of the fallopian tubes. To do so, sperm must traverse the cervix at the junction of the vagina and uterus. For most of the menstrual cycle, fluid produced by glands in the cervix is thick and too dense for sperm to penetrate. (Thick cervical mucus also prevents microorganisms from entering the uterus.) Near ovulation, however, the cervical mucus becomes less dense, taking on the consistency of egg white. It also becomes organized into channels that help sperm move from the vagina into the uterus.

**ovulation** release of a mature, fertilizable egg from the ovary

Within seconds after ejaculation in the vagina, some sperm move through the cervix and into the uterus, but the majority of sperm become trapped in semen that coagulates in the upper portion of the vagina. After about 20 minutes the coagulated semen liquefies and sperm move into microscopic folds in the tissue of the cervix.

Weak or abnormal sperm are unlikely to move beyond the cervix. Healthy sperm, in contrast, tend to be released into the uterus continuously over the ensuing 48 hours.

## Preparation of Ova for Fertilization

During each of a woman's menstrual cycles, several ova approach full maturation. However, usually only one ovum (sometimes more, thus establishing the possibility for twin and higher-order pregnancies) completes the process to become fertilizable and is released from the ovary; the other maturing ova degenerate. An ovum matures in a bed of nutrient- and hormone-producing cells called a **follicle**.

**follicle** a bed of nutrient- and hormone-producing cells in the ovary in which an egg matures

As an ovum matures, its associated follicle cells produce increasing amounts of a special fluid. As the middle of the menstrual month approaches, the amount of luteinizing hormone (LH) from the pituitary gland increases, rising to a peak about 36 hours before the ovum is released (the "LH surge"). This hormone causes the progressive degradation of the cells surrounding the follicle, and eventually the follicle ruptures and the ovum and a few dozen follicle cells lift off from the surface of the ovary.

Once freed from the ovary, the ovum can survive for about 24 hours. If it is fertilized during that time, a pregnancy may ensue. If it is not fertilized, the ovum degenerates and a potential pregnancy must await a new menstrual cycle.

After ovulation, the ruptured, now eggless, follicle turns into a structure called the *corpus luteum* that secretes the hormone progesterone. The progesterone circulates through the woman's body and prepares it to nurture an embryo should fertilization occur.

## Ovum Transport

An ovum released from the ovary is suspended in the small space between the ovary and the open end of the adjacent fallopian tube. It is captured and ushered into the tube by currents created by fingerlike folds on the ends of the tube, called *fimbriae*, which sweep across the surface of the ovary. The rhythmic motion of the tube itself and thousands of tiny hairlike projections on the inner lining of the tube promote ovum capture and move the ovum and its surrounding follicle cells toward the uterus.

## Sperm Penetration of the Ovum

Although many millions of sperm are deposited in the vagina during sexual intercourse, only a few hundred survive the journey to the fallopian tube to potentially fertilize a mature ovum. As the sperm travel to the fallopian tube, fluids in the cavity of the uterus prepare sperm for penetrating the layer of follicle cells that surrounds the ovum. About 20 sperm may eventually approach an ovum; however, only one succeeds in getting through the ovum's outer membrane (**FIGURE 4.3**). When it does, entry of all other sperm into the ovum is blocked by (1) the release of granules that surround the inner circumference of the ovum, (2) changes in the electrical charge on the ovum's surface, and (3) structural changes in the ovum's surface that prevent the binding of additional sperm to the ovum.

After it enters the ovum, the fertilizing sperm loses its tail, and its nucleus enlarges to become what is called the *male pronucleus*. The ovum's nucleus chang-

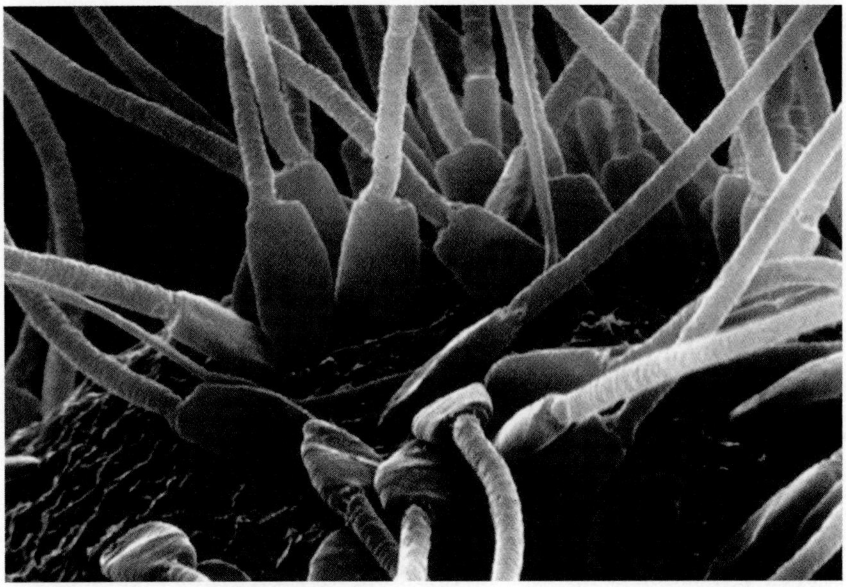

FIGURE 4.3 **Sperm Penetrating an Ovum.**

**zygote** the fertilized egg

es to become what is called the *female pronucleus.* At this point the fertilized ovum is called a zygote.

Each pronucleus contains 23 chromosomes. During the next several hours the chromosomes in each pronucleus replicate, and about 20 hours after fertilization the membrane of each pronucleus breaks down and the 92 chromosomes (46 paternal and 46 maternal) meet in the center of the zygote. After they meet, the zygote immediately divides into two attached cells, each with 46 chromosomes, 23 maternal and 23 paternal.

Additional replications occur at about daily intervals, eventually creating a ball of cells, which is moved toward the uterus by the thousands of fingerlike cilia on the inner walls of the fallopian tube (FIGURE 4.4). By about the fourth day after fertilization, the zygote is a ball of between 50 to 100 cells arranged as a fluid-filled sphere (*blastocyst*). Most of the cells of the blastocyst are destined to form the placenta. A small number of cells clustered at one pole of the blastocyst, the inner

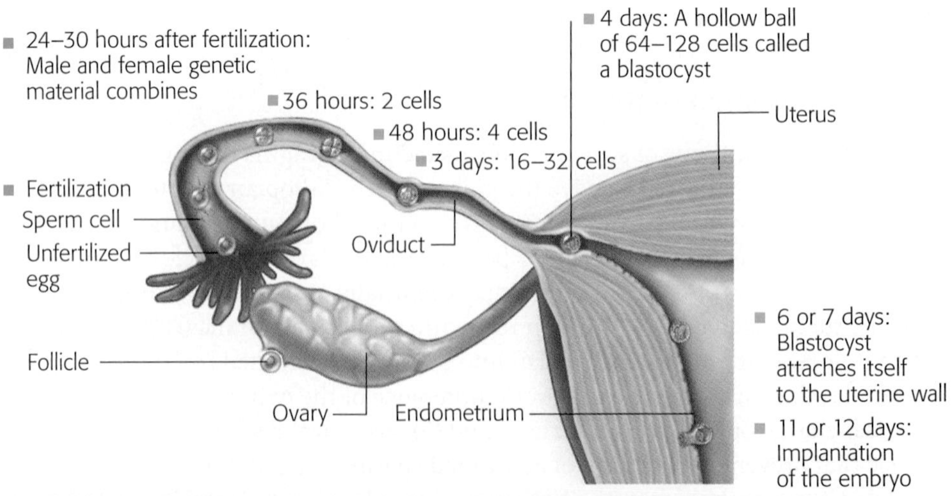


FIGURE 4.4 **Fertilization and Early Development of the Embryo.** A sperm penetrates an egg to form a zygote. The zygote undergoes a series of cell divisions to form a hollow ball of cells (blastocyst), which implants in the uterus about seven days after fertilization.

cell mass, are the first cells of what is to become the child's body. At this stage, the developing child is referred to as an embryo.

**embryo** the earliest stage of intrauterine development, from fertilization to week 10

**human chorionic gonadotropin (hCG)** a hormone produced by the embryo that signals the mother's body that a state of pregnancy exists

## Implantation

On about the sixth day after fertilization, the embryo is a large ball of several hundred cells. Its outer covering becomes "sticky" so it can attach to the lining of the uterus, usually near the upper portion.

Shortly after attaching, the embryo begins to burrow into the uterine lining by secreting enzymes that break down uterine tissue. Eventually, the burrowing embryo comes into contact with nutrient-filled glands in the lining of the uterus, which it taps into for further growth. Material in the uterine fluids and tissue debris from the breakdown of the uterine lining also provide nutrients for the embryo.

During the next few days the embryo burrows deeper into the uterus by sending out fingerlike projections, called *chorionic villi*, into the endometrium. Eventually the tips of the advancing chorionic villi come upon maternal blood vessels and break them open. This allows the embryo to acquire nutrients from the mother's blood. More and more chorionic villi form, so more and more maternal blood vessels are tapped.

## Cessation of Menstruation

Soon after it implants in the uterus, the embryo produces a hormone unique to pregnancy, called human chorionic gonadotropin (hCG), which is secreted into the maternal bloodstream. This hormone stimulates the mother's ovaries to increase the production of estrogen and progesterone, which, in turn, prevent the next menstrual period. If there were no way for the embryo to signal the mother's body of its presence in the uterus, a menstrual period would occur and the pregnancy would end.

Besides preventing the next menstrual period, estrogen and progesterone bring about the first noticeable signs of pregnancy: occasional nausea and vomiting referred to as "morning sickness," enlarged and tender breasts, increased frequency of urination, and enlargement of the uterus.

Both clinical and home pregnancy tests are based on analyzing a woman's urine for the presence of hCG. Home pregnancy tests are quite accurate if carried out several days after a missed menstrual period. If the test is done too soon, the tests are likely to indicate a woman is not pregnant when, in fact, she is ("false negative"). Anyone with a positive test should redo the test in a few days or get a pregnancy test from a health professional.

# Pregnancy

Occasionally, implantation occurs outside the uterus. This is called an *ectopic pregnancy*. Although in very rare instances, they occur on the outer layer of the uterus or the bowel, ectopic pregnancies most often occur in a fallopian tube (called *tubal pregnancies*) where passage of the embryo is blocked by tubal malformation or by scarring or twisting from a prior infection, often gonorrhea or chlamydia. If a tubal pregnancy remains undiscovered, the embryo will become too large for the fallopian tube and the tube will burst, creating internal bleeding and a critical medical situation. Some women are forewarned of tubal rupture by a sharp stabbing pain, cramps, or a constant dull pain and are able to seek medical attention before the tube ruptures.

## Fetal Development

**fetus** the stage of intrauterine development from about the tenth week after fertilization to birth
**amnion** a saclike structure in which the fetus develops
**placenta** an organ unique to pregnancy that transports oxygen and nutrients from the mother to the fetus and waste products from the fetus to the mother
**umbilical cord** a structure that transports blood from the fetus to and from the placenta

After implantation, the placenta continues to enlarge and the embryo begins to develop organs. At this time the embryo is called a **fetus**. By the tenth week after fertilization nearly all of the fetal body is formed and the fetus weighs about 1 gram. During the rest of development, the fetal body grows and most of the organs become functional. At birth an average fetus weighs almost 3000 grams (about 7 pounds).

Fetal development and growth take place within a fluid-filled membranous sac called the **amnion**, which lies within the uterus (**FIGURE 4.5**). By developing in the *amniotic fluid* the fetus grows unimpeded by the mother's internal organs and is protected from potentially damaging jolts when the mother changes her body position. The amnion ruptures just before birth, which is sometimes called "breaking of the bag of waters."

### The Placenta

The **placenta** is an organ unique to pregnancy. It develops from the chorionic villi, and thus is composed of fetal tissue. Its functions are to transport oxygen and nutrients from the mother to the fetus and waste products from the fetus to the mother. Nutrients move from maternal blood vessels into fetal blood vessels within the chorionic villi. Waste products are transferred from the fetal blood to the mother's blood in the opposite manner. At no time do the fetal and maternal bloodstreams mix. Blood flows from the fetus to and from the placenta through the **umbilical cord**. The placenta also manufactures many hormones unique to pregnancy.

Because every individual's cells have their own unique chemical identity, a pregnant woman's immune system can potentially respond to fetal cells as "foreign" by attacking them. This does not occur, however, because the fetus produces chemicals that protect it from the mother's immune system.

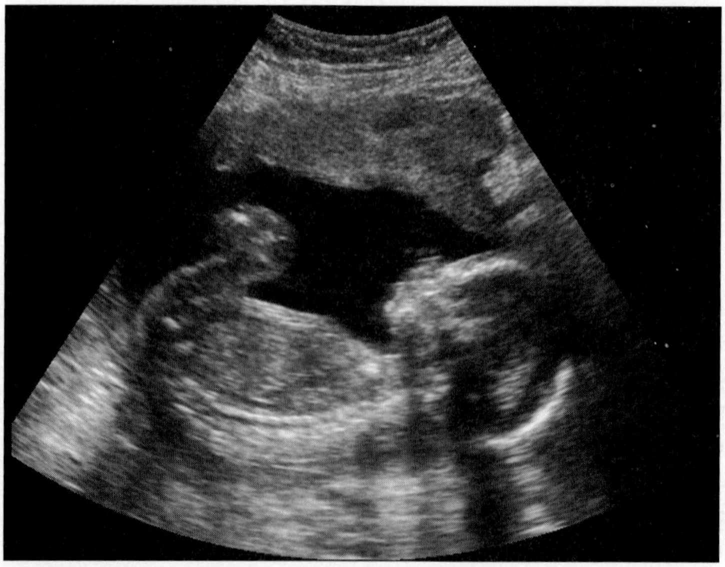

Image of a fetus obtained by ultrasound scan.

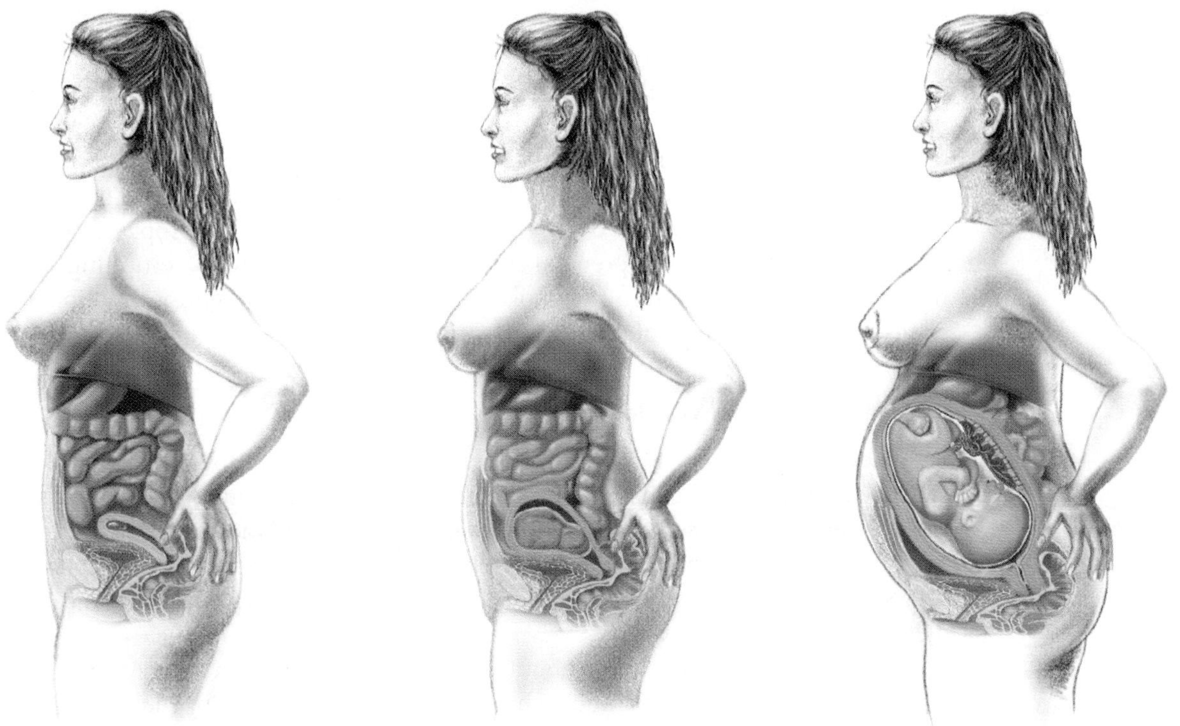


FIGURE 4.5 **Growth and Development of a Human Fetus.** Through the three trimesters of pregnancy, the fetus develops inside the fluid-filled amnion.

## Pregnancy

### The Duration of Pregnancy

It takes at least 266 days for a fertilized human ovum to develop fully into a fetus ready for birth. The average pregnancy, however, is 280 days (40 weeks, or 10 lunar months). The apparent discrepancy arises because the beginning of pregnancy is marked by doctors as the first day of flow in the menstrual cycle during which conception occurred rather than the day of fertilization. Uncomplicated pregnancies can range from 260 to 315 days.

During pregnancy many changes occur in a woman's body. For example, the blood plasma increases in volume by as much as 50% over her nonpregnant levels; the heart beats 10% faster and with 20% to 30% greater output of blood per minute, the number of red blood cells increases, and breathing becomes deeper and slightly faster. One of the most striking changes during pregnancy is the growth of the uterus. The nonpregnant uterus is approximately 7–8 centimeters long and weighs about 60–100 grams; by the end of pregnancy the uterus is approximately 30 centimeters long and weighs nearly 1000 grams.

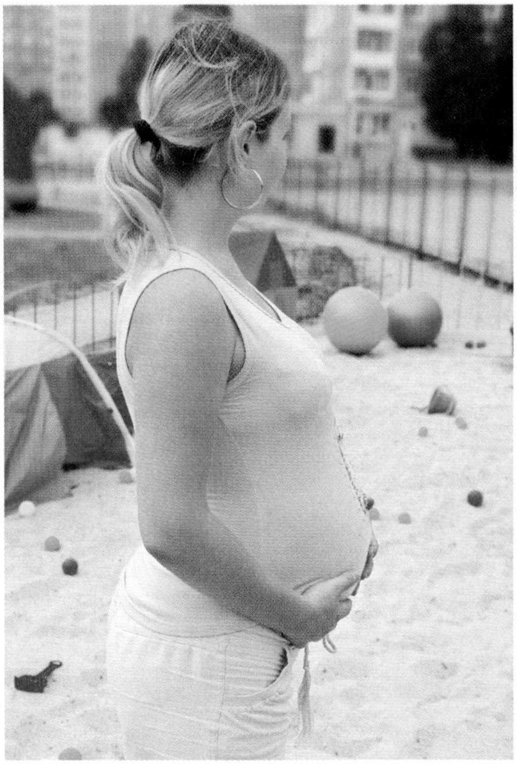

### Health Habits During Pregnancy

Every child deserves to be born as healthy as possible. It is only fair to the unborn child—who did not ask to be conceived—that all the genetic potential to develop a healthy body and brain be given the opportunity to be fully expressed. If a developing baby could talk, he or she might say, "Mom, my lifelong health and well-being are in your hands right now. I know that nine months is a long time to be concerned about doing the right things, but it's important to me that you try. That way, I'll get the best chance to become the best person I can be and you'll stay healthy so we can share a lot of good times after I'm born." Factors that deserve attention during pregnancy include ensuring proper nutrition, obtaining professional prenatal care, getting enough exercise, refraining from smoking and consuming alcohol and other drugs, and accepting emotional changes as a normal part of pregnancy.

## Nutrition During Pregnancy

Fetal development requires an ample supply of all nutrients necessary for growth so that new cells and organs can develop optimally. All fetal nutrients come from the mother via the placenta, so a mother must "eat for two," meaning that she must ensure that her diet contains adequate nutrients for herself and the fetus (**Table 4.1**). Some pregnant women are advised to supplement a generally well-balanced diet with iron and folic acid.

Many women are concerned about weight gain during pregnancy. Although it is never good to weigh too much, an increase of 25–30 pounds by the end of pregnancy is all right, most of which comes in the last two-thirds of pregnancy: 7 pounds in fetal weight; 2 pounds in enlarged uterus; 1 pound for placenta; 1 pound for amnion and amniotic fluid; 4–8 pounds of fluid for additional blood and fluids; and 4 pounds of body fat.

**Table 4.1** Recommended Daily Dietary Reference Intakes (DRI) for Nonpregnant, Pregnant, and Lactating Women, Ages 25–50

| | Nonpregnant | Pregnant | Lactating |
|---|---|---|---|
| Protein (g) | 46 | 71 | 71 |
| Carbohydrate | 130 | 175 | 210 |
| Vitamin A (μg) | 700 | 770 | 1300 |
| Vitamin D (μg) | 5 | 5 | 5 |
| Vitamin C (mg) | 75 | 85 | 120 |
| Thiamine (mg) | 1.2 | 1.1 | 1.4 |
| Riboflavin (mg) | 1.1 | 1.4 | 1.6 |
| Niacin (mg) | 14 | 18 | 17 |
| Vitamin $B_6$ (mg) | 1.3 | 1.9 | 2.0 |
| Folate (mg) | 400 | 600 | 500 |
| Vitamin $B_{12}$ (mg) | 2.4 | 2.6 | 2.8 |
| Calcium (mg) | 1000 | 1000 | 1000 |
| Phosphorus (mg) | 700 | 700 | 700 |
| Iron (mg) | 18 | 27 | 9 |
| Zinc (mg) | 8 | 11 | 12 |
| Iodine (mg) | 150 | 220 | 290 |

Data from Food and Nutrition Board, Institute of Medicine, National Academy of Sciences. (2004). *Dietary reference intakes.* Washington, DC: National Academies Press.

## Prenatal Care

Pregnancy involves extensive and profound biological changes in both fetus and mother. These significant biological changes carry some health risks, which is the reason mothers-to-be are advised to obtain professional prenatal care. Women who receive competent, professional prenatal care are more likely to have a successful pregnancy and give birth to a healthy child than those who do not. Prenatal care can detect and lessen the consequences of diseases specific to pregnancy; manage problems resulting from a malfunctioning placenta; reduce the risks of birth defects; educate the mother and her family about proper nutrition and not smoking, drinking alcohol, or taking other drugs during pregnancy; and educate and prepare the mother and her partner for childbirth, breastfeeding, and post-birth care of the baby.

Professional prenatal care has contributed to a dramatic reduction in the risk of death in pregnancy and childbirth. In 1920 the maternal mortality rate in the United States was 690 per 100,000 births. By 1955 the rate had fallen to 50 per 100,000 births. Now, the maternal mortality rate is about 8 per 100,000 births, because about 90% of pregnant women obtain an average of 12 prenatal visits.

## Physical Activity and Exercise

Physical activity and exercise—particularly gentle exercise—are generally beneficial during pregnancy. The degree of physical activity during pregnancy depends on a woman's desires and abilities. Some women engage in physical activity almost to the day of delivery. Women who are not routinely athletic are wise to begin a program early in pregnancy to maintain correct posture; strengthen bones and abdominal muscles; improve breathing; reduce backaches, constipation, bloating, and swelling; and sleep better and relax.

## Emotional Well-Being

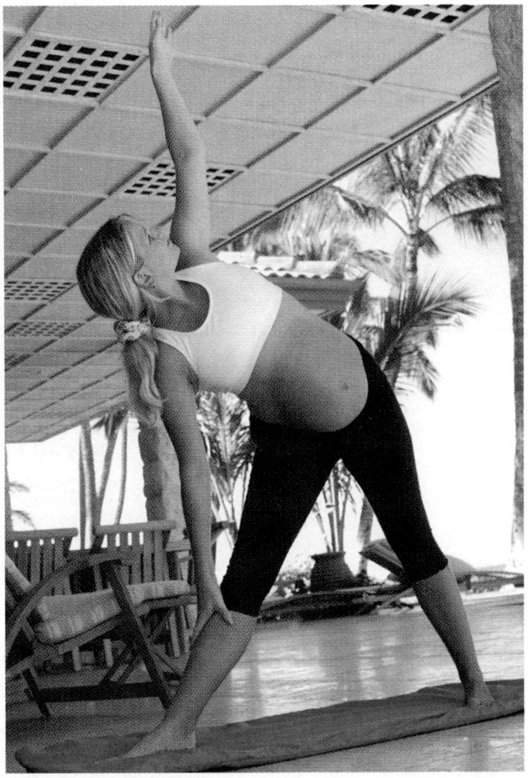

Pregnancy can be a time of intense feelings, not only for the mother-to-be but also for her partner and others who are close to her. Enthusiasm, excitement, anticipation, fear about the baby's condition, uncertainties about one's suitability as a parent, and a desire for more (or less) love, affection, and support are all natural.

As at other times of life, intense feelings during pregnancy can be accepted and managed by taking time each day to quiet the mind and body by engaging in mediation, yoga, or other relaxation methods. Massage also is beneficial, and it may fulfill the desires of those who feel more sensual during pregnancy. Some couples have increased desires for sexual intercourse during pregnancy, which is all right unless a medical problem that would be worsened by sex is evident.

## (No!) Smoking During Pregnancy

Smoking cigarettes during pregnancy reduces the amount of oxygen available to the fetus and floods the fetal body with the 4000-plus chemicals that are in tobacco smoke, 43 of which are known to cause cancer. A pregnant woman who smokes cigarettes increases the risk of birth defects, including an abnormal heart or brain, cleft lip or palate, retarded fetal growth, spontaneous abortion, death of the fetus, and a smaller-than-normal infant at birth. If she continues to smoke after the baby is born, a woman increases the risk of shortening her own life by 11 years from lung cancer, heart attack, or other deadly illness and contributing to respiratory problems in her child.

### (No!) Drinking Alcohol During Pregnancy

The alcohol a pregnant woman drinks easily gets into the fetus's body and reaches a level equal to that of the mother. Because the fetal body is small and its drug-detoxifying systems are immature, alcohol remains in the fetal bloodstream long after it has disappeared from the mother's blood. This puts the fetus at risk for a variety of mental and physical defects from *fetal alcohol spectrum disorder* including its most severe form, *fetal alcohol syndrome* (see Chapter 7). Women should *never* drink alcohol if pregnancy is a possibility. Sexually active women who do not use a birth control method should *not* drink alcohol because alcohol in the bloodstream can affect fetal brain development well before a woman realizes that she is pregnant.

## Sexual Interaction During Pregnancy

Compared with prepregnancy, the desire and frequency of sexual intercourse generally diminishes during pregnancy and soon after childbirth, although for some couples they stay the same or increase, especially during the first trimester. In the vast majority of American women, sexual desire and activity decline considerably during the month prior to childbirth and six to eight weeks thereafter.

Diminishing sexual desire and activity during pregnancy often arise from fears that sexual intercourse will harm the fetus or jeopardize the pregnancy. Also, a woman may feel uncomfortable, nauseous, or exhausted while pregnant. Breast-feeding and attending to the needs of an infant can reduce a woman's desire for sex, as can postpartum depression. Because infant care is demanding and tiring, after the baby is born one or both parents may be too tired for intense sex; cuddling, gentle touching, and talking may be preferable.

Unless there is some physical problem that would be worsened by sex, sexual intercourse and orgasm are permissible during pregnancy. As pregnancy progresses, the man-on-top position may not be feasible or desirable, and couples can employ other positions for intercourse (e.g., side-by-side, woman-on-top, rear-entry). If intercourse is not desired, closeness and sexual arousal may still occur through touching, holding, showering or bathing together, massage, mutual masturbation, and oral sex. A woman's breasts will be enlarged and tender, so she may not want them stimulated or stimulated in new ways. It is recommended that couples refrain from sexual intercourse for several weeks following childbirth to allow an episiotomy or tears to heal, to let the uterus and vagina return to pre-pregnancy sizes, and to become fully capable of sexual responsiveness.

## Childbirth

After about 266 days of intrauterine life, the fetus is physiologically ready to leave the mother's body and face the outside world. No one knows for sure what a person feels when being born, but many believe the feelings are intense. Frederick Leboyer, a French physician, developed a birthing procedure involving dim lighting, soft music, and the delivery of the baby into a bath of warm water to try to minimize the presumed psychic trauma of birth.

For the newborn's parents, childbirth can bring great joy, relief that the pregnancy is ended, and surprise at the baby's appearance. For onlookers and family members, childbirth may elicit wonder, reverence, and concern for the conditions of the mother and baby.

A few weeks before childbirth, the fetus becomes positioned for birth by descending in the uterus. This is called *lightening*. In about 95% of births, the fetus is in a head-down position. When not head-down, the fetus may be head-up or lying sideways. In nearly all instances the fetus's legs are tucked up against the abdomen in the "fetal position."

**labor** the expulsion of the fetus from the mother's body

Childbirth or **labor** (also called *parturition*) involves the forceful expulsion from the uterus of the fetus, amniotic fluid, and the placenta via strong, rhythmic contractions of the muscle layer of the uterus (FIGURE 4.6). Labor usually begins with roughly minute-long contractions coming at approximately 10- to 20-minute intervals. As labor progresses, these regular contractions usually become more intense, frequent, and of longer duration, perhaps up to 90 seconds. Voluntary

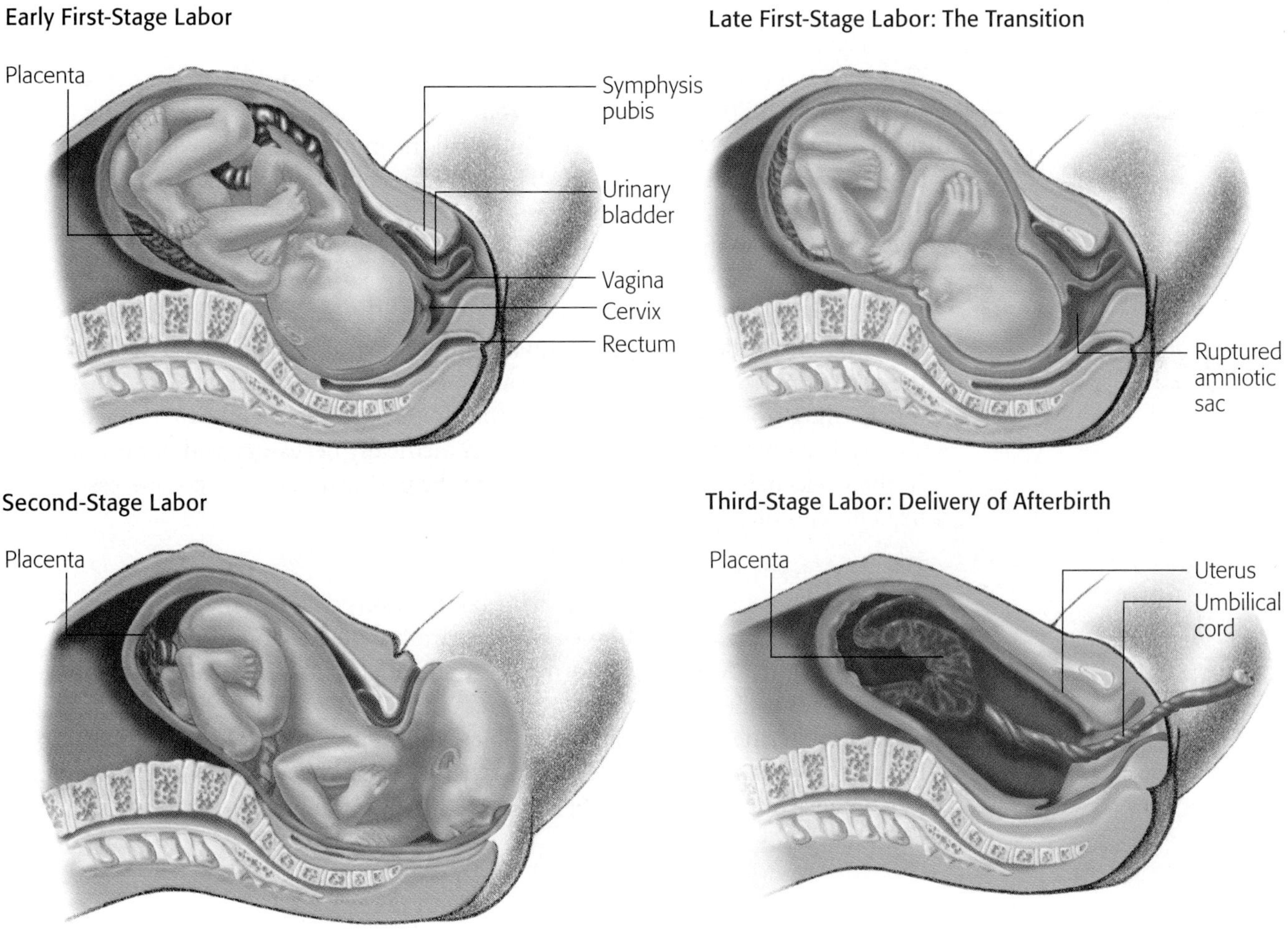


**FIGURE 4.6 Childbirth.** The stages of labor. (a) Early first stage: The cervix is dilating. (b) Late first stage (transition stage): The cervix is fully dilated and the amniotic sac has ruptured, releasing amniotic fluid; the fetal head bends forward, bringing the chin to the upper chest. (c) Second stage: the birth of the baby. As the fetus moves toward the outside, its body turns sideways, then the head rotates from a sideways position to facing forward, and finally the head extends upward to permit easier exit from the body. After emergence of the head, the body turns sideways again to facilitate delivery of the shoulder and the rest of the body. (d) Third stage: delivery of the placenta (afterbirth).

contractions of the abdominal muscles also help expel the uterine contents. During the last half of pregnancy a woman may have intermittent uterine contractions (Braxton–Hicks contractions). These can be distinguished by their occurrence at irregular intervals and rather short duration.

Childbirth occurs in three stages:

1. *First stage:* Dilation (widening) of the cervix, also called *effacement*
2. *Second stage:* Expulsion of the fetus from the mother's body
3. *Third stage:* Delivery of the placenta and fetal membranes (*afterbirth*)

### The First Stage of Labor: Cervical Effacement

This stage of childbirth is usually the longest, typically lasting eight to 12 hours; sometimes longer for first-time mothers and sometimes shorter for women who have given birth before. It begins with the onset of uterine contractions and ends when the cervix is fully dilated. During this stage the opening of the mother's cervix enlarges from 1 centimeter to about 10 centimeters. This stage may be initiated by "breaking of the bag of waters," disruption of the amniotic sac and the loss via the vagina of about a liter of amniotic fluid, and "bloody show," the discharge of a mucous plug from the cervix. Sometimes the first stage of labor is slow to begin or slows after starting, in which case any of a variety of medical and nonmedical interventions can be employed to induce labor.

### The Second Stage of Labor: Birth of the Baby

This stage, which lasts from 30 minutes to two hours, begins when the cervix is fully dilated and the fetus descends from the uterus into the vagina. During this stage involuntary contractions continue and the mother also can voluntarily contract her abdominal muscles ("push") with each contraction to help expel the baby. The official time of birth is when the entire fetal body is clear of the mother's body.

Occasionally, emergence of the fetus slows or stops because the head is too large for the vaginal opening, the fetus is in an irregular position, or the perineum cannot stretch sufficiently. When delivery slows, the baby may have trouble breathing or otherwise be in danger. In this circumstance, an **episiotomy**, an incision in the perineum from the vagina to the anus, can be performed to enlarge the opening. Healing from the episiotomy can take two to six weeks and can be uncomfortable, so it should be performed only when medically necessary and not routinely. In the weeks before childbirth, massaging the perineal region often can lessen the need for episiotomy.

**episiotomy** an incision in the perineum from the vagina to the anus

### The Third Stage of Labor: Delivery of the Placenta

This stage lasts 15–30 minutes. Uterine contractions dislodge the placenta and remnants of the fetal membranes from the wall of the uterus and expel them from the vagina. A blood clot forms at the site of placental attachment to prevent bleeding. Over the next two to three hours the uterus continues to contract. This constricts uterine arteries and lessens bleeding, and it helps restore the uterus to its pre-pregnant size. Breastfeeding also helps return the uterus to its pre-pregnant size because oxytocin, one of the hormones involved in breastfeeding, stimulates contractions of the uterus.

## Relief of Discomfort and Pain

Discomfort or pain can be associated with labor, especially in the later phases of the first stage and the early stages of the second, due to stretches and strains as the fetus emerges from the vagina. A variety of methods are available to lessen discomfort and pain during labor, including hypnosis, warm baths, walking, massage, deep breathing, meditation, sterile-water injections, and the administration

## Dear Penelope . . .

***I'm late. Do home pregnancy tests really work?***
***— Needs to Know***

*Dear Needs to Know,*

Home pregnancy tests are fairly reliable if you use them correctly and repeat the test. If, however, you want the results to be as accurate as possible, get tested by a professional at your student health center, your doctor's office, or a family planning clinic.

Virtually all tests for pregnancy, whether self- or clinic-administered, analyze a woman's blood or urine for a hormone specific to pregnancy (because it is produced by the fertilized egg) called human chorionic gonadotropin (hCG). This hormone begins to appear about eight to 10 days after fertilization; the amount doubles every couple of days.

A pregnancy test can be wrong if it indicates that a woman is pregnant when she isn't ("false positive") or if she is not pregnant when she actually is ("false negative"). A false positive is usually discovered when the woman seeks prenatal care. A false negative can go undetected until signs and symptoms of pregnancy appear. Reasons for false negatives are that (1) the amount of hCG in the test fluid is too small to be detected or (2) the test is carried out incorrectly. For these reasons, it is recommended at any negative result be retested in a week. Despite claims by product manufacturers, a scientific study comparing accuracy among home pregnancy tests showed that only one test was nearly 100% accurate; it was also the easiest to interpret correctly. Other brands could be accurate the first time about 70% of the time, with accuracy improving to 90% by the fifth test. All at-home pregnancy test products have extensive Web sites that describe how to conduct the test with the least likelihood for errors.

Courtesy of the UC Davis *Aggie*

of pain-relieving medications that leave the mother conscious so she can actively participate in expelling the fetus and that have a low risk of harming the fetus. General anesthesia (complete unconsciousness) is used only in cases of very difficult births.

Social and psychological support also contribute to lessening labor pain and discomfort. Women who expect to be able to manage childbirth successfully generally have less discomfort and require less pain medication than those who are fearful. This is one reason pregnant women are encouraged to take childbirth preparation classes. Also, women who have continuous emotional support during childbirth generally need less pain medication. Support can come from a father or other family member, a trained labor assistant called a *doula*, or a nurse or other obstetric professional. Giving birth in a homelike setting and with caregivers in attendance whom the mother knows also contribute to a more positive birthing experience.

## Cesarean Births

In situations of difficult birth, the fetus can be delivered surgically via a procedure called a **cesarean section (C-section)**. This involves anesthetizing the mother and making an incision through her abdomen and the uterus to free the baby. Medical indications for cesarean include the woman having had a prior cesarean, the baby being too large to be born vaginally, the baby being positioned in the uterus such that a difficult labor is expected, a slow fetal heart rate or other signs of fetal distress, active genital herpes, and other medical problems (FIGURE 4.7). For both mother and baby, cesareans are less safe than uncomplicated vaginal deliveries, and they cost more.

**cesarean section (C-section)** surgical delivery of the fetus via incision in the mother's abdomen

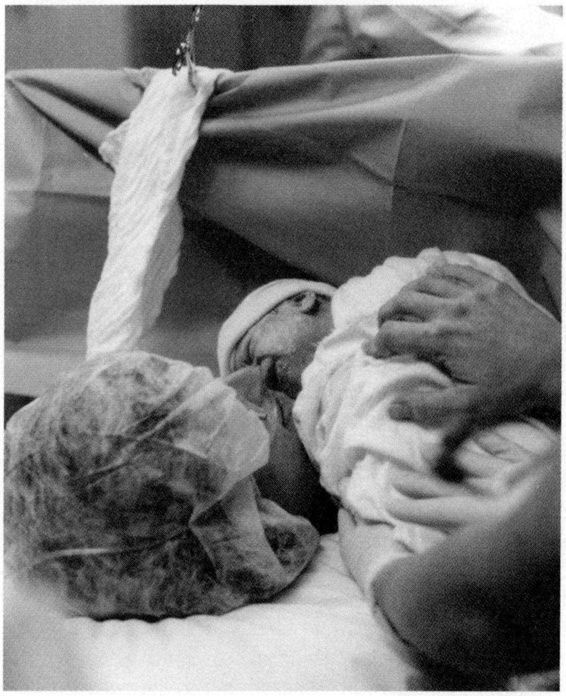

FIGURE 4.7 **Reasons for Cesarean Delivery.** Reasons include labor progresses slowly or stops; baby may have difficulty breathing; baby lies feet first or sideways in the uterus and cannot pass through the vagina; baby's head is turned; mother has active genital herpes lesion; placenta detaches early; placenta covers the cervix; baby is large; mother's pelvis is small; and mother has health or developmental problems.

In the United States today, nearly 28% of births are by C-section. In 1970 only 5% of births were cesarean. Among the reasons offered for this increase are parents' and/or physicians' desire for a convenient delivery. Also, the physician and hospital may not want to risk a difficult labor that might harm the baby or trigger an expensive lawsuit subsequently. Parents understandably expect their newborn to be healthy and well. If a birth is difficult and a child is harmed, parents may blame the physician for not performing a cesarean or not performing one quickly enough to avoid trouble during labor. Obstetrical malpractice lawsuits are the most common among medical subspecialties, and obstetrical liability insurance rates also are the highest among primary care practitioners.

## Premature Births

Normal pregnancies are supposed to last about 40 weeks, but in the United States, 12% of babies are born before 37 weeks of pregnancy (described as *preterm infants* or "premies"). The number of preterm births in the United States has increased by about 27% since 1980. Similar increases are reported in Australia, Canada, New Zealand, and the United Kingdom.

Although intensive medical care can help them survive, preterm infants are at high risk for many disabilities, including mental retardation, cerebral palsy, lung and gastrointestinal problems, and vision and hearing loss. It is estimated that the medical and nonmedical expenses associated with premature births exceed those of any other disease or disability. Babies delivered at 22 to 25 weeks are extremely underdeveloped and vulnerable. By school age, at least 80% of them show severe cognitive deficiencies and neurological problems.

HEALTHY SEXUALITY

### Infant Mortality

The first year of any infant's life can be risky, especially if there is an insufficient health care system to intervene when a pregnant woman, an infant, or an infant's mother gets sick. The worldwide infant mortality rate (the rate at which babies die before their first birthday) is 42 deaths per 1000 live births. This means that worldwide, 7.1 million infants die each year.

There is an enormous disparity in infant mortality among countries. The infant mortality rates (deaths per 1000 live births) around the world include:

| | |
|---|---|
| Sweden | 2.75 |
| Japan | 2.79 |
| France | 3.33 |
| Germany | 3.99 |
| United Kingdom | 4.85 |
| New Zealand | 4.92 |
| Canada | 5.04 |
| United States | 6.22 |
| Chile | 7.71 |
| Panama | 12.67 |
| China | 20.25 |
| Indonesia | 29.97 |
| *World* | *44.13* |
| Bolivia | 44.46 |
| Pakistan | 67.36 |
| Chad | 98.69 |
| Afghanistan | 153.14 |
| Angola | 180.21 |

Data from *The World Fact Book*. Washington, DC: Central Intelligence Agency, 2009. Complete list of 224 countries available at: https://www.cia.gov/library/publications/the-world-factbook/rankorder/2091rank.html. Accessed October 6, 2010.

When mothers and babies have access to good health care, infant mortality is caused by serious birth defects, preterm delivery and low birth weight, automobile accidents, sudden infant death syndrome (SIDS), and infections, including HIV. When mothers and babies do not have access to health care, infants die because of complications surrounding childbirth, malnutrition, infection (e.g., HIV, malaria), unsanitary conditions, and absence of the mother or other caretaker.

The overall U.S. infant mortality rate is 6.3 deaths per 1000 live births. The U.S. rate is higher than in other industrialized countries because many Americans do not have access to health care. The U.S. infant mortality rate varies by race. The rate for non-Hispanic Caucasians is 5.76 deaths per 1000 live births; African Americans, 13.63; Hispanics, 5.8; American Indians and Alaskan natives, 4.9; and Asian/Pacific Islanders, 8.06.

To reduce the rate of infant mortality in the world, the World Health Organization wants to increase the availability of health services to all mothers. To reduce the rate of infant mortality in the United States, the Department of Health and Human Services wants to increase the proportion of mothers getting early prenatal care; decrease the incidence of SIDS; lessen the percentage of pregnant women who smoke cigarettes, drink alcohol, and take other drugs; and reduce the number of low-birth-weight infants.

The age of the mother, infertility treatments, maternal illness (e.g., diabetes, high blood pressure), and infection can lead to premature birth. Also, personal health behaviors (e.g., smoking, drug use, malnutrition, overweight) and social/environmental factors (e.g., poverty, overwork, lack of prenatal care, stress) may be involved in premature birth.

About 50% of pregnant women who show signs of premature labor actually deliver early. But since there is no way to distinguish between the women who will proceed to term and those who will not, women at risk are given drugs to stop premature contractions.

## The Postpartum Transition

After the child is born, the mother goes through several weeks of postpartum transition called the *puerperium*. During this time, the physiological changes of pregnancy slowly reverse and the vagina and surrounding structures recuperate from labor. Uterine tissue (called *lochia*) that is no longer needed is discharged for the first month or so after childbirth. Following childbirth, estrogen and progesterone levels, which were high during pregnancy, drop to extremely low levels within 72 hours.

During the puerperium, the mother and her partner begin to adjust to demands of their new living situation. Childbirth and infant care can be exhausting. Many women experience the "baby blues," which are transitory mood changes involving tiredness, depression, loneliness, and fear. These feelings usually abate in a few weeks, but about 13% of women experience postpartum depression severe and disabling enough to require professional help. Postpartum mood changes are so common that they are thought to be related to the massive drop in hormone levels after birth. Besides changes in hormone levels, childbirth also brings many psychological and social changes for the mother, her partner, and other family and household members.

## Sudden Infant Death Syndrome

**sudden infant death syndrome (SIDS)** the sudden unexpected death of an infant for no known reason

**colostrum** a yellowish precursor to mature mother's milk

**Sudden infant death syndrome (SIDS)** is the sudden death of an infant less than 1 year of age that occurs during sleep. Each year about 2300 infant deaths occur in the United States. The cause of SIDS is unknown; babies who succumb to SIDS do not show any abnormality that can be discovered at autopsy. The best advice for parents of newborns is to put infants to sleep on their backs to avoid the risk of an infant suffocating while lying on its stomach.

## Breastfeeding

The breasts become prepared for nursing in the early weeks of pregnancy with an increase in the number of milk ducts and the deposition of fat in the breast tissue. The nipples and areola generally enlarge and often deepen in color. These changes cause the breasts to become tender early in pregnancy.

About midway in pregnancy the breasts begin to manufacture **colostrum**, a yellowish precursor to mature milk. For the first few days after birth, colostrum is the major nutrient supplied by the breasts. As the newborn nurses, colostrum is drained from the breasts and is replaced by milk. Colostrum contains nutrients and is especially high in maternal antibodies that protect the infant against infection.

Mother's milk contains specific milk proteins, antibodies, the milk sugar *lactose*, fat, and water. Milk production is controlled by the pituitary hormone *prolactin*, the levels of which rise during pregnancy and remain high as long as the woman nurses.

Insertion of the nipple into the baby's mouth activates the baby's sucking reflex. When the baby sucks, nerve impulses are transmitted from the breast to the mother's brain, which triggers the release of the hormone *oxytocin* from the mother's posterior pituitary gland. Oxytocin circulates through the mother's bloodstream to the breasts, where it causes the muscle cells that line the milk ducts to contract and eject milk from the nipple.

As long as the baby continues to nurse and the breasts are regularly drained of milk, the hormonal stimulation of milk production continues and the baby can be nursed for many months. Without such stimuli, milk production stops. Poor nutrition, stress, fatigue, and lack of social support also can stop milk production. As long as the mother continues to nurse, she is highly unlikely to become pregnant because the hormones that support milk production and nursing almost always prevent ovulation and the occurrence of menstrual cycles as long as the baby is breastfeeding.

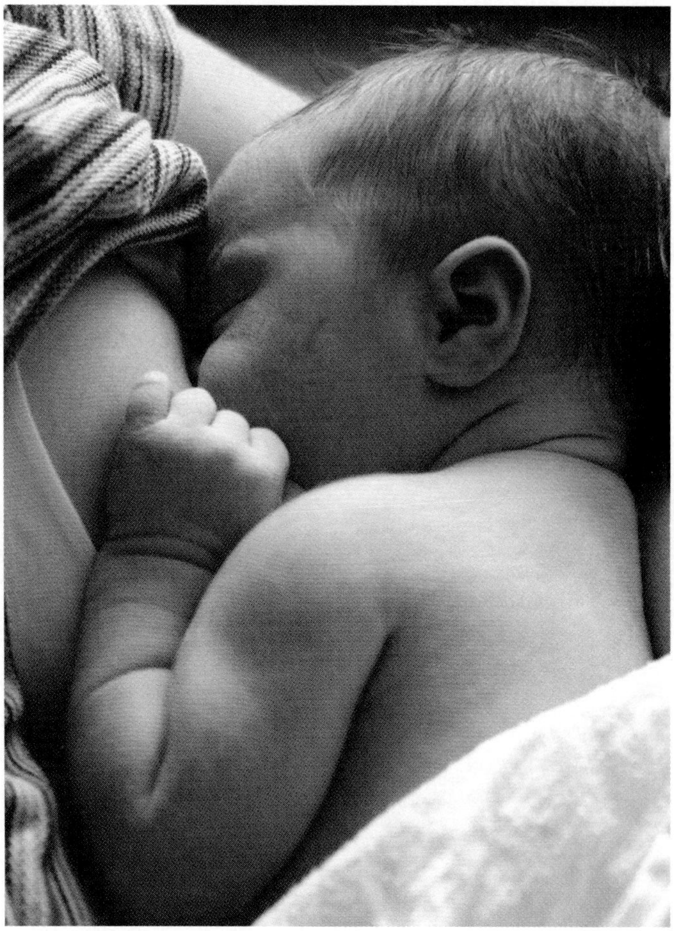

Occasionally, pleasurable feelings accompanying breastfeeding can have an erotic tone, possibly producing genital sensations and even occasionally orgasm. These feelings and responses are normal and natural, and a woman should not feel guilty or distressed by them.

Breastfeeding may take place for several weeks, months, or even years and replaced gradually by bottle-feeding until the child is weaned (stops nursing altogether). A nursing mother can use a breast pump to put her own milk into bottles for the baby to consume when she is not available.

The many advantages of breastfeeding include:

1. It is economical, is readily available, and eliminates the effort involved in purchasing, preparing, and heating bottles and formula.
2. It transfers immunity (protection against infections) from the mother to the infant, and breast milk itself and the act of nursing stimulate the development of the infant's own immune defenses.
3. Breast milk promotes the development of the infant's digestive system.
4. Breastfed babies have fewer allergies, less diarrhea, fewer dental problems, and less colic (stomachache).
5. Breast milk is nutritionally balanced for human infants; formulas containing cow's milk are not nutritionally identical to human milk, although they are nutritionally adequate.
6. Breastfeeding may increase the psychological attachment between mother and infant (called bonding).
7. The hormones involved in the production and release of milk cause uterine contractions, which help the uterus return to its normal size. During the first week or so after childbirth these contractions may be intense and even painful. Thereafter some women describe them as pleasurable, sensual, or erotic.
8. Many women find that breastfeeding allows them to have the opportunity to sit down, relax, and have a pleasurable experience with their babies.

The many advantages of breastfeeding do not mean that bottlefeeding is not wholesome. There are many healthy, well-adjusted people who were bottlefed infants. Some women are physically unable to breastfeed. Some mothers choose not to breast feed because work, family, and other responsibilities make it inconvenient; breastfeeding in public or at work is still not accepted in many communities or places of employment. Some women choose not to breastfeed because they fear that changes in the shape of their breasts will lower their sexual attractiveness. Also, bottlefeeding allows the father to take an active role in infant feeding. More important than whether the milk comes from the breast or a bottle is the physical contact and loving the infant receives while being fed.

## Infertility

**infertile** not able to conceive a child after one year of trying
**sterility** permanently infertile

Approximately 7% of American married couples of childbearing age are **infertile**. This means that they are unable to become pregnant after a year of trying. Problems with a male partner's reproductive biology are responsible for infertility in about 40% of infertile couples; female factors are responsible in another 40% to 50%. In about 10% of infertile couples, no cause can be determined. With professional help, about half of all infertile couples can eventually have children. A significant number of couples medically determined to be infertile eventually have children without medical interventions. Permanent infertility is called **sterility**.

In both sexes, infertility can be caused by a variety of conditions that adversely affect the functioning of an otherwise normal reproductive system. For example, ill health, cigarette smoking, chronic alcohol use, marijuana and other drug use, exposure to radiation or toxic chemicals, malnutrition, anxiety, stress, and fatigue can lessen a person's reproductive capabilities. Medical treatment or changes in lifestyle often restore fertility. Age also plays a role. Women in their 20s conceive more readily than women in their late 30s and early 40s do.

Because sperm and ovum production and the functioning of male and female reproductive tracts are dependent on adequate hormone production, hormonal problems are a common cause of infertility in both men and women. Infertility can result from underproduction of GnRF, FSH, LH, testosterone, estrogen, or progesterone. Augmenting inadequate hormone production with natural hormones or synthetic fertility drugs can restore fertility. Fertility drugs, however, increase the chances of having twins or multiples.

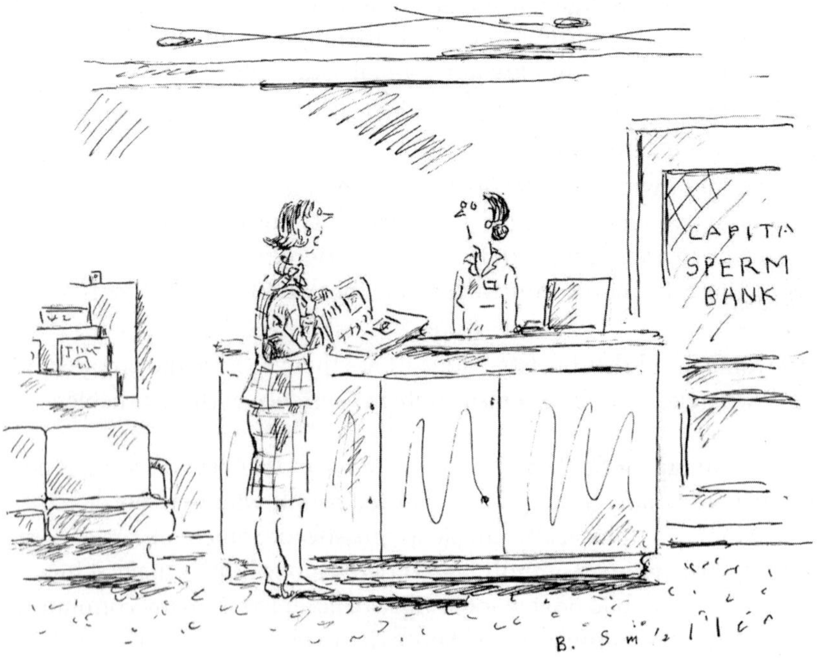


*"If he's so smart, why does he have to sell his sperm?"*

Infertility can also be caused by anatomical abnormalities or damage to female or male reproductive systems. For example, chlamydia and gonorrhea infections can scar or damage the fallopian tubes or epididymides. Growths and tumors in the reproductive tract can block the movement of sperm and ova. Sometimes surgical repair of damaged reproductive organs can restore fertility.

Problems with insemination and sperm transport also can cause infertility. For example, a man may have difficulty getting and maintaining an erection or ejaculating into the vagina. A woman may produce very thick or voluminous cervical mucus, which can block entry of sperm into the uterus. Sometimes infertility is caused by not having intercourse at or near the time of ovulation. A procedure called *intrauterine insemination* (IUI) can be used to increase the number of sperm that reach the fallopian tubes and thereby increase the chance of fertilization. With this method, the ejaculate is collected, the sperm are washed, and then the sperm are placed directly into the uterus using a syringe with a thin tube (catheter). The sperm donor can be a male partner or a donor male. Each year in the United States, about 10,000 babies are conceived by IUI.

## Enhancing Fertility Options

Several medical procedures, referred to as **assisted reproductive technologies**, are available to help infertile couples become pregnant. These methods involve removing ova from a woman's ovaries, combining them with sperm in a laboratory dish, and returning them to the woman's body or that of another woman. These methods include the following:

**assisted reproductive technologies** medical procedures that involve removing ova from a woman's body, combining them with sperm in the laboratory, and returning them to the woman's body or that of another woman

1. IVF (*in vitro fertilization*). In this method, a donor woman is given hormones to induce release of several ova, which are collected surgically. The ova are fertilized in a laboratory dish by sperm from the partner or a donor. Usually several of the resulting embryos are placed into the uterus of the donor woman or a surrogate (if the donor cannot or does not wish to have the child). Successful pregnancy and childbirth occur in about 50% of procedures. About one-third of IVF pregnancies produce one child, one-third produce fraternal twins, and one-third triplets or more. Multiple births are associated with lower birth weights and higher rates of birth defects. Multiple births also endanger the mother by increasing her risks for high blood pressure, anemia, premature labor, and cesarean section. Multiple births also can impose financial and psychological burdens on parents.
2. GIFT (*gamete intrafallopian transfer*). GIFT involves obtaining ova from a fertile woman and sperm from a partner, and then placing the ova and sperm in each of the fallopian tubes, where fertilization can take place.
3. ZIFT (*zygote intrafallopian transfer*). ZIFT involves collecting ova and sperm from partners, allowing fertilization to occur in a laboratory dish, and then placing a fertilized egg (*zygote*) in a fallopian tube.

Employing any medical procedure to become pregnant can be an intensely emotional, physically arduous, and expensive procedure. Most couples find it difficult to consider the chances for success realistically without dampening the drive that allows them to undertake these procedures.

## SEXUALITY IN REVIEW

- People choose to have children for a variety of reasons.
- Sperm are transferred from male to female during sexual intercourse.

- In adult females, ova (eggs) are produced regularly in ovaries and are transported to fallopian tubes to be fertilized.
- Only one sperm out of millions in ejaculate penetrates and fertilizes an ovum.
- Pregnancy is established when a fertilized ovum implants in the uterus.
- Fetal development requires 266 days.
- Childbirth is a three-phase process.
- Breastfeeding has numerous benefits for both baby and mother.
- Infertility can sometimes be overcome through use of new medical technologies.

## CRITICAL THINKING ABOUT SEXUALITY

1. We know that drugs, alcohol, and smoking are dangerous to a developing fetus. Imagine that you are working as a server in a restaurant. What would you say or do if a pregnant customer ordered a bottle of wine? Describe the scene as you imagine it. If you would not say anything, explain your reasons.
2. What are the benefits and drawbacks of being a parent? Explain your reasoning.
3. Comment on this point of view: People have been having babies "naturally" for thousands of years. Nowadays, however, childbirth is entirely too medicalized, with birth classes, hospital delivery rooms, anesthesia, fetal monitoring, episiotomy, labor induction, cesareans, circumcision of male infants, and bottle feeding.
4. Extremely premature babies (fewer than 25 weeks' gestational age) can be kept alive with intense (and very expensive) medical intervention, although it is almost certain that they will have serious health and mental problems later on in childhood. Just because this kind of technological intervention is possible, do you believe its application is wise?

## REFERENCES AND RECOMMENDED RESOURCES

### References

Chiras, D. G. (2008). *Human biology.* Sudbury, MA: Jones & Bartlett Learning.

Dwyer, T., & Ponsonby, A. L. (2009). Sudden infant death syndrome and prone sleeping position. *Annals of Epidemiology, 19*, 245–249.

Jones, R. E. (2006). *Human reproductive biology, 3rd ed.* San Diego: Academic Press.

U.S. Centers for Disease Control and Prevention. Assisted reproductive technology (ART). Available at: http://www.cdc.gov/art. Accessed May 3, 2010.

Women's Health. Healthy pregnancy. Available at: http://www.womenshealth.gov/pregnancy. Accessed April 27, 2010.

### Recommended Resources

Lamaze International. (2010). Available at: http://www.lamaze.org/ChildbirthProfessionals/ResourcesforProfessionals/CarePracticePapers/tabid/90/Default.aspx. Information on healthy birth practices.

March of Dimes. (2010). Preterm labor. Available at: http://www.marchofdimes.com/pnhec/188_1080.asp. Details on preterm labor.

Mayo Clinic. (2004). *Mayo Clinic guide to a healthy pregnancy.* New York: Harper. A precise, accurate information from a reputable source for parents.

Mayo Clinic. Available at: http://www.mayoclinic.com/health/postpartum-depression/DS00546. Information on postpartum depression.

MedlinePlus. (2010). Available at: http://www.nlm.nih.gov/medlineplus/ency/article/001191.htm. More information on infertility.

Murkoff, H., & Mazel, S. (2008). *What to expect when you're expecting, 4th ed.* New York: Workman. One of the most widely read books about pregnancy and parenting.

Vohr, B. R., & Allen, M. (2005). Extreme prematurity: The continuing dilemma. *New England Journal of Medicine, 352*, 71–72.

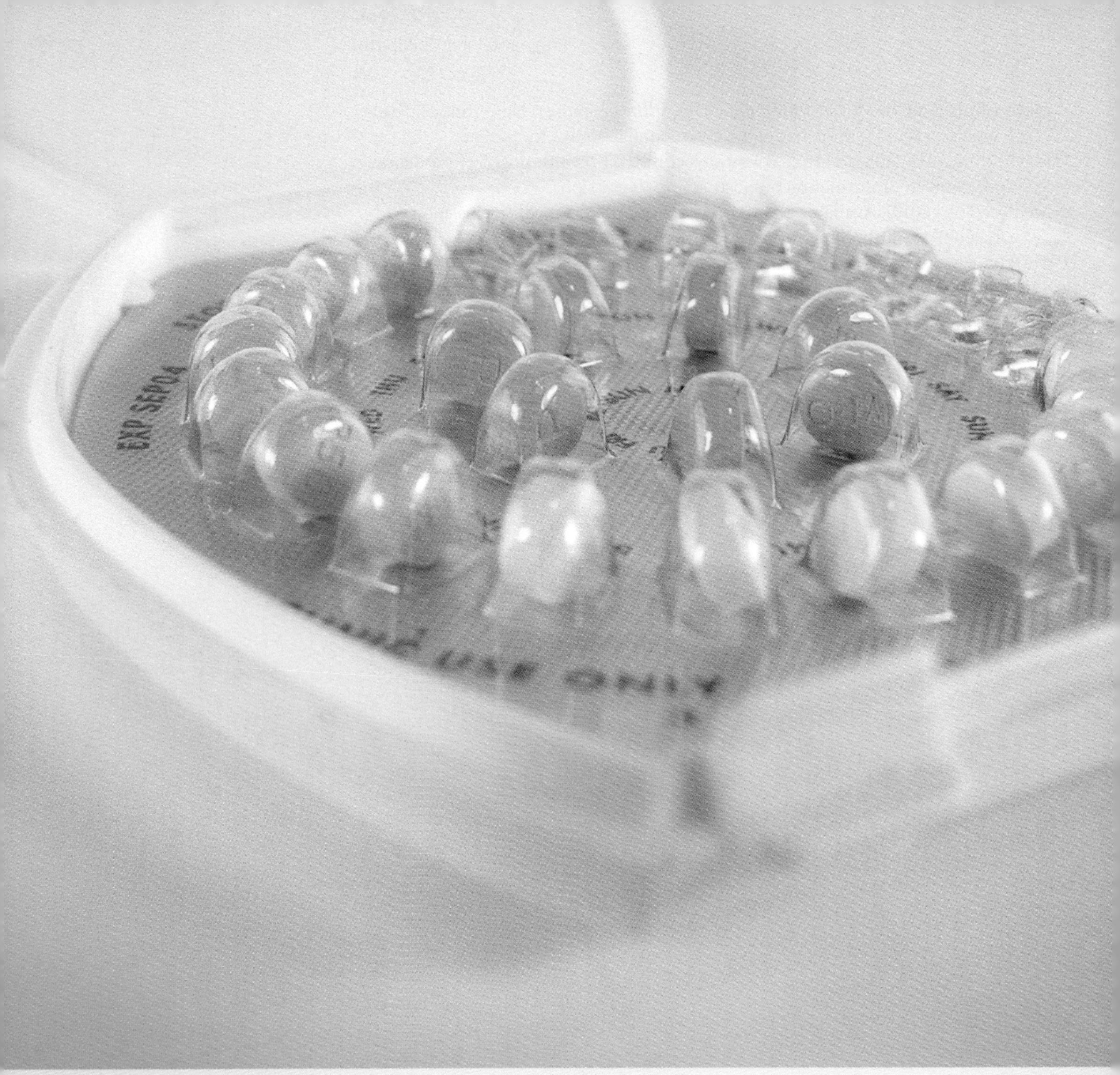


*Tenderness and kindness are not signs of weakness and despair, but manifestations of strength and resolutions.*

— Kahlil Gibran

CHAPTER 5

# Fertility Control and Abortion

## Student Learning Objectives

1. Define typical and lowest observed failure rate for fertility control methods
2. List and describe four methods of combination hormonal contraception
3. Describe two types of progestin-only contraception
4. Describe five fertility awareness methods of contraception
5. List and describe six barrier methods of contraception
6. Explain how an IUD is used to prevent pregnancy
7. Describe female and male methods of contraceptive sterilization
8. Give at least three reasons why many people do not use fertility control methods
9. Define emergency contraception
10. Describe surgical and medical methods of abortion

Because humans have sexual intercourse for a variety of reasons other than to produce children, people have been attempting to control their fertility for thousands of years. The ancient Egyptian Ebers Papyrus (~1550 BCE) advised women to make a paste consisting of bark from the acacia tree, dates, and a bit of honey, then dip a ball of wool into the paste and place it in the vagina. Other ancient methods include douching with water, vinegar, or mixtures of plant and animal substances; drinking potions; having the woman jump or sneeze after intercourse; and placing a paste made of honey and crocodile or elephant dung in the vagina. Some methods still in use today include not ejaculating (called *coitus reservatus*), not ejaculating in the vagina (called *coitus interruptus*), and prayer.

In the past 150 years, scientific knowledge of human reproductive biology and modern biotechnology have produced an array of relatively safe, reliable methods to help control fertility and reduce the risk of unintended pregnancy (**Table 5.1**). Some fertility control methods work prior to fertilization (*contraceptives*). Other methods work after fertilization (*postconception methods*).

## Fertility Control Effectiveness

A healthy, fertile couple having sexual intercourse about twice a week without trying to prevent pregnancy has an 85% chance of getting pregnant within 12 months. Nearly half of the 6.5 million U.S. pregnancies each year are unintended. About half of those pregnancies occurred because a fertility control method failed or was used improperly. Approximately 50% of American women aged 15–44 have experienced at least one unintended pregnancy.

Avoiding unintended pregnancy requires weighing the benefits and drawbacks of each fertility control method and choosing one or more that both partners are comfortable using properly *each time* sexual activity takes place. Even a technologically perfect method can fail when it is not used properly and consistently. Individuals and couples in industrialized countries have available to them a

**Table 5.1** Modern Fertility Control Methods Work at Different Steps in the Reproductive Process

| Step | Contraceptive Method |
|---|---|
| Maturation of Egg | Fertility awareness methods help determine when an egg is (or was) fertilizable. |
| Egg Release (*ovulation*) | Combination hormonal contraceptives inhibit the release of eggs from the ovary. |
| Tubal Transport | Tubal ligation blocks the pathway of the egg in the fallopian tube. |
| Sperm Transport in the Male (*emission*) | Vasectomy blocks the movement of sperm from the testes to the penis. |
| Insemination | Male condom, female condom, penile withdrawal, and vaginal douching provide physical barriers. |
| Sperm Passage in the Female | Vaginal spermicides, the contraceptive sponge, the diaphragm, and the cervical cap block sperm passage in the female. |
| Tubal Transport of Embryo | The intrauterine device and progestin-only pills and injections create a biological imbalance in the uterus so that implantation is not possible. |

**Table 5.2** Effectiveness of Common Contraceptives

| Method | Typical Failure Rate (%) | Lowest Observed Failure Rate (%) |
|---|---|---|
| No Method (Chance) | 85.0 | 85.0 |
| Withdrawal | 19.0 | 4.0 |
| Combination Birth Control Pill | 6–8.0 | 0.1 |
| Contraceptive Patch | N/A | 0.3 |
| Vaginal Ring | N/A | 0.3 |
| Combination Injection | N/A | 0.05 |
| Progestin-Only Pill | 5.0 | 0.5 |
| Copper-T IUD | 0.8 | 0.6 |
| Male Latex Condom | 14.0 | 3.0 |
| Female Latex Condom | 21.0 | 5.0 |
| Diaphragm | 16.0 | 6.0 |
| Spermicides | 29.0 | 15.0 |
| Fertility Awareness | 20.0 | 1–9.0 |
| Tubal Ligation | 0.5 | 0.5 |
| Vasectomy | 0.15 | 0.1 |

Data are percentage of women becoming pregnant using a method for one year. Typical failure rate means the method was not always used correctly. Lowest observed failure rate means the method was always used correctly and with every act of sexual intercourse.

variety of contraceptive methods that are effective, safe, affordable, easy to use, reversible, and protect against sexually transmitted infections.

The effectiveness of a fertility control method is estimated in terms of its **failure rate**, which is the percentage of women who are likely to become pregnant during the first year of using that method. Fertility control methods are evaluated in terms of two failure rates (**Table 5.2**):

1. The **lowest observed failure rate** estimates how well a method performs when used as intended and consistently.
2. **Typical user failure rate** estimates how well a method performs when all of the errors and problems that people typically encounter with a method are taken into account.

**failure rate** a measure of contraceptive effectiveness, given as the percentage of women who are likely to become unintentionally pregnant using a particular method during the first year of use

**lowest observed failure rate** the effectiveness of a contraceptive method when used properly

**typical user failure rate** the effectiveness of a contraceptive method that takes into account all of the errors when in general use in a population

## Penile Withdrawal

**Penile withdrawal** (also called *coitus interruptus*) requires the man to withdraw his penis from the vagina before ejaculation. This method is among the least effective methods of fertility control, principally because many men are unable to exercise sufficient control and restraint in order to remove the penis in time. Also, semen deposited on the woman's genitals or abdomen, or on clothes or bed linen, can enter the vagina by contact with the vulva. Withdrawal also has the disadvantage of potentially diminishing a couple's sexual pleasure. When the partners are focused on whether the man will withdraw in time, neither is free to experience fully the pleasure of sexual interaction.

**penile withdrawal** withdrawing the penis from the vagina before ejaculation in order to prevent insemination

## Douching

**douching** rinsing the vagina with fluid (water, diluted vinegar, commercial douches)

Douching, rinsing the vagina with fluid (water, diluted vinegar, commercial douches) after sexual intercourse, is a time-honored yet ineffective method of contraception. After ejaculation in the vagina, thousands of sperm move through the cervix and enter the uterus within a few seconds. There isn't time to flush out sperm from the vagina before a significant number enter the uterus. Furthermore, the force from the spray of the douche may propel sperm into the uterus, aiding conception rather than preventing it.

## Hormonal Contraceptives

In May 1960, the U.S. Food and Drug Administration (FDA) approved the use of hormonal contraceptives for women. Since that time, millions of American women and hundreds of millions of women worldwide have used a variety of hormonal contraceptives because of their convenience, low cost, reversibility, tolerable side effects, and effectiveness. Two forms of hormonal contraception are available: combination estrogen–progestin and progestin-only.

### Combination Hormonal Contraceptives

**combination hormonal contraceptives** contraceptives containing estrogen and progestin

In the United States, combination hormonal contraceptives are the most popular reversible method of fertility control, accounting for nearly 25% of contraceptive use among all women who contracept and about 40% of women under 30 years old who contracept. Combination hormonal contraceptives contain two chemicals that in many ways mimic the actions of a woman's naturally occurring ovarian hormones, estrogen and progesterone.

Unpleasant side effects that are associated with the use of hormonal contraceptives, many of which lessen or disappear after a few cycles, include nausea, breast tenderness, increased breast size, cyclic fluid retention, headaches, increased appetite or weight gain, depression, fatigue, decreased sex drive, acne or oily skin, and loss of interest in sex. Some beneficial side effects include diminution or disappearance of menstrual cramps, a reduction in the number of bleeding days and blood loss, the ability to regulate the menstrual cycle, which can be important to travelers and athletes, and lower risk for pelvic inflammatory disease, benign (noncancerous) breast disease, ovarian cysts, ectopic pregnancy, and iron-deficiency anemia.

Combination hormonal contraceptives do not increase the likelihood of developing breast cancer. However, users of this method who are over 35 years old and who smoke cigarettes are at risk for fatal blood clots and should stop smoking. High blood pressure, diabetes, and other health problems may make hormonal contraception unsafe. Experiencing severe abdominal pain, severe chest pain, severe headaches, unusual eye problems (e.g., blurry vision, "flashing lights," temporary blindness), or severe thigh pain is reason to consult a physician or health clinic immediately.

Combination hormonal contraceptives are available as pills, a skin patch, a vaginal insert, and by injection.

#### The Pill

Combination hormonal contraceptive pills ("birth control pills") generally come in packets of 21 or 28 pills. A 91-day, extended-use pill also is available, which has

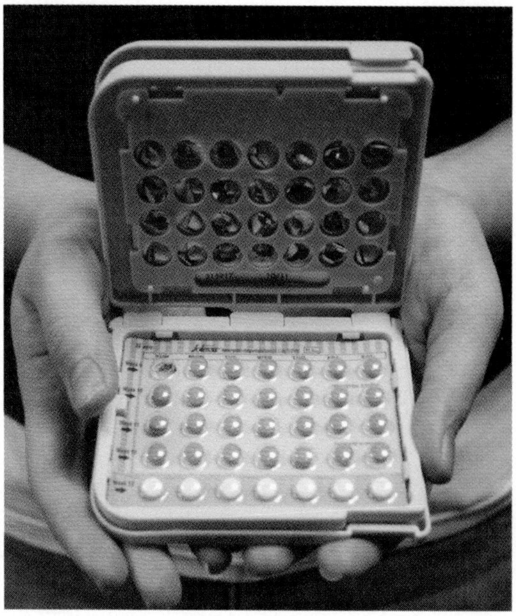

the advantages of fewer menstrual cycles per year and less opportunity to forget starting up a new packet of pills after a menstrual period.

In the 21-pill packet, all the pills contain specific amounts of hormone. In the 28-pill packets, 21 of the pills contain hormones; the other seven (called "reminder pills") are inert or contain iron to help prevent iron-deficiency anemia. In some pill regimens the amount of estrogenic and progestogenic hormones vary to mimic the variations in hormone levels in a woman's menstrual cycle.

The first pill in a packet is taken on a predetermined day, and one pill is taken each day thereafter. Approximately two days after the twenty-first pill is taken, a menstrual period occurs. (After several months on the pill, some women experience little or no menstrual bleeding. This circumstance is not harmful. Any concerns, however, should be conveyed to a health professional.)

A pill should be taken at the same time each day to increase its effectiveness. A woman should associate pill-taking with a routine activity, such as going to bed or teeth-brushing, to lessen the risk of forgetting to take it. Forgetting near mid-cycle when an egg is available for fertilization can result in a pregnancy.

Long-term fertility is not lessened by using the pill. Some women, however, experience menstrual irregularities in the first few months after discontinuing the method. Even so, they can still become pregnant soon after discontinuing the pill. There is no association between pill use and subsequent birth defects in children born to pill users, unless a woman ingests pills while she is pregnant (e.g., becoming unintentionally pregnant while taking the pill). In this case, birth defects are possible because the hormones in the pills may damage the embryo and fetus.

### Skin Patch

The contraceptive skin patch is applied to the lower abdomen, buttocks, or upper body (not the breasts) and releases hormones slowly. Each patch is worn continuously for one week and then replaced with a new patch on the same day of the week for a total of three weeks. The fourth week is patch-free. This is when menstruation occurs. In general, the patch's side effects are similar to the pill's.

Because there are no pills to forget taking, the patch tends to be slightly more effective than pills. Occasionally, the patch does not stay attached to the skin and contraceptive effectiveness is lost. Also, some women experience skin irritation at the site of application and discontinue the patch. The product may be less effective in women weighing more than 200 pounds.

### Vaginal Ring

The contraceptive vaginal ring is a flexible device about 2 inches in diameter containing synthetic hormones that are similar to the active ingredients in hormonal contraceptive pills. A woman inserts the ring herself. After the ring is inserted, the hormones are continuously released. A ring is used for three weeks, then it is removed. After seven days, during which time a menstrual period occurs, a new ring is inserted.

The ring is highly effective and has the same side effects as hormonal contraceptive pills. One additional caution is that the ring can be expelled before the three weeks are over. If the ring has been out of the vagina for more than three hours, an additional method of contraception (male condom or spermicide) must be used until the ring has been back in place for seven days. Other side effects of the vaginal ring include vaginal discharge, vaginitis, and irritation.

## Dear Penelope . . .

***I have no sympathy for women who complain that they don't have multiple orgasms. Hey, I'm still waiting for my first! I'm not hung up on sex, and I'm healthy. What am I supposed to do? Go through life ignoring it? Faking it? Should I take lessons?***
***— Feeling Sexually Incomplete***

*Dear Feeling,*

Your frustrations are certainly understandable. This column gets a lot of questions about female orgasm. Oddly enough, a hundred years ago, when women weren't supposed to be interested in sex, orgasm was considered inappropriate for a woman. Now we have the opposite; female orgasm has become a symbol of sexual competence for both sexes. A woman's orgasm proves that she is a complete sexual being and that her partner is an accomplished lover.

Concern about sexual adequacy and performance distracts a person from full engagement in sexual experience. When people stop thinking about their sexual performance and allow themselves to fully experience sexual sensations and pleasure, orgasm often follows naturally. A person may require some sexual experience to learn how to "let go" of concerns and other mental distractions and to focus on increasing sexual pleasure instead. Orgasm can be one of the pleasurable and wonderful parts of sex. However, it is not everything there is to sex. More important is mutual pleasuring and not accomplishing some performance goal.

As for multiple orgasms: Many people think that if one orgasm per sexual episode is good, more must be better. "More is better" thinking turns sex into work. Save that kind of thinking for making money. In sex, it may be better not to think at all.

Courtesy of the UC Davis *Aggie*

#### Injectable Contraceptives

Injections of the same hormones that are in contraceptive pills last nearly 90 days. The injection is administered during menstruation in the buttocks, thigh, or upper arm. The effectiveness, side effects, and risks of this method are similar to those of other combination hormonal contraceptives.

### Progestin-Only Contraceptives

**progestin-only contraceptives** contraceptives for women that contain only a synthetic version of the natural hormone progesterone

**Progestin-only contraceptives** are available as pills and injectables. These methods work by inhibiting ovulation, thickening cervical mucus to make sperm passage into the uterus more difficult, and changing the uterine environment so that pregnancy is less likely. Side effects may include menstrual irregularities, weight gain, depression, fatigue, decreased sex drive, acne or oily skin, and headaches. The FDA warns that long-term use of the progestin-only injectable (Depo-Provera) increases the risk of irreversible bone loss.

## Fertility Awareness Methods

**fertility awareness methods** contraceptive methods that rely on estimates of when an ovum is fertilizable or when ovulation has occurred

**unsafe days** when using fertility awareness methods, the days in the menstrual month when fertilization is likely

**Fertility awareness methods** (also called *natural family planning*, the *rhythm method*, or *periodic abstinence*) attempt to determine the days in a woman's menstrual cycle when an ovum has been released from the ovary and is capable of being fertilized. These methods *estimate* when ovulation is most likely to occur or indicate when ovulation *has already* taken place.

Knowing when ovulation is likely to occur or that it has already taken place tells a couple the days in the menstrual cycle not to have unprotected sexual intercourse, called the **unsafe days**. On unsafe days, a couple should use an alternative method of avoiding pregnancy, such as condoms, a diaphragm, or spermicides; enjoy ways of sexual pleasuring other than sexual intercourse; or abstain from sexual contact altogether.

The days in the menstrual cycle when a woman is least likely to be fertile are the safe days. Even on the **safe days**, however, fertilization is possible because of natural variations in a woman's reproductive processes. Therefore, safe days are really "relatively safe days."

**safe days** when using fertility awareness methods, the days in the menstrual month when fertilization is unlikely

**calendar rhythm** estimating the "safe days" by charting menstrual cycle length on a calendar

Fertility awareness offers the advantages of being safe and inexpensive, and religious convictions make it the only acceptable fertility control method for many. However, the method is among the least effective. Failures occur because people do not keep careful records, they find the intervals of abstinence during the unsafe days too long, or they find having to plan sex only for the safe days a hindrance to spontaneous lovemaking.

There are five techniques for practicing fertility awareness.

1. *Calendar rhythm*. The **calendar rhythm** method estimates the most likely fertile, or unsafe days, in a woman's menstrual cycle by assuming that:
   - A fertilizable egg is released from an ovary 14 days (plus or minus two days) prior to the onset of the next menstrual flow. In a 28-day cycle, this would be the midcycle day, or the fourteenth day from the onset of the previous menstrual period.
   - An ovum is capable of being fertilized for 24 hours after release from the ovary.
   - Sperm deposited in the vagina remain capable of fertilization for up to five days.

   Using calendar rhythm effectively requires knowledge of the female fertility cycle and instruction in doing the calculations correctly (**FIGURE 5.1**). Family planning agencies, women's health clinics, and books on fertility awareness methods can be helpful in learning the method.

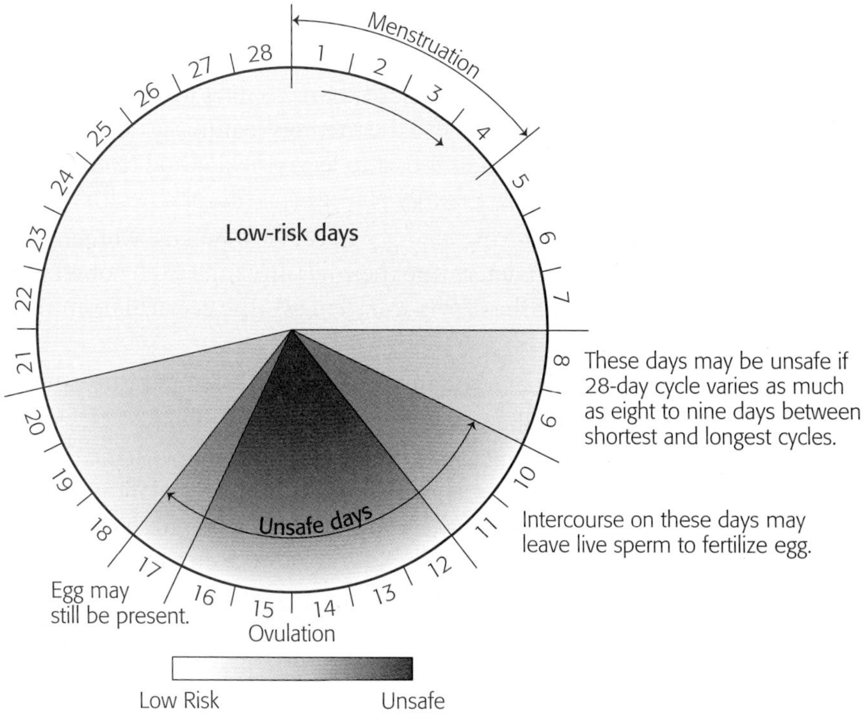


**FIGURE 5.1 Calendar Rhythm Method of Contraception.** The calendar rhythm method is based on avoiding intercourse when sperm can fertilize an ovum. Unsafe days for intercourse in this chart are days 12 to 16.

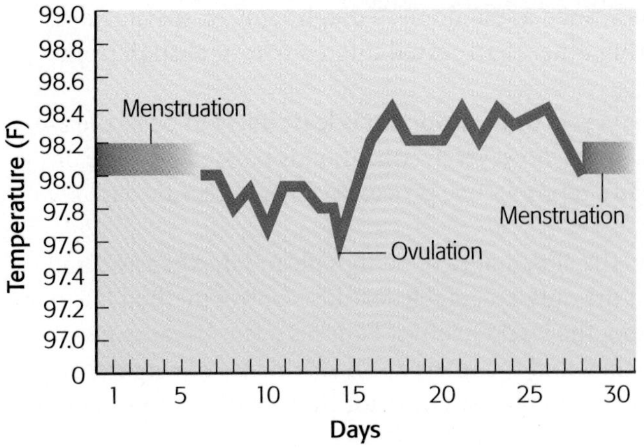


FIGURE 5.2 **Basal Body Temperature Method of Contraception.** A woman's body temperature rises about 1°F during the days following ovulation. Once the BBT has risen for three consecutive days, assume that ovulation has taken place and that the rest of the days in that menstrual cycle are safe for unprotected intercourse. To use the BBT method, a woman must record her basal body temperature each morning before engaging in *any* activity. Temperature measurement should last at least five minutes.

2. *Temperature method.* The basal body temperature (BBT) is the lowest temperature in a healthy person during waking hours. In over 70% of women the BBT rises approximately one degree after ovulation (FIGURE 5.2). By keeping a daily record of the BBT, a woman can determine when ovulation has occurred and therefore the unsafe and safe days for unprotected intercourse until the beginning of the next menstrual cycle. The BBT method cannot predict when ovulation will occur, so a woman must still estimate with calendar rhythm or other method the safe and unsafe days before ovulation.
3. *Mucus method.* Certain hormone-sensitive glands in the cervix produce mucus that changes in amount, color, and consistency during different phases of the menstrual cycle. Observing changes in cervical mucus can help determine when ovulation occurs, and safe and unsafe days for intercourse can be planned accordingly. Success with the method requires learning to read the changes in cervical mucus. It is best to learn the method from an experienced (and successful) user, a family planning clinic, or a health center.

   In conjunction with monitoring changes in cervical mucus, women adept at vaginal self-exam can determine their fertility interval by observing changes in the opening of the cervix (*cervical os*). The cervical opening expands just prior to ovulation.
4. *Sympto-thermal method.* This method involves using the temperature and mucus methods simultaneously.
5. *Hormonal methods.* Hormonal methods measure in a woman's urine the amount of the pituitary hormone, LH, which peaks at the time of ovulation. Ovulation predictor kits to measure the levels of LH can be purchased in pharmacies. Manufacturers claim that the kits are 85% accurate.

**barrier methods** contraceptive methods that physically or chemically block the pathway of sperm into or inside the female reproductive tract
**spermicide** a chemical capable of killing sperm

## Barrier Methods

Barrier methods of fertility control block the movement of sperm in the female reproductive tract and/or bring sperm into contact with a sperm-killing chemical (spermicide). They include the male condom, the female condom, the diaphragm, the cervical cap, the contraceptive sponge, and spermicidal contraceptives (foams, gels, and creams).

## The Male Condom

The **male condom**, or rubber, is a membranous sheath that covers the erect penis and catches semen before it enters the vagina (FIGURE 5.3). Currently, over 90% of condoms are made of latex; nearly all of the rest are made of polyurethane. A very

**male condom** a latex rubber sheath that covers the erect penis

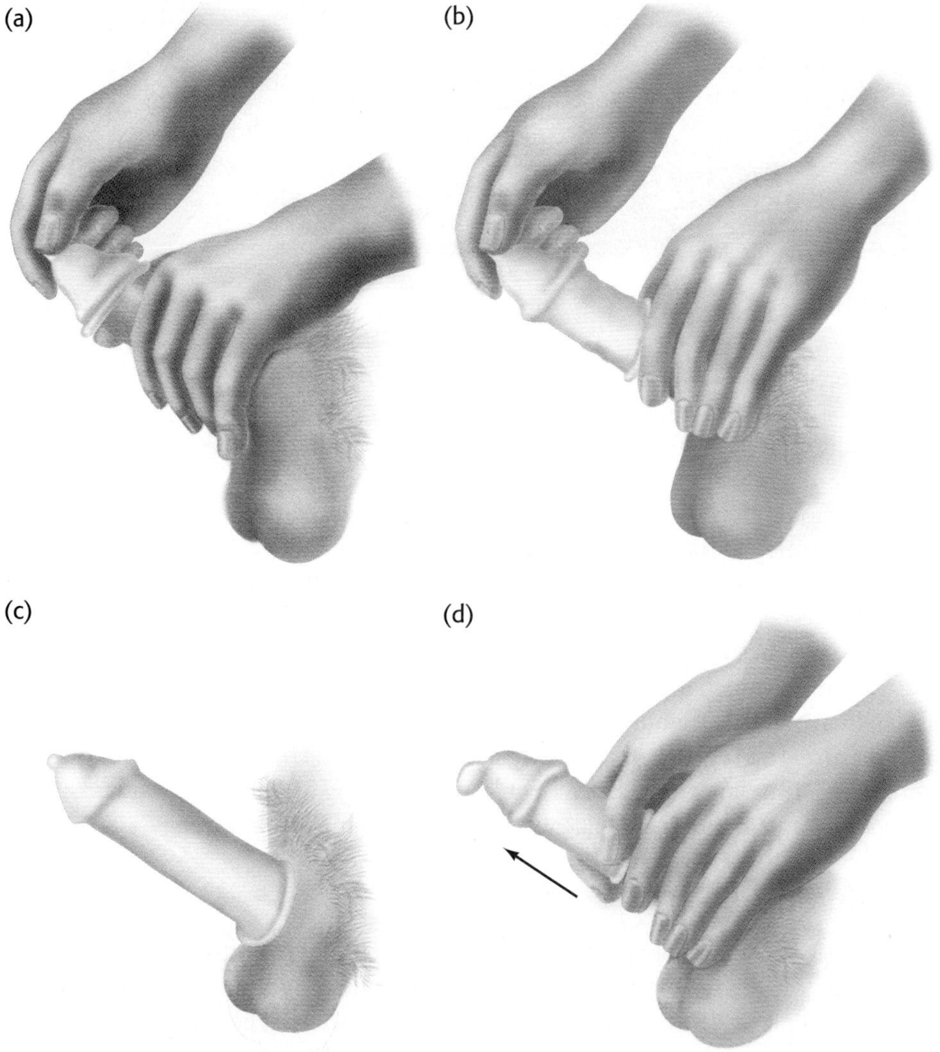


FIGURE 5.3 **Using a Male Condom.** Take the condom out of its package carefully so as not to damage it (no teeth, no fingernails). If there are holes or breaks, or if it's sticky or brittle, toss it out and use another. Put the condom on the erect penis before intercourse begins. Interrupting intercourse to put on a condom increases the chances of pregnancy because the man might not be able to control ejaculation. Also, putting on the condom at the beginning offers best protection against STDs. (a) Unroll the condom onto the erect penis (pull back the foreskin). (b) Leave about one-half inch at the tip to catch semen. Some condoms have specially designed (reservoir) tips for semen collection. (c) The tip of the condom should be pressed free of air to prevent breakage after ejaculation. Do not use Vaseline or mineral oil as a lubricant. They will destroy the latex. If a lubricant is desired, use a water-based lubricant such as K-Y jelly or a spermicide. (d) After ejaculation, withdraw the penis before it becomes soft—otherwise, the condom might slip off. When removing the penis, hold the condom on the penis to be sure it does not slip off. Check the condom for holes or breaks. If any appear, spermicidal foam or jelly should be put into the vagina immediately, and emergency contraception ("morning-after pill") should possibly be sought. Condoms should be used only once and then discarded.

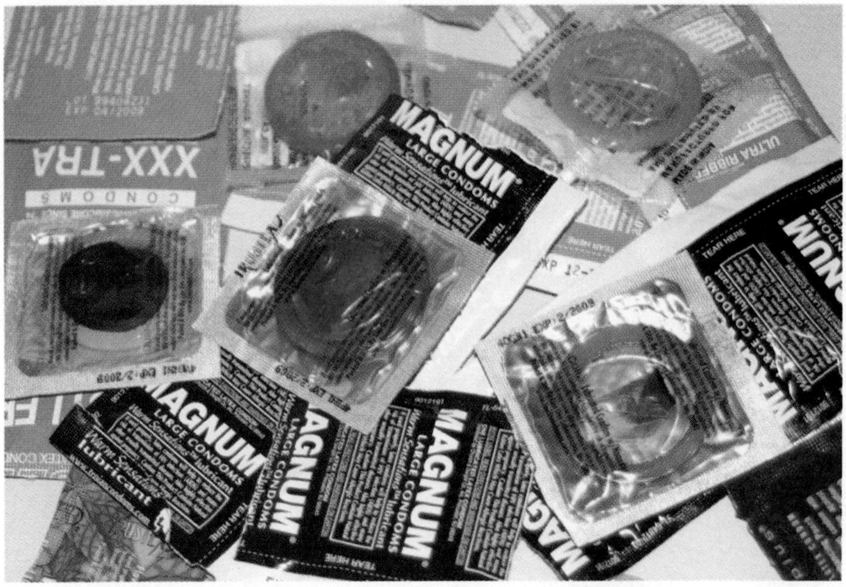


small percentage are so-called "skin" condoms, which are manufactured from lamb intestines.

Condoms are easy to obtain, inexpensive, free of medical risk (on rare occasions a man or a woman may be allergic to latex, a lubricant, or a spermicide), reliable, and moderately effective. Used in conjunction with another barrier method, such as spermicidal foam, condoms are nearly 100% effective. Condoms precoated with spermicide are available. Stored in a cool, dry place, condoms retain their effectiveness for up to five years. In a warm environment, such as a wallet or the glove compartment of a car, the latex deteriorates.

A condom can change tactile sensations, but it does not totally block them, which, in any event, are only one of many factors that contribute to sexual arousal and pleasure. Having a negative attitude about condoms may diminish pleasure far more than a thin layer of latex ever could. When using a condom, consider ways to incorporate putting on the device without interrupting lovemaking.

## The Female Condom

**female condom** a polyurethane sheath that fits into the vagina

**diaphragm** a dome-shaped, latex cup that is coated with a spermicide-containing gel or cream and placed in the vagina to cover the cervix

The female condom is a polyurethane, tubelike pouch that fits into the vagina (FIGURE 5.4). At the upper, closed end is a ring that helps with insertion and holds the device in place. The open end, which covers the external genitalia, also has a ring. The device can be inserted prior to intercourse, thus not becoming a barrier to sexual spontaneity.

The female condom is resistant to damage by oil-based lubricants and heat. Disadvantages include discomfort and difficulties with insertion, positioning, and remaining in place. There are no serious side effects or allergic reactions with use. That the female condom covers the cervix, vagina, and external genitalia contributes to protection against the transmission of sexual infections.

## The Diaphragm

The diaphragm is a dome-shaped, latex cup that is coated with a spermicide-containing gel or cream and placed in the vagina to cover the cervix. It is effective if used correctly and every time a woman has intercourse. Other than the rare

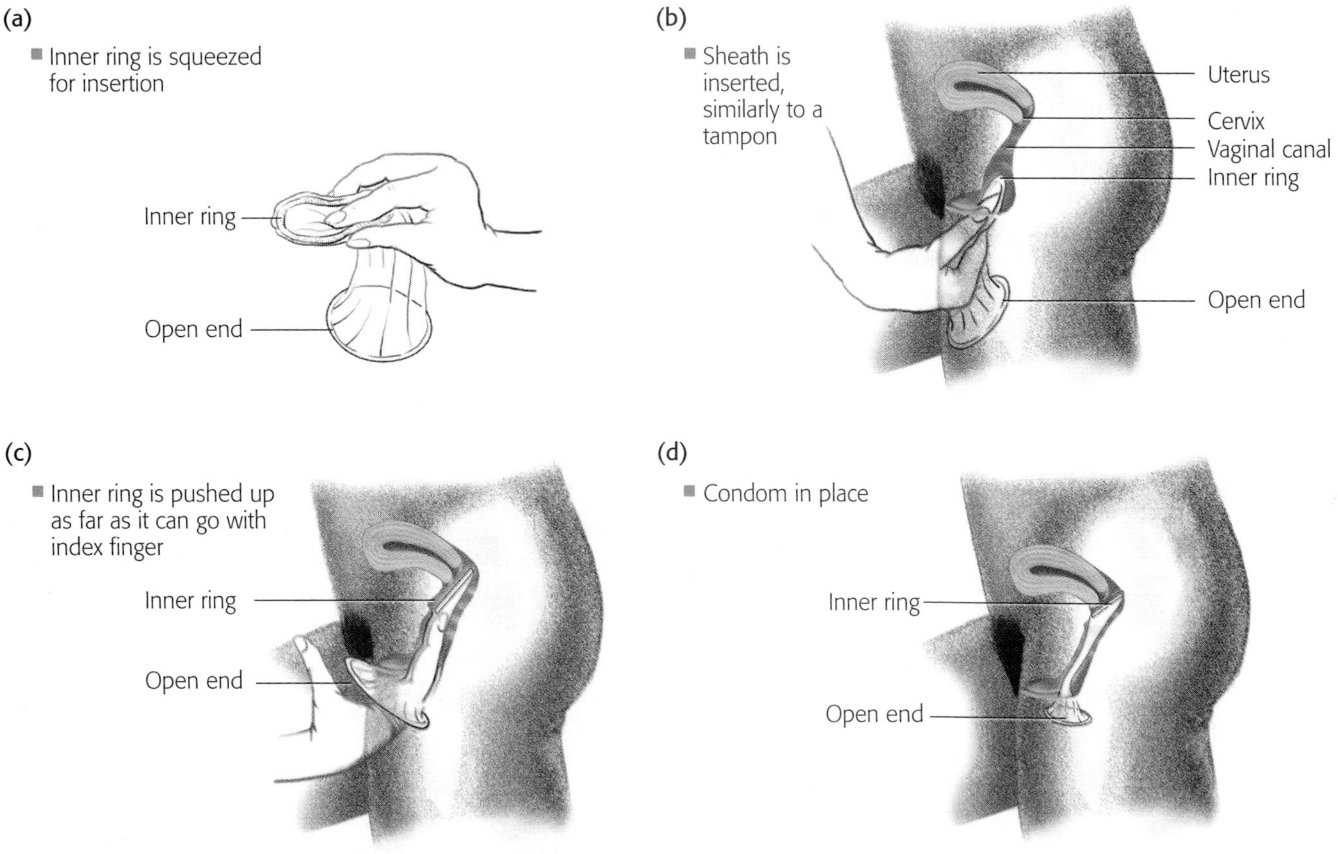


FIGURE 5.4 **Female Condom Insertion and Positioning.**

occurrence of *toxic shock syndrome*, few major medical problems are associated with its use. Women with a history of toxic shock syndrome are advised to use a different fertility control method. Very few women or their partners may be allergic to the latex or the spermicide. Some women may experience discomfort with the diaphragm in place. Changing brands or getting a better-fitting diaphragm often solves these problems.

Each woman must be fitted (by a family planning professional or a physician) with a diaphragm that is the correct size for her. The need to be fitted properly is one reason that diaphragms are available only by prescription. Any change in a woman's body size from a gain or loss of several pounds, pregnancy, or pelvic surgery is reason to have the fit of the diaphragm checked by a professional and a new diaphragm prescribed if necessary. A woman should not use another woman's diaphragm because the fit might be wrong, which lowers the device's effectiveness.

Only rarely will a man feel the diaphragm during sexual intercourse if the device is inserted properly. Sometimes a man may feel the rim of the diaphragm when vaginal penetration is very deep. If either the man or the woman experiences unusual sensations or discomfort during intercourse, then the diaphragm may not be inserted correctly, it may have become dislodged during intercourse, or it may be the wrong size.

Besides use as a contraceptive, the diaphragm can be used as a barrier to menstrual flow, which can make sexual intercourse during menstruation more acceptable for some couples.

**cervical cap** a rubber, thimble-shaped contraceptive that fits on the cervix (bottom part of the uterus)
**contraceptive sponge** a nonprescription contraceptive device that is inserted into the vagina
**vaginal spermicides** foams, gels, creams, and suppositories that contain a spermicide
**intrauterine device (IUD)** a fertility control method involving the placing of a small, plastic T-shaped object in the uterus

## The Cervical Cap

The **cervical cap** is a cup-shaped rubber device that snugly covers the cervix similar to the way a thimble fits on a finger. Like a diaphragm, a cervical cap is coated with spermicide, but unlike a diaphragm, a cervical cap remains in place for one or two days. Cervical caps come in several sizes and must be fitted by a health professional for each woman. The major disadvantages of the cervical cap are difficulty with insertion and removal, occasional discomfort during intercourse, dislodgment during intercourse, and possibly irritation of the cervix.

## The Contraceptive Sponge

The **contraceptive sponge** is made of a compressible spongy synthetic material in the shape of a mushroom cap. The sponge is impregnated with spermicide and works by destroying sperm, absorbing ejaculate, and blocking the entrance to the uterus. Sponges are available without a doctor's prescription.

Among women who have never had a child, the lowest observed failure rate is 14% and the typical failure rate is 18%. The lowest and typical failure rates among women who have had children are 28%. Allergies to the device or the spermicide can cause vaginal and/or penile irritation. Toxic shock syndrome is also a risk, especially if the device is left in the vagina for over 24 hours. Information about toxic shock syndrome is included in the package inserts.

## Vaginal Spermicides

**Vaginal spermicides** consist of a spermicidal chemical, usually nonoxynol-9, and an inert substance that transports and retains the spermicide in the vagina. They include foams, gels, creams, and vaginal suppositories and films (devices placed in the vagina that dissolve to release the spermicidal chemical). These methods are available without a doctor's prescription. Although often displayed in stores with feminine hygiene products, vaginal spermicides should not be confused with douches, deodorant products, or lubricants, none of which are contraceptives.

The effectiveness of vaginal spermicides depends on a sufficient quantity of sperm-killing chemical bathing the cervix at the time of ejaculation. Users must put the spermicide (regardless of type) in the vagina *immediately before every act of intercourse* and *before each subsequent intercourse in the same sexual encounter.* Furthermore, the foam must be made frothy and bubbly by shaking the container about 20 times before filling the applicator. Keep a spare container on hand because there is no way to know how much foam remains in a container.

Suppository users must place the suppository as far back in the vagina as possible so that when it dissolves, the spermicidal chemical covers the cervix. Allow from 10 to 30 minutes for the suppository to dissolve completely before each act of intercourse.

Vaginal spermicides tend to be gooey and slippery, which occasionally can be a nuisance, but the moisture can augment a woman's natural vaginal lubrication and enhance sensation. The methods can be a hindrance to oral–genital stimulation. In rare instances someone may be allergic to a particular product. Changing brands may alleviate this problem.

## The Intrauterine Device

An **intrauterine device (IUD)** is a small plastic object that is placed inside the cavity of the uterus to prevent pregnancy by killing or weakening sperm, altering the timing of the ovum's or embryo's movement through the fallopian tube, and/or

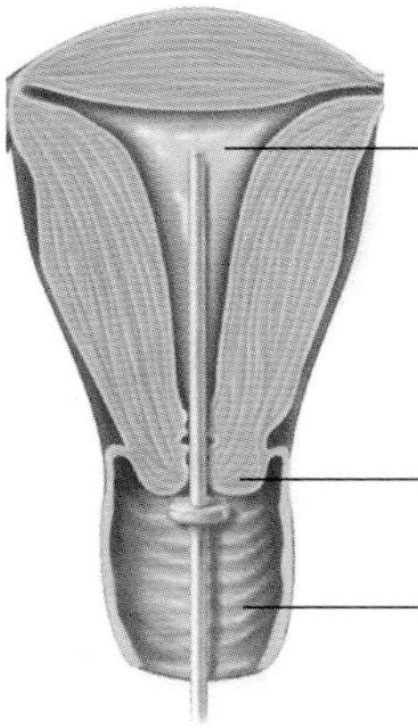


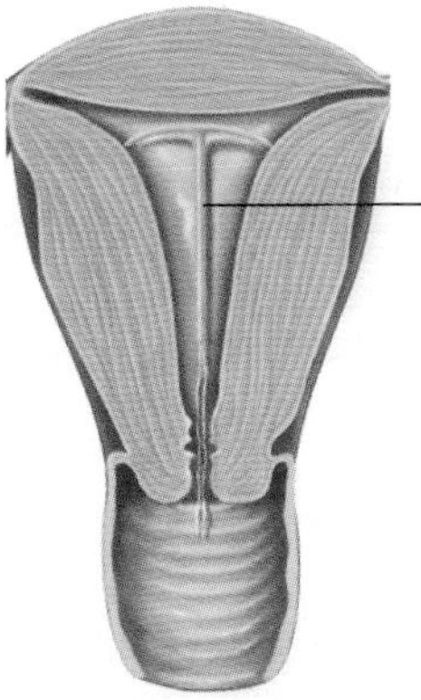


FIGURE 5.5 **The Intrauterine Device (IUD).** The IUD is inserted past the cervix into the uterus. Prior to insertion the length of the uterus is measured with an instrument called a sound. Upon insertion the arms of the IUD gradually unfold. Once the inserter is removed, the threads attached to IUD will be clipped to extend into the vagina through the cervical opening.

inhibiting implantation of the embryo in the uterine lining (FIGURE 5.5). An IUD remains in place for as long as a woman desires, even for months or years. An IUD has a short string that hangs into the vagina, where it cannot be seen but can be felt to ensure proper placement. The string also aids removal.

IUDs available in the United States are flexible plastic devices shaped like a "T." One type is impregnated with hormone (progesterone or a synthetic progestin). Another type is wrapped with fine copper wire that slowly dissolves and releases copper ions. Both the hormone and copper augment an IUD's effectiveness by slowing sperm migration in the woman and preventing implantation of an embryo. Some IUD users experience heavier menstrual flow or menstrual cramps. IUD use is associated with an increased risk of pelvic inflammatory disease, uterine perforations, and ectopic pregnancy.

## Sterilization Methods

**sterility** the condition of being biologically incapable of having children

**Sterility** refers to being permanently unable to have children; it applies to both males and females. Surgical methods that render a person sterile but have no effect on her or his ability to engage in or enjoy sex are very popular among couples who are certain that they do not want children, or, as is more often the case, no more children. The popularity of sterilization stems from its nearly 100% effectiveness, relative safety, and relatively low one-time cost. Female sterilization methods

(a)

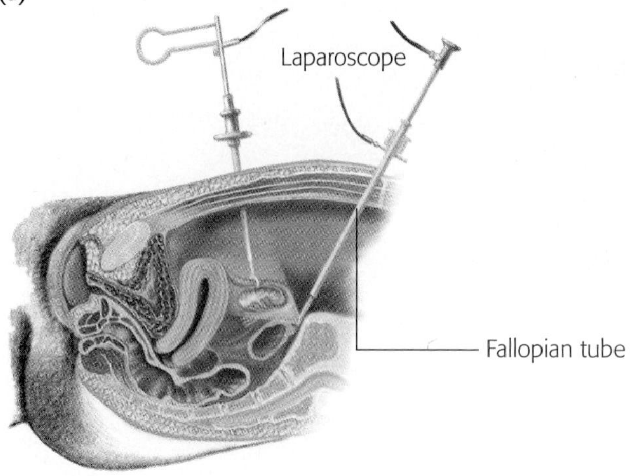


(b)

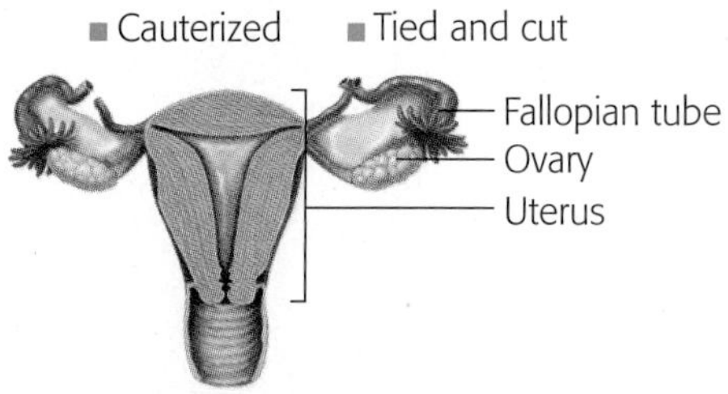


FIGURE 5.6 **Tubal Ligation.** Female sterilization by laparoscopic ligation. (a) Side view. The tubes are located using a laparoscope and cut, tied, or cauterized through a second incision. (b) Front view. The tubes after ligation.

include tubal ligation and hysterectomy. The male sterilization method is the vasectomy.

## Tubal Ligation

**tubal ligation** the cutting or blocking of the fallopian tubes so a woman can no longer get pregnant
**hysterectomy** surgical removal of the uterus

Tubal ligation involves blocking of the fallopian tubes by cutting and tying, sealing, or closing them with clips, bands, or rings (FIGURE 5.6). Most tubal ligations are performed under local anesthesia in a clinic or doctor's office. The procedure involves entering the abdominal cavity through a small incision and inflating the cavity (with carbon dioxide or nitrous oxide gas) so the doctor can locate and block the tubes.

Usually one or two incisions about an inch long are made at the pubic hair line and/or belly button. Alternatively, an incision is made in the back of the vagina (*culpotomy*). The incidence of postoperative complications is very low and is due more to the doctor's skill than the procedure itself.

Although tubal ligation is intended to be a permanent method of fertility control, accidental pregnancies occasionally occur because a blocked tube spontaneously reopens. In about half of cases these accidental pregnancies are ectopic (within the tube). Surgical reversal of tubal blocking is possible, with a success rate (as measured by becoming pregnant) of 50% to 70%.

## Hysterectomy

Hysterectomy is surgical removal of the uterus. Most experts do not recommend hysterectomy solely for sterilization purposes because the chances of postoperative complications are high, the operation is expensive compared with other steriliza-

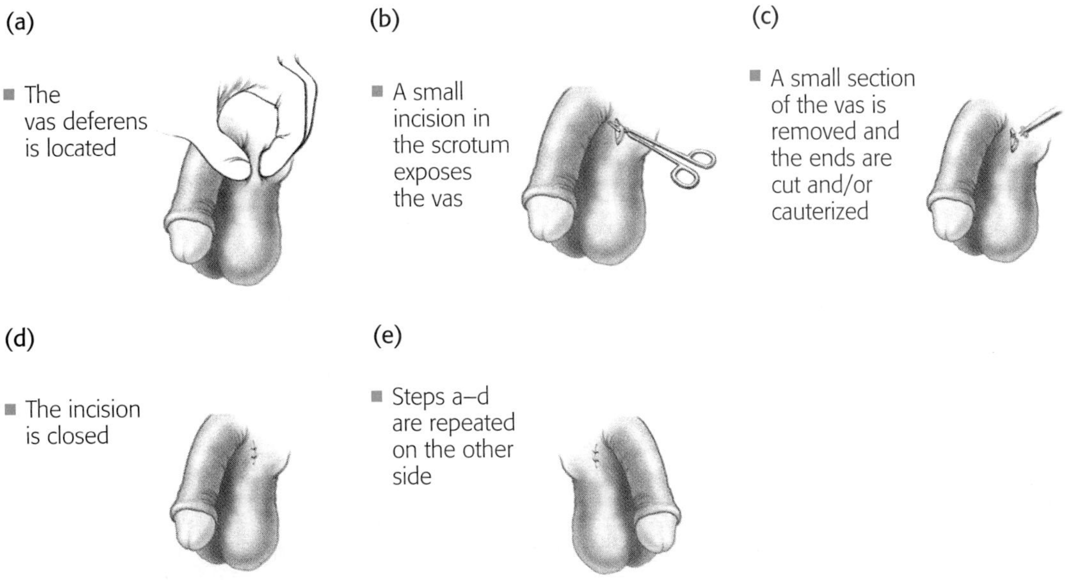
(a)
■ The vas deferens is located
(b)
■ A small incision in the scrotum exposes the vas
(c)
■ A small section of the vas is removed and the ends are cut and/or cauterized
(d)
■ The incision is closed
(e)
■ Steps a–d are repeated on the other side

FIGURE 5.7 **Vasectomy.**

tion techniques, and for some women the uterus contributes to sexual pleasure. As a sterilization method, hysterectomy is generally performed when a woman is already in a hospital after having just given birth and she is certain that she wants no more children.

## Vasectomy

A **vasectomy** is a form of voluntary male sterilization. It involves severing and/or blocking each of the two vas deferens, which prevents sperm from exiting the man's body (FIGURE 5.7). Because the cut is made "upstream" from the organs that produce seminal fluid, a man ejaculates spermless fluid. And since sperm make up no more than 5% of the volume of semen, neither a man nor his partner is aware of any change.

**vasectomy** the cutting or blocking of the pair of vas deferens to make a man incapable of fertilization

A vasectomy has no effect on a man's hormone production, his ability to get and maintain an erection, or his ability to engage in and enjoy sexual relations. The procedure is usually carried out under local anesthesia in a doctor's office or clinic in about 20 minutes. The incidence of postoperative complications is very low, and within a week most men can return to normal activities. However, a man can be fertile for several weeks after the procedure because the sperm ducts contain sperm that were present before the vasectomy took place. Once these are ejaculated, the man is sterile. About one-half to two-thirds of vasectomized men develop antibodies to sperm, but this is not harmful.

Vasectomy is supposed to be permanent, but, very rarely, the cut ends of a vas deferens spontaneously rejoin and an unintended pregnancy results. Surgical reversal of vasectomy is sometimes possible, with a success rate (measured by the ability to have children) of about 50%.

# Why People Do Not Use Fertility Control

Despite a presumed and sometimes stated desire not to become pregnant, approximately 5% percent of married couples and 15% of nonmarried sexually active individuals use no fertility control method. About 20% of nonmarried American women between the ages of 20 and 29 do not use contraception during their most recent intercourse. About 40% of American college students do not use a fertility control method regularly.

Some of the reasons that people do not use fertility control even if they do not want to become pregnant include low motivation, lack of knowledge about conception and contraception, negative attitudes about contraception, ambivalence about being sexual, and relationship factors. Satisfactory contraceptive behavior can also be impaired by the use of alcohol and other drugs.

## Low Motivation

People who know that they want children soon, who have mixed feelings about avoiding pregnancy, or who are indifferent about becoming pregnant are less motivated to use fertility control. For example, a couple that has decided that they want to have a child "sometime in the near future" but are unconcerned as to exactly when are likely to be less motivated to use fertility control than is a couple that is absolutely certain that they do not want to have a child until some specified time, or at all.

## Lack of Knowledge

Not knowing the facts about conception and how to prevent pregnancy can lead to a false perception of risk for becoming pregnant. For example, some people believe the myths that pregnancy is not possible if a woman has an orgasm, if she urinates after intercourse, or if she is having sexual intercourse for the first time. Sometimes a fertility control method is believed to be more effective than it really is, or it may be used incorrectly. For example, some people erroneously believe that a woman is most fertile during the bleeding days of the menstrual cycle, and thus practice fertility awareness incorrectly. Some couples lose, misplace, or run out of their primary contraceptive and do not have a backup method available.

## Negative Attitudes About Fertility Control

Some people believe that controlling fertility is immoral, a hassle, unromantic, or harmful. One's own attitudes about fertility control, or the perceived or fantasized attitudes of others, such as a sexual partner, peers, or parents, can inhibit sexually active individuals from using fertility control. People may use their beliefs to avoid seeing doctors or going to clinics, or they may be too shy to buy over-the-counter contraceptives.

## Ambivalence About Being Sexual

Some people are unable to "plan ahead" with respect to fertility control because they cannot admit to themselves and others that they are sexually active. Ambivalence among women may arise from the conflict of desiring sex yet fearing being labeled "easy" or "a slut" by planning for it. Negative attitudes about sex and guilt about being sexual inhibit both learning about contraception and using methods correctly.

### Relationship Issues

Individuals in committed relationships are better contraceptors than individuals who are not in such relationships. Involvement with a committed partner tends to lessen guilt associated with being sexual, and hence improves attitudes about contraceptive practice. People in a committed relationship tend to have sexual intercourse more often and regularly, which gives the couple opportunities to talk about contraception and to find and become adept at using method(s) that they prefer. Individuals with irregular sexual contact, either because of geographical separation or relationship problems, may have difficulties in establishing a contraception regime. In new or casual sexual relationships, not using an effective fertility control method at first intercourse is common.

## Sharing the Responsibility for Contraception

The responsibility for contraception has two components:

1. Choosing a method, taking into account the nature of an individual's (or couple's) sexual activities, the frequency of intercourse, future plans regarding having children, and personal and religious values.
2. Using a chosen method (or methods) consistently and correctly.

Although it may seem logical that the responsibility for contraception rests with the partner for whose body a particular method is designed, in actuality, sharing the responsibility for contraception improves sexual interaction and relationships. With shared responsibility, partners are more likely to use their chosen method(s) properly, which makes contraception more effective; the fear of pregnancy is reduced, which makes sex more enjoyable; resentment for shouldering all the responsibility is reduced, which strengthens the relationship; and mutual decision-making involved in choosing and using a method leads to better couple-communication.

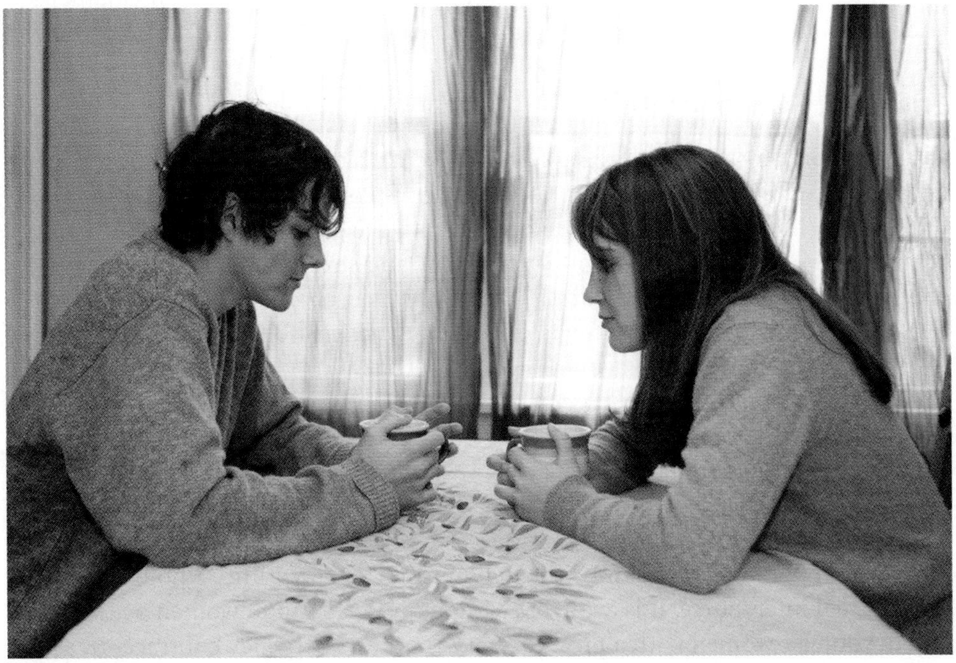

Sharing the responsibility for contraception means talking about it, which some people find embarrassing or awkward. Talking about contraception implies that sex is going to take place, which may force an individual to face personal ambivalence about engaging in sex. Also, some people assume that talking about contraception will hinder sexual spontaneity, whereas the opposite is true. Once concerns about contraception (and preventing sexually transmitted diseases) are addressed, couples can feel freer to express themselves sexually. Furthermore, some partners who are sexual with each other intermittently or for the first time may not discuss contraception before sex because they fear "spoiling the mood."

The best time to discuss contraception is before sexual intercourse begins. A partner can say something like, "I would really like to make love (have sex) with you, and I want to be sure we're protected." That kind of introduction can be followed by a statement of preference and personal responsibility, such as "I prefer to use condoms" or "I'm on the pill," or asking a question, such as "What birth control method do you prefer?" or "What are we going to do about birth control?"

Because many contraceptives are designed for use in the female, a man who is very interested in and concerned about preventing an unintended pregnancy may not discuss contraception, feeling embarrassed or afraid to appear ignorant or unmanly. Many women, however, welcome a man who discusses contraception. Discussions of contraception enhance communication about other sexual matters, too, such as the role of sex in a relationship, likes and dislikes, and preventing sexually transmitted diseases.

## Abortion

**abortion** the intentional, premature termination of pregnancy

**Abortion** is the intentional, premature termination of pregnancy. It is one of the oldest and most widely practiced methods of fertility control. Chinese medical writings dating from 2700 B.C. recommended abortion. A cross-cultural study found that all but one of 300 ancient societies had used abortion to control the size of families. Currently in the United States, approximately 1.5 million abortions are performed annually. This number represents about one-fourth of all pregnancies and about one-half of all unintended pregnancies.

### Emergency Contraception

**emergency contraception (EC)** either drug or IUD methods to prevent pregnancy if fertilization might have occurred

**Emergency contraception (EC)** is designed to prevent pregnancy if fertilization *might* have occurred. Situations that warrant emergency contraception include having unprotected intercourse, misusing a contraceptive (e.g., forgetting to take birth control pills, condom breaking or slipping off), and sexual assault. Emergency contraception is not intended to be a primary birth control method. As the name implies, it is intended for unanticipated, emergency situations. There are two forms of emergency contraception:

*Hormonal emergency contraception* consists of taking the same kinds of hormones that are in contraceptive pills. One type contains both an estrogen and a progestin. It is taken in two large doses 12 hours apart within 72 hours of unprotected intercourse.

Another type of EC consists of a progestin-only pill. One product contains levonorgestrel; it is called Plan B. This pill must be taken within 72 hours of unprotected intercourse. It is available without prescription to women over 18 and to younger women with a prescription. Another emergency contraceptive pill

### HEALTHY SEXUALITY

#### Contraceptive Availability Reduces Abortions

The World Health Organization estimates that 125 million women in the world, most of them in developing countries, are not using effective fertility control methods in spite of their stated desires to space or limit the number of children they have. The family planning needs of these women are unmet because of limited or no access to quality health services, limited availability of a variety of contraceptive methods, lack of birth control information, concerns about safety and side effects, and cultural factors such as social, religious, or partner disapproval.

Because so many women lack access to modern contraceptives, about 38% of all pregnancies worldwide are unintended, and about 60% of these result in an induced abortion. Moreover, about 20 million of these abortions are unsafe—that is, carried out by persons lacking the necessary skills or in an environment lacking the minimum medical standards, or both. Lacking quality care, about 80,000 women die of unsafe abortion every year, more than 200 per day.

Choosing when to become pregnant (and avoiding abortion) enhances a woman's health and well-being, which, in turn, enhances the health and well-being of her family and community.

containing ulipristal, called ellaOne, can be taken up to five days after unprotected intercourse.

These methods are very effective, reducing the chances of pregnancy by 90%. Side effects can include nausea and vomiting and possible adverse effects on the hormones on the developing fetus should the method fail and the pregnancy continues. These forms of emergency contraception block ovulation and thus are not regarded as methods of abortion.

*IUD emergency contraception* involves inserting a copper-T IUD up to five days after unprotected intercourse. This method is more effective than the hormonal methods, reducing the risk of pregnancy by more than 99% following unprotected intercourse.

## Surgical Abortion

There are three kinds of surgical abortion:

1. *Manual vacuum aspiration (MVA)* is performed as soon as pregnancy is confirmed up to the tenth week after fertilization. A local anesthetic is given, the cervix is gradually widened, and the uterus is emptied with the gentle suction of a manual syringe. The procedure takes about 10 minutes. It is extremely safe and effective.
2. *Dilatation and suction curettage* is performed between the sixth and fourteenth weeks of pregnancy. Local anesthesia is used and the cervix is dilated. The uterus is then emptied with gentle, machine-operated suction. A curette (narrow metal loop) may be used to clean the walls of the uterus.
3. *Dilatation and evacuation (D&E)* is performed after the fifteenth week of pregnancy. The cervix is dilated and the uterus is emptied with medical instruments, suction, and curettage. After the twentieth week, abortion is very rare.

## Medical (Chemical) Abortion

There are two forms of medical (chemical) abortion: early and late.

*Early medical abortion* is carried out prior to the seventh or eighth week after fertilization. It is generally a two-phase procedure.

*Phase 1*: *Methotrexate* or *mifepristone* (also called *RU 486*) are given to a pregnant woman to stop the pregnancy. These chemicals block the action of the naturally occurring hormone progesterone, which is essential for successful implantation and continuation of pregnancy. Blocking progesterone's actions in the early phases of pregnancy causes a miscarriage.

*Phase 2*: After the progesterone-blockers, *misoprostol* (a type of hormone called a *prostaglandin*) is given to induce contractions of the uterus and facilitate expulsion of the uterine contents within hours or days.

Medical abortion can be performed as soon as pregnancy is confirmed and is effective up to 63 days after the last menstrual period. Medical abortion with methotrexate is about 90% effective; with mifepristone (RU 486), between 92% and 95% effective. Millions of women have safely used these forms of medical abortion in the past 20 years.

These chemical abortions are overseen by trained medical personnel in a clinic over the course of a week, after which time a menstrual period occurs, which ends the pregnancy. Methotrexate and misoprostol may cause serious birth defects if the pregnancy continues. If a medical abortion is unsuccessful, a surgical abortion usually follows.

*Late medical abortion* is carried out after the twelfth week of pregnancy. This method involves infusing saline (salty water) or urea into the uterus to kill the fetus and prostaglandin to induce uterine contractions to empty the uterus.

## Aftereffects of Abortion

Despite the fact that abortion in the United States is legal and that nearly 1 million American women annually receive medically safe abortions, the decision to terminate a pregnancy voluntarily is rarely an easy one. Most women are ambivalent about abortion, as are many men.

A variety of studies on women's psychological responses to legal abortion suggest that the time between the confirmation of pregnancy and receiving an abortion is generally emotionally trying, with most women experiencing anxiety and some depression. After the abortion, symptoms of anxiety or depression are less prevalent, although a woman may experience anger or disappointment. The predominant feeling of most women is relief that the abortion had been performed successfully. Several months after their abortion, some women resolve upsetting feelings about the abortion and some continue to be troubled by the experience or consider it too upsetting to think about.

## Moral and Legal Aspects of Abortion

Abortion as a socially sanctioned method of birth control has been debated in Western societies for centuries. For example, over 2000 years ago the Greek philosophers Aristotle and Plato supported abortion, whereas Hippocrates, the founder of modern medicine, forbade it. Throughout the Middle Ages and the Renaissance, abortion was common, although various religious leaders objected to the practice on ethical grounds.

At the time the U.S. Constitution was ratified, and for several decades thereafter, abortion was legal if it took place before the time of *quickening*—when a woman could feel fetal movements. Quickening usually occurs near the sixteenth week of pregnancy. The first statutes regulating abortion were enacted in the 1820s in Connecticut and New York. By the end of the Civil War more states had enacted restrictive abortion legislation, not only to preserve the health and life of a pregnant woman but also to encourage American-born women to have children and to discourage nonreproductive sex. By 1900, abortion was illegal in all U.S. jurisdictions, and it remained so for over 60 years.

However, laws did not stop women from having abortions. In the first decades of the twentieth century, millions of women obtained illegal abortions. Those with money could travel to other countries where abortion was legal and performed in a hospital with trained personnel, or they could afford a clandestine abortion performed by an American physician who accepted the risk of prosecution. Most women, however, had to obtain abortions from nonmedical practitioners who often performed the procedure using coat hangers, spoons, disinfectant, or lye. Many women were maimed or killed by such procedures. The psychological trauma even of a successful procedure was enormous. By the 1950s, an estimated 200,000 to 1 million women were getting illegal abortions annually.

By the 1960s, people began to take into account the social and psychological costs of illegal abortion and, on January 22, 1973, the U.S. Supreme Court, in *Roe v. Wade*, declared that states could not make laws prohibiting abortion on the ground that they violated a woman's right to privacy—in this case, the right to decide about the outcome of a pregnancy.

Although abortion is legal, many people have mixed feelings about it. Because there is no universally accepted scientific definition of when a life begins, many individuals question whether abortion is murder. Some opponents of abortion believe that its availability encourages irresponsible sexual behavior. Some see abortion as a threat to family life and values. Even the staunchest proponents of abortion would prefer that it never occur, but they argue that women must have the right to control their bodies, and they believe that abortion is needed as a last resort if contraception fails, if a woman is pregnant because of rape or incest, if the child may suffer a serious birth defect, or if the woman's life and health are jeopardized by pregnancy or childbirth.

## SEXUALITY IN REVIEW

- Many fertility control methods are available for both men and women, including hormonal, barrier, and sterilization.
- The effectiveness of fertility control methods is measured in terms of typical and user failure rates.
- Negative attitudes about fertility control can lead to using a method improperly or not at all.
- Fertility control methods differ widely in their effectiveness and ease of use.
- If a woman has had unprotected intercourse or has been raped, emergency contraception (EC) can prevent a pregnancy; these should be used with medical supervision.
- Abortion is the intentional premature termination of a pregnancy and can be accomplished by a variety of techniques.

## CRITICAL THINKING ABOUT SEXUALITY

1. Consider the fact that 50% of pregnancies among married couples are unplanned and unintended. Discuss what measures you think could be taken by our society to reduce the number of unintended pregnancies by both married and unmarried couples. Consider as many different possibilities as you can think of.
2. In choosing a contraceptive method for themselves, a couple based their decision on a method's lowest observed/theoretical failure rate. Discuss why it would be better for them to use the typical/actual failure rate in making their decision.

3. A woman goes to a pharmacy to receive contraceptives prescribed by her doctor. The pharmacist refuses to fill the prescription because, she says, birth control violates her moral and religious principles. Proponents of allowing healthcare providers to refuse services to patients on moral grounds say that no one should be forced to do something against their ethical beliefs. Opponents of refusing services argue that as long as a service is legal, a health practitioner does not have the right to impose her or his moral beliefs on another and, furthermore, that health practitioners are licensed by civil authority and hence cannot impose personal convictions in the performance of their public duties. What is your stand on this issue?
4. John was stunned by the doctor's suggestion that Melanie stop taking birth control pills. Until now he had given little thought to birth control because Melanie had always taken care of it, but now he would have to assume some of the responsibility. Melanie's reaction to the doctor's suggestion was mixed. She was glad to avoid the possible health risks associated with hormonal contraception, but she also realized that other contraceptive methods were not as convenient. And although she had resented slightly having to be completely responsible for birth control, now she was not sure if she wanted to share that control. If you were Melanie's doctor, what factors would you suggest that Melanie and John consider when choosing another form of contraception? Do you think Melanie's hesitation about relinquishing control over contraception is justified? How much influence do you think men should have in contraceptive decisions?

## REFERENCES AND RECOMMENDED RESOURCES

### References

Charles, V. E. (2008). Abortion and long-term mental health outcomes: A systematic review of the evidence. *Contraception, 78*, 436–450.

Cohen, A. L., et al. (2007). Toxic shock associated with *Clostridium sordellii* and *Clostridium perfringens* after medical and spontaneous abortion. *Obstetrics and Gynecology, 110*, 1027–1033.

Trussell, J., & Wynn, L. L. (2008). Reducing unintended pregnancy in the United States. *Contraception, 77*, 1–5.

### Recommended Resources

Blumenthal, P. D., & Edelman, A. (2008). Hormonal contraception. *Obstetrics and Gynecology, 112*, 670–684. A thorough update of the various forms of hormonal contraception.

Eldridge, L. (2010). *In our control: The complete guide to contraceptive choices for women.* New York: Seven Stories Press. Discusses the pros and cons of the major birth control methods.

Hatcher, R. A., et al. (2008). *Contraceptive technology, 19th ed.* New York: Thompson Reuters. The most comprehensive discussion of contraception and abortion available, written by world-renowned experts in the field.

MedlinePlus. (2010). Available at: http://www.nlm.nih.gov/medlineplus/birthcontrol.html. Complete information on birth control from the National Library of Medicine.

Planned Parenthood. (2010). Available at: http://www.plannedparenthood.org. The most well-known provider of family planning information and services in the world.

Public Broadcasting Service. (1999–2002). The Pill. Available at: http://www.pbs.org/wgbh/amex/pill/index.html. The history of oral contraception from antiquity to the present.

Trussell, J., & Raymond, E. G. (2010). Emergency contraception: A last chance to prevent unintended pregnancy. Available at: http://ec.princeton.edu/questions/ec-review.pdf. Provides a detailed scientific discussion of the medical and social science literature about emergency contraception.

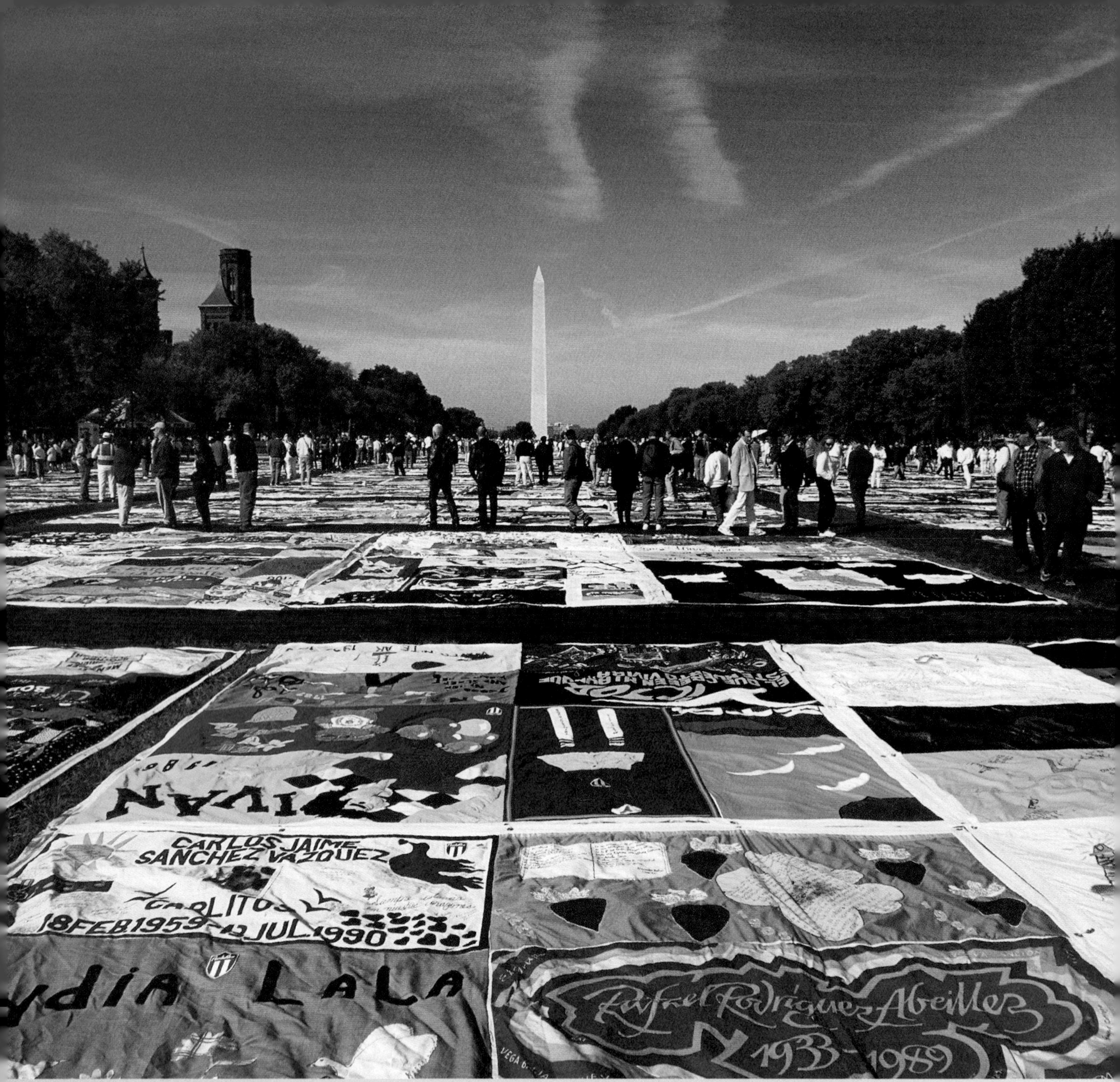


*“It is with our passions, as it is with fire and water, they are good servants but bad masters.”*

— Aesop

CHAPTER 6

# Avoiding Sexually Transmitted Diseases and AIDS

## Student Learning Objectives

1. List the nine risk factors for acquiring an STD
2. Describe how to practice safer sex and some common barriers to practicing it
3. List the 11 infections in North America that are most commonly transmitted by sexual contact
4. Identify the causative agents, symptoms, and treatments for the following STDs: trichomoniasis, gonorrhea, chlamydia, genital herpes, and anogenital warts
5. List the risk factors for HIV/AIDS
6. Describe HIV testing

Throughout the world, about 25 different diseases can be passed from person to person via sexual contact; 11 are common in North America (**Table 6.1**). The World Health Organization estimates that each year 500 to 600 million people in the world acquire a sexually transmitted disease (STD), also referred to as a sexually transmitted infection (STI). In North America, the number of annual STD infections approximates 19 million, a rate second only to the common cold (**FIGURE 6.1**). About half of these infections occur in people under age 25.

STDs have been afflicting humans for thousands of years. Ancient Chinese medical writings describe diseases of the genitalia that were probably syphilis. The ancient Egyptians described genital diseases that were probably gonorrhea. The Old Testament and Talmudic writings describe a condition called *ziba*, which was associated with the emission of fluid, referred to as *issue*, from the nonerect penis or the vagina. *Ziba* was probably gonorrhea, and *issue* was probably the discharge

**Table 6.1** Common Sexually Transmitted Diseases in the United States

| STD | Symptoms | Treatment |
|---|---|---|
| HIV/AIDS | Flulike symptoms followed by any of a number of diseases characteristic of immunodeficiency | Drugs may retard viral reproduction temporarily; opportunistic infections can be treated to some degree |
| Chlamydia | If present, usually occur within three weeks: infected men have a discharge from the penis and painful urination; women may have a vaginal discharge | Antibiotics |
| Genital Warts | If present, usually occur within one to three months: small, dry growths on the genitals, anus, cervix, and possibly mouth | Podophyllin |
| Gonorrhea | Usually occur within two weeks: discharge from the penis, vagina, or anus; pain on urination or defecation or during sexual intercourse; pain and swelling in the pelvic region; genital and oral infections may be asymptomatic | Antibiotics |
| Hepatitis B | Low-grade fever, fatigue, headaches, loss of appetite, nausea, dark urine, and jaundice | Rest, proper nutrition; vaccination for hepatitis B |
| Genital Herpes | Usually occur within two weeks: painful blisters on site of infection (e.g., genitals, anus, cervix); occasionally itching, painful urination, and fever | None; acyclovir relieves symptoms |
| Molluscum Contagiosum | Smooth, rounded, shiny, whitish growths on the skin of the trunk and anogenital region | Surgical removal of growths |
| Pubic Lice | Usually occur within five weeks: intense itching in the genital region; lice may be visible in pubic hair; small white eggs may be visible on pubic hair | Gamma benzene hexachloride |
| Scabies | Tiny, itchy lesions caused by mites burrowing into the skin | Topical insecticides |
| Syphilis | First stage occurs within three weeks: a chancre (painless sore) on the genitals, anus, or mouth; secondary stage, skin rash (if left untreated); tertiary stage includes diseases of several body organs | Antibiotics |
| Trichomoniasis | Yellowish-green vaginal discharge with an unpleasant odor; vaginal itching; occasionally painful intercourse | Metronidazole |

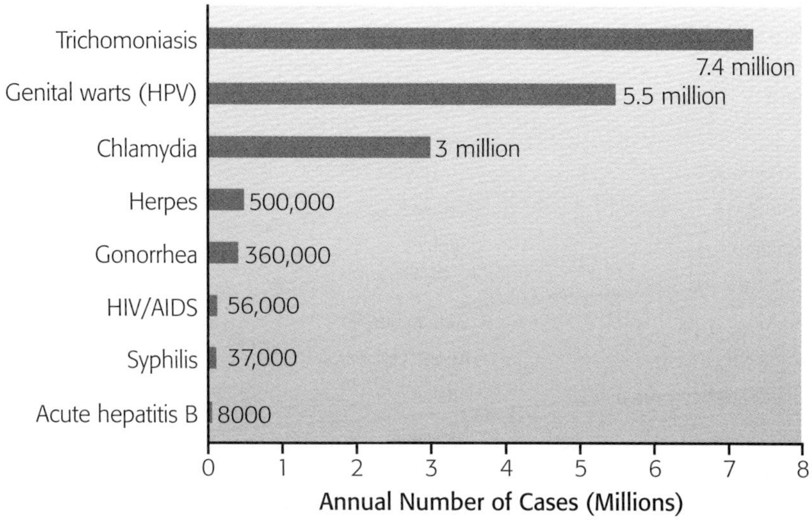


FIGURE 6.1 **Estimated Yearly Number of STDs in the United States.**

associated with the infection. Many famous historical figures are thought to have had sexually transmitted diseases (FIGURE 6.2).

The social and human costs of STDs are enormous. In the United States, the direct and indirect economic costs of the major STDs and their complications total $20 billion a year. The human suffering and economic costs wrought by AIDS are well documented. Less well known are the disappointment and suffering of thousands of women who are left infertile after a serious STD-related pelvic infection. Also, women who acquire a human papillomavirus infection (anogenital warts) are predisposed to cervical cancer. Fortunately, a vaccine to prevent human papillomavirus (HPV) infection is now available. And the 500,000 Americans who acquire genital herpes each year are likely to be infected for the rest of their lives, since this virus cannot be eliminated from the body once a person has become infected.

Abraham
Job
Dürer
Gauguin
Sarah
King David
Schubert
Boswell
Julius Caesar
Cleopatra
Molière

Goethe
Charlemagne
Napoleon
Van Gogh
Oscar Wilde
Henry VIII
Columbus
Nietzsche
Goya
Peter the Great
Catherine the Great

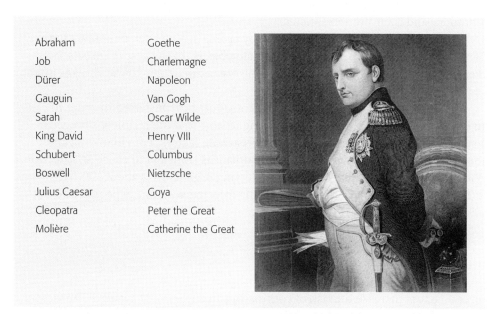

FIGURE 6.2 **Famous People Who Are Thought to Have Had an STD.** No one knows for sure, but many historians think these famous people were infected.

**Table 6.2** Agents That Cause the More Prevalent STDs

| Infectious Agent | Disease |
|---|---|
| Bacteria | |
| *Chlamydia trachomatis* | Chlamydia |
| *Neisseria gonorrhoeae* | Gonorrhea |
| *Treponema pallidum* | Syphilis |
| Viruses | |
| Herpes simplex virus, types 1 and 2 | Genital herpes |
| Human papillomavirus | Anogenital warts |
| Human immunodeficiency virus (HIV) | AIDS |
| Hepatitis B virus | Hepatitis |
| Molluscum contagiosum virus | Molluscum contagiosum |
| Protozoa | |
| *Trichomonas vaginalis* | Trichomoniasis (vaginitis) |
| Insects | |
| *Phthirus pubis* | Lice ("crabs") |
| *Sarcoptes scabiei* | Mites ("scabies") |

## What Is a Sexually Transmitted Disease?

**sexually transmitted disease (STD)** an infection or infestation caused by a biological agent (e.g., virus, bacterium, insect) that is transferred from person to person by sexual interaction

A **sexually transmitted disease (STD)** is an infection that is transmitted by sexual contact, usually sexual intercourse. Human STDs are caused by viruses, bacteria, protozoa, worms, and insects (**Table 6.2**).

STD-causing agents can enter the body (1) through breaks in the skin; (2) through the wet surface layers, or *mucous membranes*, of the body's orifices: nose and mouth, penis, vagina, urethra, and anus; and (3) the blood, either by injection or during sexual activity by means of tiny microscopic abrasions on the penis, in the vagina, the anus, or in the mouth. Once inside the body, STD-causing agents reproduce and their numbers increase.

In general, STDs are not transferred by animals, air, water, or contact with doorknobs, toilet seats, and other inanimate objects. In the case of insects, however, contact with any surface on which the organisms, their larvae, or eggs might be present may cause an infection.

A certain number of STD-causing agents must be transferred in order to cause an infection. This number varies according to how well the recipient's body can defend itself and a variety of specific host–parasite factors. For chlamydia and gonorrhea, the transfer of about 1000 organisms is sufficient to cause an infection. With syphilis, the requisite number of infecting organisms is about 100. With gonorrhea and chlamydia, the risk of becoming infected with one exposure is about 60% to 90% in men and 20% to 35% in women.

## Risk Factors for STDs

Several factors increase the risk of contracting an STD. Being aware of the factors can help decrease the risk of acquiring an STD and also support community-wide STD prevention.

## Multiple Sexual Partners

Many individuals have several lifetime sexual partners because they become sexually active in late adolescence and may not marry until their mid- to late 20s or 30s. About 20% of unmarried adults have more than one sex partner in a year. Also, many people in a supposedly sexually exclusive relationship have sex with other partners, generally without the "exclusive" partner's knowledge. Individuals who know that their partners have sexual relations with others have lower rates of STDs than individuals who do not know.

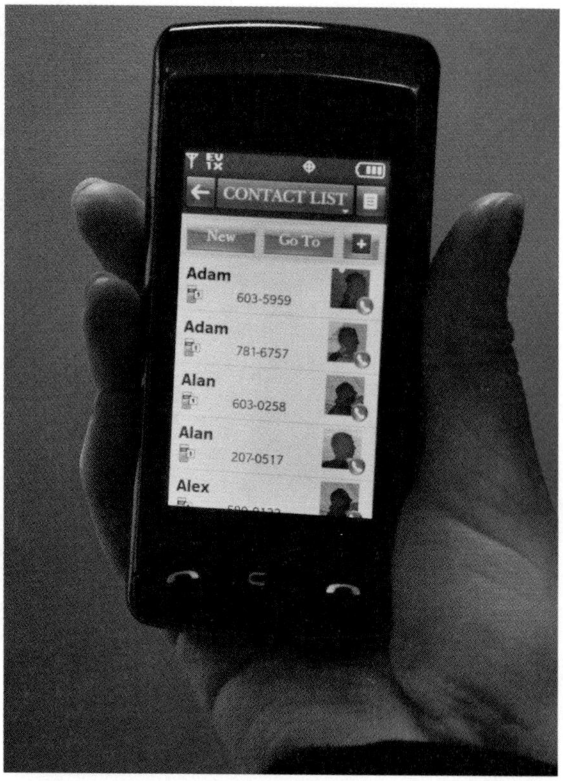


Multiple partners is a major risk for STD transmission.

## False Sense of Safety

Using hormonal contraceptives may reduce the use of condoms because people mistakenly equate protection from pregnancy with prevention from STDs. Also, the availability of anti-STD medications such as antibiotics creates the false assumption that all STDs are curable, which facilitates STD-risky behavior.

## Absence of Signs and Symptoms

Some STDs have mild or no symptoms, so an infection can worsen and unknowingly be passed to others. Among U.S. young adults aged 18–26, nearly 5% are infected with chlamydia and do not know it because of a lack of symptoms.

## Untreated Conditions

Some individuals do not know the signs and symptoms of STDs, may not have access to medical care, or may not comply with treatment regimens. Each of these factors contributes to an infected individual remaining infected and contagious.

## Impaired Judgment

Drug- and alcohol-impaired individuals are less likely to use condoms and may have sex with people they do not know, thus putting them at risk for contracting an STD. Studies show that higher alcohol taxes and increases in the legal drinking age are associated with decreased rates of gonorrhea, which suggests that alcohol consumption contributes to acquiring this infection, probably through having unprotected sex with unfamiliar partners.

## Lack of Immunity

Some STD-causing organisms can escape the body's immune defenses, causing individuals to remain infected and transmit the infection, often for life. Human immunodeficiency virus (HIV) and herpes viruses are examples of such infections.

**human immunodeficiency virus (HIV)** the cause of AIDS

## Body Piercing

Wounds from piercing give infectious organisms direct access to the bloodstream. Nipple, tongue, and lip jewelry may increase the risk of infections from oral contact. People who have had their bodies pierced should follow aftercare instruc-

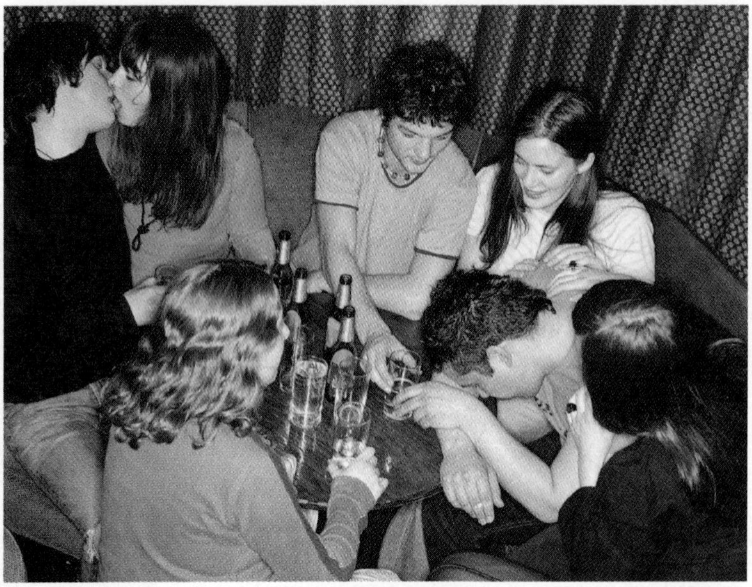

Drunkenness at parties can impair judgement.

tions faithfully to prevent infection. They should refrain from sexual contact in the pierced region until the hole is completely healed, which may take three to six months.

### Value Judgments

Negative and moralistic attitudes about STDs prevent people from getting tested, contacting partners after a positive diagnosis, and talking to new partners about previous infections.

### Denial

"It can't happen to me," "He's too nice to have an STD," and "She's too pretty to have an STD" are fictions.

## Preventing Sexually Transmitted Diseases

Vaccines are the most safe and efficient way to prevent several STDs. Unfortunately, vaccines are available only for hepatitis B and human papillomavirus (HPV). Until other vaccines are developed, preventing STDs requires that societies provide consistent public health programs and services for STD education, prevention, and treatment. Infected individuals need to seek treatment and take responsibility for not infecting other partners. Individuals who practice "safer sex" reduce their risk of infection (**Table 6.3**).

### Barriers to Practicing Safer Sex

In most instances, guidelines for safer sex are guidelines for sensible and better sex, whether one is concerned about STDs or not. Yet, people do not use safer sex methods routinely because they are not accustomed to doing them and because of social and psychological barriers, such as:

- Assuming that STDs happen only to "dirty," "promiscuous," and "immoral" people. Believing one's sexual partners are "clean" and "nice" makes getting an STD seem impossible.

**Table 6.3** Practicing Safer Sex

| |
|---|
| **Abstain from Sexual Activity** |
| The surest way to reduce the risk of acquiring a sexually transmitted disease is to abstain from body-to-body sexual interaction. This does not mean that one has to give up sexual interaction altogether. Sex does not equal intercourse. There are many nonintercourse ways of giving and receiving sexual pleasure: touching, kissing, exchanging a massage, and sleeping together without intercourse. |
| **Know Your Partner's Sexual History** |
| This means knowing if your partner has engaged in STD-risky activities. This kind of information is difficult to acquire early in a relationship, because exchanging information about sexual histories requires a certain level of trust, which takes some time to develop. |
| **Use Condoms** |
| Latex condoms protect against acquiring STDs even if another form of birth control is employed. Keep in mind that hormonal contraceptives ("the pill") offer no protection against STDs. Sexually active women and men should accept as standard practice with new partners the use of condoms, carry condoms whenever the possibility for sex exists, and expect a partner's cooperation with using condoms. |
| **Be Selective (and Careful)** |
| Urges and pressures for partners to be sexual before they know each other well enough to talk about their past sexual experiences forces them to deny there is a risk of contracting an STD. They may tell themselves, "There's nothing to worry about, this person is too nice to have an STD," even though they know there is a potential risk. Postpone sexual interaction with a new partner and say something like, "I'd like to be close to you, but I'm not ready to have sex until we get to know each other better." "Not yet" and "maybe" are options when considering an invitation to be sexual. |
| **Talk** |
| Tell a new partner about any prior exposure to an STD. Ask first-time partners about their possible prior exposure to STDs. Start by saying, "I want to be sure we are both safe from sexual infections." |

- Assuming that generally good health habits protects against STDs. Telling oneself, "I eat right. I exercise. I can't get an STD," is denying the real risk.
- Believing that a campus community isolates students from the risk of STDs. Many college students are sexually active before they enter college. Also, sexually active students going home on vacations may bring STDs back to campus. On many campuses, students in the same living groups and student organizations have sex with one another.
- Feeling guilty and uncomfortable about being sexual. This prevents individuals from planning sex, carrying condoms, and talking about possible risks with new partners.
- Social and peer pressure to be sexual, which encourages people to be sexual in situations that are potentially STD-risky, such as one-night stands and brief sexual relationships. The risk of infection is lessened when individuals resist social pressures to have sex with a stranger and ask themselves, "Is this the right partner?," "Is this the right relationship?," "Am I going to feel OK about this afterward?"
- Thinking about STDs in moral terms—that is, associating them with dirtiness and immorality instead of considering them as we do other infectious diseases—makes people reluctant to think and talk about them, and makes society ignore STDs until they reach epidemic levels.
- Fear of rejection. To have to tell a partner that you have an infection, or to say that you once had an infection and are now all right, can bring feelings of guilt and shame, which can prevent the discussion altogether. To ask about a partner's possible or actual previous STD exposure may be interpreted as accusing the partner as being sexually "loose" or immoral. Rather than risk an angry response or a rejection, the topic is avoided.

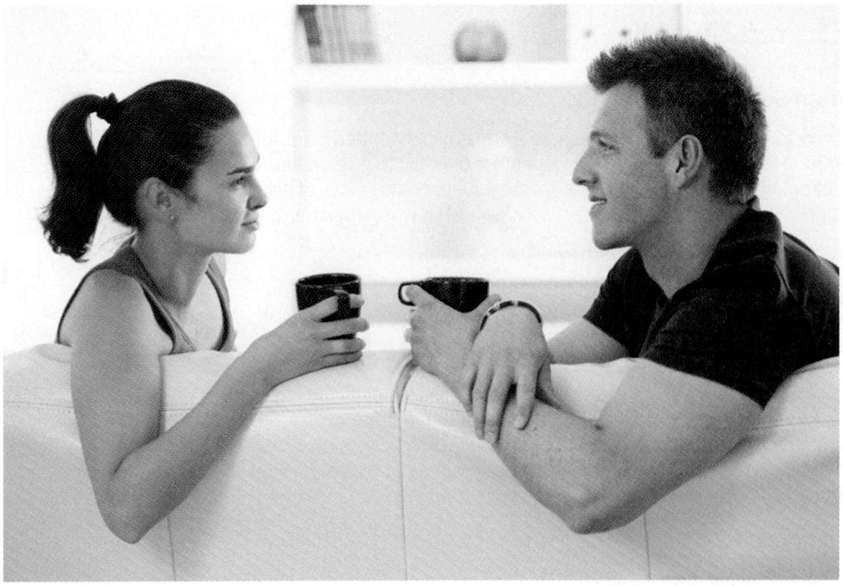

### Talking About Possible STD-Exposure with a Sexual Partner

Verbally addressing one's possible exposure to STDs can be difficult (especially with a new partner) because of the fear of being rejected, offending the partner, or spoiling an erotic mood. Disclosing one's discomfort about talking about sexual interaction is one way to relieve anxiety about it.

A conversation could begin with one partner saying, "There's something I want us to talk about, and I feel sort of uncomfortable about it, but I think it's important to both of us, so here goes." After that introduction, the individual can offer information about him or herself by saying something like, "We don't know each other very well; I'm concerned about sexual diseases. I want you to know this about me." That person should offer all of the information that he or she would like to be told. After hearing the disclosure, the other person is likely to respond in kind. And if more information is desired, one could say something like, "Thanks for telling me all of that. I'd feel more comfortable if I knew a little more about . . ." whatever it is. What if the other person gets offended or won't talk about this subject? Or what if the other person can't be trusted? If partners cannot carry on a discussion about something as serious as STDs, postponing sexual interaction until the relationship has progressed to a greater level of trust is prudent. Potential sexual partners should keep in mind that being under the influence of alcohol or other drugs can affect one's judgment in making decisions about what is safe and what is not safe.

## Protozoal and Bacterial STDs

**trichomoniasis** vaginal infection caused by the protozoan *Trichomonas vaginali*

### Trichomoniasis

Although not often regarded as sexually transmitted, vaginal infections caused by the protozoan *Trichomonas vaginalis* are transmissible by sexual intercourse. Symptoms of **trichomoniasis** tend to occur in women (vaginal itching and a cheesy, odorous discharge from the vagina), but the organisms can survive in the urethra of the penis and under the penile foreskin. A man who harbors these organisms can infect other sexual partners or even reinfect the partner who transmitted the organisms to him.

About 7 million new cases of trichomonas are diagnosed in the United States each year. Clinically, a diagnosis is made by collecting fluid from the vagina and testing for the presence of trichomonas microorganisms. Medications are available to treat these infections successfully. An infected woman's male partner(s) should also undergo testing and treatment.

## Bacterial Vaginosis

The vagina normally contains a variety of bacteria that support a healthy vaginal environment. However, overgrowth of certain types of bacteria (generally *Gardnerella vaginalis*) can cause an infection called **bacterial vaginosis (BV)**, which can be transmitted via sexual intercourse. Symptoms of BV include vaginal discharge, which may have a "fishy" smell, particularly after intercourse. Sometimes BV has no symptoms.

**bacterial vaginosis (BV)** a vaginal infection, often caused by *Gardnerella vaginalis*
**chlamydia** a sexually transmitted bacterial infection of the genitals, anus, mouth, eyes, and occasionally the lungs

## Chlamydia

**Chlamydia** is caused by the bacterium *Chlamydia trachomatis*, which specifically infects certain cells that line the mucous membranes of the genitals, mouth, anus, rectum, the conjunctiva of the eyes, and occasionally the lungs. The chlamydia organisms bind to the surfaces of host cells and induce the host cells to engulf them. After gaining entrance to the cell, these organisms resist the host cell's defenses and "steal" from the host cell the biochemical substances required for their own survival and growth. The chlamydia organisms ultimately destroy the host cells.

In the United States each year, approximately 3 million Americans are *reported* to have contracted chlamydia, a figure that public health experts estimate represents only one-third of all cases that actually occur. In as many as half of all cases, chlamydia occurs simultaneously with gonorrhea. Besides adults, newborns are susceptible to chlamydia infection if their mothers are infected at the time of birth. The most common complications of chlamydia infection in newborns are conjunctivitis (eye infection) and pneumonia.

One reason that chlamydia infections are so prevalent is that 75% of infected women and 50% of infected men have extremely mild or no symptoms. Thus, infected individuals can unknowingly transmit the infection to new sex partners. When symptoms occur, they include pain on urination in both men and women (*dysuria*) and a whitish discharge from the penis or vagina. Symptoms generally appear within seven to 21 days after infection.

Chlamydia can be treated successfully with *antibiotics*, drugs that kill bacteria. Left untreated, chlamydia organisms can multiply and cause inflammation and damage of the reproductive organs in both sexes. In men, untreated chlamydia can result in inflammation of the epididymis (*epididymitis*), which is characterized by pain, swelling, and tenderness in the scrotum, and sometimes a mild fever. Damage to the tissues in the epididymis can eventually lead to sterility. In women, untreated chlamydia infections can lead to infections of the cervix, uterus, Fallopian tubes, and peritoneum. Chlamydia infections of the female reproductive tract often produce no symptoms until the infection is quite advanced. In these instances a woman may experience chronic pelvic pain, vaginal discharge, intermittent bleeding from the vagina, and pain during sexual intercourse (*dyspareunia*). Infection of the Fallopian tubes can produce scar tissue that damages the tubes' lining and/or partially or completely blocks the tubes. These conditions may render a woman infertile. In the United States, about 10,000 cases of female infertility per year are due to damage from chlamydia infection. Chlamydia infection can also increase the risk of ectopic pregnancy.

Chlamydial infections induce an immune response in the host, but for unknown reasons infected individuals do not build an immunity to future chlamydia infections. This means that individuals can be reinfected upon repeated exposure to the organisms.

## Gonorrhea

**gonorrhea** a sexually transmitted bacterial infection of the genitals, anus, mouth, and eyes
**syphilis** a sexually transmitted bacterial infection caused by the bacterium *Treponema pallidum*
**chancre** a painless sore that is one of the first signs of a syphilis infection

**Gonorrhea**, also known as "the clap," is caused by the bacterium *Neisseria gonorrheae*. Gonorrheal organisms specifically infect the mucous membranes of the body, most often the genitals, reproductive organs, mouth and throat, anus, and eye. *Neisseriae* cannot survive on toilet seats, doorknobs, bed sheets, clothes, or towels. Transmission in adults almost always occurs by genital, oral, or anal sexual contact; infection of the eyes occurs by hand (usually through self-infection). Each year about 300,000 American adults are infected with gonorrhea.

Newborn babies exposed to gonorrheal organisms during vaginal birth may develop gonorrhea infection of the eyes. Most states require that antibiotics or a few drops of silver nitrate be put into the eyes of babies immediately after birth to kill gonorrhea bacteria and prevent possible blindness.

Although the bacteria causing them are quite different, the symptoms of gonorrhea and chlamydia infections are very similar. Like chlamydia, many people infected with gonorrheal organisms do not develop symptoms, and thus their infection goes unnoticed. If the infection progresses, men may develop epididymitis and women may develop infections of the uterus, Fallopian tubes, and pelvic region. Untreated infections may cause sterility. When symptoms appear, they include painful urination in both sexes and a yellowish discharge from the penis or vagina. Occasionally, there is pain in the groin, testes, or lower abdomen. The first symptoms of gonorrhea usually appear within seven to 10 days after exposure.

Gonorrhea can be successfully treated with antibiotics. However, antibiotic-resistant strains of the organism are prevalent. In nearly half of all cases of gonorrhea, chlamydia also is present. Individuals undergoing examination for gonorrhea should also be tested for chlamydia.

## Syphilis

**Syphilis** is caused by spiral-shaped bacteria called *Treponema pallidum*. These organisms are transmitted from person to person through microscopic breaks in the skin. The organisms can be transmitted through genital, oral, and anal contact as well as by direct transfer into the blood. Syphilis can also be transmitted from an infected mother to her fetus, perhaps as early as the ninth week of pregnancy.

The first noticeable sign of syphilis is a painless open sore called a **chancre** ("shanker"), which can appear any time between the first week and third month after infection. If the infection is not treated within that time, the chancre will heal and the disease enters a "secondary stage" characterized by a skin rash, loss of hair, and the appearance of round, flat-topped growths on most areas of the body. Left untreated, the signs of the secondary stage also disappear, and the infection enters

HEALTHY SEXUALITY

### The Tuskegee Syphilis Study: A Tragic Chapter in American History

To study the progression of untreated syphilis, in 1932 the U.S. Public Health Service began a disgraceful, unethical study involving nearly 400 poor African American men with syphilis from Macon County, Alabama.

The men in the study were never told they had syphilis, nor were they told the real purpose of the study. Instead, they were told they were being treated for "bad blood," a local term used to describe several illnesses, including syphilis, anemia, and fatigue. For participating in the study, the men were given free medical exams, free meals, and burial insurance.

The study was to last six months, but it continued for 40 years. Even though penicillin became available to cure the disease in 1947, the drug was withheld from the study subjects. At no time were the study subjects told they could receive treatment that might cure their disease. The researchers wanted to see how the disease progressed and produced death.

In the early 1970s, public health workers leaked the story to the media, and in 1972 the U.S. government stopped the study and agreed to pay for medical care and burial insurance for all surviving participants. On behalf of the nation, in 1997 President Bill Clinton apologized for the study, its inherent racism, and the unnecessary harm it caused.

For information, refer to the following resources:

Jones, James H. (1993). *Bad blood: The Tuskegee syphilis experiment.* New York: Free Press.

Bad Blood. A historical exhibit about the Tuskegee Syphilis Study from the University of Virginia Library. Available at: http://www.healthsystem.virginia.edu/internet/library/historical/medical_history/bad_blood.

U.S. Centers for Disease Control and Prevention. Tuskegee Syphilis Study. Available at: http://www.cdc.gov/nchstp/od/tuskegee/index.html.

a symptomless (latency) period during which the syphilis organisms multiply in many other regions of the body, eventually damaging vital organs, such as the heart or brain, and causing severe illness or death. Syphilis can be treated successfully with antibiotics at any stage of the infection.

## STDs Caused by Viruses

### Herpes Simplex Virus

**herpes** a sexually transmitted viral infection of the genitals, anus, mouth, and eyes, characterized by the appearance of wet, open, painful sores at the site of the infection

Herpes infections of the anogenital region are caused by either of two strains of *herpes simplex virus* (HSV), HSV-1 and HSV-2. HSV-1 is frequently associated with cold sores on the mouth ("fever blisters"), whereas HSV-2 is generally associated with lesions on the penis, vagina, vaginal labia, rectum, and the skin of the genital, pelvic, and anal regions. Each year between 500,000 and 1 million American adults acquire a genital herpes infection. As many as 40 million American adults have been and remain infected with HSV, as the organism cannot be eliminated from the body.

A herpes lesion on the genitals usually appears within two to 20 days after exposure to HSV. The major symptoms of genital herpes infection are the presence of one or more blisters, which eventually break to become wet, painful sores that last about two to three weeks; fever; and occasionally pain in the lower abdomen. Eventually, these initial symptoms disappear but the herpes virus remains dormant in certain areas of the body's nerve cells, permitting periodic recurrences of symptoms, called "flare-ups," at or near the site(s) of the initial infection. It is thought that stress, anxiety, poor nutrition, sunlight, and skin irritation can bring on recurrences. Flare-ups may be "telegraphed" by a tingling or itching in the genital region or pain in the buttocks or down the leg. Visible lesions may or may not appear, so people anticipating a flare-up should be cautious about transmitting HSV to a partner.

Herpes infection is extremely contagious when a sore is present. People with open lesions should not have skin contact with others until the lesions heal completely. Transmission is possible, although much less likely, even if no sore is present through the "shedding" of virus particles from the skin. Indeed, infections with HSV-2 often have no symptoms; nevertheless, infected persons are contagious.

Whereas genital herpes infections are most frequently caused by HSV-2 and oral herpes infections by HSV-1, both HSV-2 and HSV-1 can cause genital and oral infections with identical symptoms. Thus, people with oral herpes can transmit the infection to partners via oral sex. And they can transmit it to themselves through masturbation if they have touched a sore on their mouth.

Herpes viruses can infect the eyes, leading to impairment of vision and even blindness. If the virus is present in the birth canal, newborn babies can be infected, often resulting in brain damage and abnormal development. Two-thirds of babies with untreated herpes infections die. Pregnant women who have had herpes should tell their health providers of previous infection in order to prevent possible transmission of HSV to their babies.

There is no cure for herpes. Infected individuals remain so for life. However, several drugs can minimize the duration and severity of the symptoms of an initial infection or a flare-up.

## Human Papillomaviruses and Anogenital Warts

**human papillomavirus (HPV)** the cause of anogenital warts and occasionally cervical cancer

Human papillomaviruses (HPV) are a group of more than 100 types of similar viruses, about 40 of which can be passed from person to person via sexual contact. About 20 million Americans are currently infected with HPV; about 6 million Americans become infected with HPV via sexual intercourse each year. Most HPV infections are symptomless and go away on their own. However, persistent infections with one or more of 10 types of HPV can cause cervical cancer in women. About 12,000 American women develop cervical cancer each year; about 4000 American women die each year of the disease.

Some types of HPV may cause visible warts (*Condylomata acuminata*) on or around the genitals or anus within three months of contact with an infected person. Other types of HPV do not cause visible anogenital warts, although they infect the vagina, cervix, penis, and the mouth and larynx (due to oral sex with an infected person). The types of HPV that cause visible warts on hands and feet are different from those that cause growths in the genital region.

Visible anogenital warts usually are raised or flat, single or multiple, small or large, sometimes cauliflower-shaped, soft, moist, pink, or flesh-colored swellings. They can appear on the vulva, in or around the vagina or anus, on the cervix, and on the penis, scrotum, groin, or thigh. The warts are contagious. Anogenital warts can be removed by self-applied medications (imiquimod cream, podophyllin or podofilox solutions). Also, they can be removed by a healthcare provider. Clinician-applied treatments include using 10% to 25% podophyllum resin, trichloroacetic acid, or bichloroacetic acid; physically excising the wart; cryosurgery (freezing); electrocautery (burning); or exposure to laser. Treatments remove the warts but not HPV in cells, so warts can reappear after treatment. Without treatment, warts may disappear or they may grow more numerous or larger.

Many genital HPV infections do not cause visible warts or symptoms even though the virus lives in the skin or mucous membranes. A health practitioner can detect invisible infections in several ways: (1) applying vinegar (acetic acid) to suspected infected regions and looking for infected cells to whiten; (2) viewing the vagina and cervix with a magnifying instrument (culposcopy); (3) removing a small amount of tissue (biopsy) for analysis of HPV DNA; and (4) perform-

## Dear Penelope . . .

***At a party not long ago I met an attractive, interesting woman. A week later I went out with her. Nice time. Passionate goodnight kiss. I didn't want her to think all I was after was sex, so I didn't push it. My roommate's girlfriend later told me that I blew it because my date was definitely signaling that she wanted to get physical. I felt like such an idiot!***

***I don't want to blow it next time. I don't want to be so polite that a woman thinks I'm a wimp, but I don't want to come on so strong and so fast that she thinks I'm Attila the Hun.***

***— Searching for a Good Line***

*Dear Searching,*

Forget the line. Go for an attitude adjustment.

This sounds like a terrific first date. Sharing a nice time and a passionate kiss hold real promise for future dates with your new friend. Even if she were signaling, what's the rush? A wise friend once told me, "Always get up from the table feeling a bit hungry. That way you'll look forward to coming back for more."

Apparently you also thought this was a good date until your roommate's friend came along. Trust your own judgment. By not "pushing it" you communicated to your date that you want to develop a relationship of mutual respect and trust. If you want a line, how about verbalizing that message with something like, "I had a great time. I'd like to see you again soon." If she is signaling, that lets her know you're interested in having her "come back to the table" soon.

Courtesy of the UC Davis *Aggie*

ing a Pap smear to look for abnormalities in cervical cells associated with HPV infection.

The types of HPV that infect the genital area are spread primarily through genital contact. Most HPV infections have no signs or symptoms; therefore, most infected persons are unaware they are infected, yet they can transmit the virus to a sex partner. Rarely, a pregnant woman can pass HPV to her baby during vaginal delivery.

There is a vaccine against two types of HPV that cause about 70% of cervical cancers and two types of HPV that cause about 90% of genital warts. The vaccine is given in a series of three injections over a six-month period. The vaccine is highly effective in preventing HPV infection in young women who have not yet been exposed to HPV. Many health professionals recommend that all young women be vaccinated against HPV before they reach the age at which they are likely to become sexually active.

Besides vaccination, infections with HPV may be prevented by avoiding sexual and other skin-to-skin contact with an infected person and using latex condoms.

## Hepatitis B

**Hepatitis B** is a disease of the liver caused by infection with hepatitis B virus (HBV), one of several types of hepatitis viruses. HBV is transmitted most often sexually and by blood. About 150,000 sexually transmitted HBV infections occur in the United States each year; worldwide, the number is estimated to be about 300 million.

**hepatitis B** a viral disease of the liver caused by hepatitis B virus (HBV) infection

About 30% of infected persons infected with HBV do not have any symptoms. When they appear, symptoms include low-grade fever, fatigue, headache, loss of appetite, nausea, dark urine, and jaundice (yellowing of the white of the eyes and skin). The first symptoms, which are flulike, appear between 14 and 100 days after infection. Signs of liver disease appear later.

No specific therapy exists for HBV infection. Rest, proper nutrition, and avoidance of substances harmful to the liver (e.g., alcohol, drugs) are required for recovery, which may take many months. Long-term liver damage is possible, including cancer of the liver, and death. A vaccine against HBV is available, and everyone is advised to be vaccinated, especially children, health workers, and others who are at high risk of exposure.

### Molluscum Contagiosum

**molluscum contagiosum** a virus-caused STD

**Molluscum contagiosum** is caused by a virus of the same name. About 100,000 infections occur in the United States each year. The infection is characterized by the appearance of freckle-sized, smooth, rounded, shiny, whitish growths on the skin and trunk and anogenital region. Generally, there are no associated symptoms. The lesions may resolve spontaneously, but it is best to have them removed by a health professional; otherwise, they may be transmitted to others or recur.

## Insects: Lice and Mites

### Pubic Lice

**pubic lice** insects that live on the hair shafts in the pelvic region

**scabies** an infestation of the skin by mites

**Pubic lice** (*Phthirus pubis*), also known as "crabs," are barely visible insects that live on hair shafts primarily in the genital-rectal region, and occasionally on hair in the armpits (axilla), the beard, and eyelashes. The organisms' claws are specifically adapted for grasping hairs with the diameter of pubic and axillary hair, which differs in diameter from the shafts of scalp hair. Thus, pubic lice are not usually found on the head. (Scalp hair is the ecological niche for the head louse, *Pediculus humanus capitis.*)

Lice feed on blood taken from tiny blood vessels in the skin, which they pierce with their mouth parts. Some people are sensitive to the bites and may experience itching, which is often the main symptom of infestation. The lice can also be seen; they look like small freckles. The eggs of lice are enclosed in small white pods (called "nits"), which attach to hair shafts. The presence of nits is also a sign of infestation.

Lice are transferred by body-to-body contact. They can also be transmitted via contact with objects on which eggs might have been laid, such as towels, bed linens, and clothes. An infestation of pubic lice can be eliminated by washing the pubic hair with liquids or shampoos containing agents that specifically kill lice (e.g., pyrethrins, piperonyl butoxide, gamma benzene hydrochloride). All of an infected person's clothes, towels, and bed linens also should be washed in hot water.

### Scabies

**Scabies** is an infestation of certain regions of the skin by extremely small (invisible to the naked eye) mites, *Sarcoptes scabiei.* The mites burrow into the skin, where they live and lay eggs. The tiny lesions produced by the mites often cause intense itching, which is the major sign of a scabies infection. The mites produce tiny burrows across skin lines, which often go unnoticed. Occasionally, an infestation will produce small, round nodules. The mites tend to live in the webs between the fingers, on the sides of fingers, and on the wrists, elbows, breasts, abdomen, penis, and buttocks. Rarely do mites live on the face, neck, upper back, palms, and soles.

Scabies can be transmitted sexually and nonsexually. All that is required is sufficient personal contact. The itching and any physical signs of the mites often take several weeks to appear. Scabies can be treated and eliminated with topical agents that also kill mites and their eggs.

## Acquired Immune Deficiency Syndrome

Acquired immune deficiency syndrome (AIDS) is caused by human immunodeficiency virus (HIV). Infection by HIV causes a variety of diseases that result from the destruction of certain cells of the body's immune system that are used to combat infections. Lack of a functional immune system makes a person susceptible to a variety of bacterial, viral, and fungal infections (called *opportunistic infections*) that a person with an intact immune system could readily ward off. Left untreated, HIV multiplies in immune system cells, the immune system progressively weakens, and infected individuals eventually become sick and die.

**acquired immune deficiency syndrome (AIDS)** a variety of infectious diseases related to weakening of the immune system due to infection with human immunodeficiency virus (HIV)

The course of an HIV infection varies greatly. Some individuals progress to full-blown AIDS and death within months of infection by HIV; others may have no symptoms for 10 years or more after the initial infection. During the symptomless period, the infected person is nevertheless contagious and can transmit HIV to others. The first signs of AIDS are usually mononucleosis-like symptoms (swollen lymph glands, fever, night sweats) and possibly headaches and impaired mental functioning. As the disease progresses, individuals often suffer weight loss, infections on the skin (*shingles*) or throat (*thrush*), lung infections, and certain kinds of cancer.

Among adults, HIV is transmitted mainly by blood, semen, or vaginal fluids of infected people (Table 6.4). HIV can also be transmitted from mother to child during pregnancy and childbirth, and via breast milk. About 35 million people in the world are currently infected with HIV. About 25 million people have died of AIDS complications since the global AIDS epidemic began around 1980. In the United

**Table 6.4** The Risk of HIV Infection from One Episode of Contact with an HIV-Positive Person

| Type of Contact | Risk (%) |
|---|---|
| Needle Sharing | 0.67 |
| Occupational Needlestick | 0.30 |
| Receptive Anal Intercourse | 0.1–5.0 |
| Receptive Vaginal Intercourse | 0.1–0.2 |
| Insertive Vaginal Intercourse | 0.03–0.14 |
| Insertive Anal Intercourse | 0.06 or less |
| Receptive Oral Male Intercourse | 0.06 or less |
| Insertive Oral Male Intercourse | Rare case reports |
| Female–Female Oral-Genital Contact | Rare case reports |

Adapted from Harvey, A., & Goldschmidt, R. H. (2005). HIV testing on demand. *American Family Physician, 71*, 1823–1825.

States, about 1 million persons are currently infected with HIV, and over 500,000 Americans to date have died of AIDS. In the United States, HIV infections occur most commonly in men and women between the ages of 20 and 60. The most common routes of HIV transmission are men having sex with men, injection drug use, and men and women having sex with infected other-sexed individuals. HIV/AIDS is not acquired from getting a blood test or donating blood. Due to careful donor screening and testing, acquiring HIV/AIDS from a blood transfusion in a hospital is highly unlikely.

There is no cure for HIV/AIDS. Treatment of the disease relies on (1) medically managing the opportunistic infections that result from immune suppression and (2) attempting to keep the HIV infection in check with anti-HIV drugs. Whereas anti-HIV drugs can be successful in reducing the levels of HIV in the body, they do not eliminate the virus completely. Without continued use of the drugs, viral levels quickly rise again. Another drawback to anti-HIV drugs is that HIV can develop resistance to them, thus reducing their effectiveness. Finally, anti-HIV drug treatment can cost $10,000 a year or more per patient, which is too expensive for 90% of the HIV-infected people in the world. Ultimate prevention of AIDS depends on development of a vaccine that would prevent HIV infection—a medical advance that has eluded HIV/AIDS researchers thus far.

## HIV Testing

When individuals first become infected with HIV, their immune systems are still intact and they produce copious infection-fighting proteins called *antibodies* that destroy HIV. Detecting anti-HIV antibodies is the basis of nearly all HIV/AIDS tests. Other HIV tests detect the genetic material in HIV particles, which is a more accurate measure of the level of infection (called the *viral load*).

Health officials do not advocate that everyone be tested for HIV. They do recommend, however, that individuals be tested routinely when they seek medical services or when they may have been exposed to HIV infection in any of the following ways:

- Injecting drugs or steroids using equipment (e.g., needles and syringes) shared with others
- Having unprotected vaginal, anal, or oral sex with men who have sex with men, multiple partners, or anonymous partners
- Exchanging sex for drugs or money
- Having been diagnosed with or treated for hepatitis, tuberculosis (TB), or a sexually transmitted disease
- Having had sex with someone whose history of sex partners and/or drug use is unknown to you
- Having sex with several partners
- Having sex with someone while drunk

HIV tests can detect antibodies to HIV within two to eight weeks (the average is 25 days) after exposure to the virus. In some individuals a test may not detect antibodies for six months or longer after exposure to HIV. If an initial HIV test was negative within the first three months after possible exposure, repeat testing should be considered to establish the negative status with certainty.

Most commonly, a blood sample is used to detect HIV infection. Tests using saliva or urine are also available. Some tests require a few days for the results; other rapid HIV tests can give results in about 20 minutes. All positive HIV tests must be confirmed by another, more definitive test (called the *Western Blot*). Results of this confirmatory test can take a few days to a few weeks.

HIV/AIDS testing requires pre- and post-test counseling by a health professional or trained HIV counselor. Pre-test counseling involves explaining the testing procedure, confidentiality issues, HIV/AIDS prevention, and the significance and choices if the result is positive. Post-test counseling involves discussing what negative or positive results mean, possible need for retesting, treatment options if the test is positive, and additional HIV/AIDS education.

HIV tests can be obtained from physicians and from a variety of health agencies. Tests can be anonymous or confidential. In anonymous tests, individuals are identified only by a self-selected number or alias, so a person's true identity is never recorded. In confidential tests, one's name is part of the medical record, which is supposed to be confidential.

An at-home HIV test kit has been approved by the U.S. Food and Drug Administration. The test procedure involves pricking a finger with a special device, placing drops of blood on a specially treated card, and then mailing the card to a licensed laboratory. Customers are given an identification number to use when phoning in for the results. Callers may speak to a counselor before taking the test, while waiting for the test result, and after the results are given. All individuals receiving a positive test result are provided referrals for a follow-up confirmatory test, as well as information about treatment and support services. Most HIV test kits sold over the Internet are unreliable. The U.S. Food and Drug Administration Web site offers updates on approved at-home HIV test kits, available at http://www.fda.gov/ForConsumers/ConsumerUpdates/ucm048553.htm.

## SEXUALITY IN REVIEW

- Approximately 19 million adults in North America are infected by 11 different sexually transmitted diseases (STDs).
- STD risk factors include not practicing safer sex, having multiple sex partners, having a false sense of security, and denying that one could be at risk.
- Some STDs produce mild or no symptoms, which means an infected person can unknowingly transmit an STD to others.
- STDs caused by bacteria include chlamydia, gonorrhea, and syphilis.
- Viruses that cause STDs include human papillomavirus, herpes viruses, hepatitis B virus, and human immunodeficiency virus (HIV), the cause of acquired immune deficiency syndrome (AIDS).
- Tests are available for detection of HIV infection. Anti-HIV drugs are also available, but there is no cure for AIDS.
- Pubic lice and scabies are sexually transmitted insect infections.

## CRITICAL THINKING ABOUT SEXUALITY

1. Research has consistently shown that a vast majority of college students know a lot about STDs and HIV/AIDS, and yet only 50% of students whose behaviors put them at risk for acquiring an STD or HIV/AIDS practice safer sex. To many observers, such risk taking is illogical, not to mention dangerous. One could postulate, however, that college students are behaving rationally (from their point of view) when they do not practice safer sex. Looking at your behavior and the attitudes of people in your peer group,

what are possible explanations for why college students do not practice safer sex? Based on your explanations, how would you advise your college to lessen the risk of STDs and HIV/AIDS among students?

2. Jason and Ilana were going to make a great couple. All of their friends thought so. But Jason was troubled. Although they agreed not to have sexual intercourse before marriage, as their intimacy deepened Ilana felt obliged to tell Jason of the genital herpes infection she acquired when she was a wild 15-year-old. "I'm not that person anymore," she said, "and it's under control. Still, you never get rid of it." Should Jason continue with this relationship? What factors should he consider in making his decision?
3. The monthly meeting of the Washington County School Board had never had so many attendees as the night of the vote on the new health curriculum for the county's middle schools. At issue was revising the module on sexual infections to include *how* such infections were actually transmitted. Some parents objected to including a discussion of STDs and HIV/AIDS, arguing that doing so only makes the students curious about sex and drugs and encourages experimentation. A second group of parents, while supporting a discussion of the causes and symptoms of the diseases, nevertheless objected to any discussion of behaviors involved in their transmission. They believed that the children ought to know about the biological aspects of the issue as a foundation for their own efforts at dissuading their children from any experimentation with unsafe sexual practices and drugs. A third group of parents argued that the only way to ensure prevention was to discuss the behaviors involved. They claimed that the children would not take the discussion seriously unless all aspects of the issue were covered, and hence would be tempted either to disregard the information or to become curious about what was not covered and put themselves at risk. If you were one of the school board members, how would you vote, and how would you justify your vote to parents?
4. Because she had consistently voted to support research on HIV/AIDS, it shocked many people when Congressmember Harmas refused to vote for a $7.8 billion appropriation to pay for protease inhibitor medicine for the medically indigent with AIDS both in the United States and around the world. "I have total compassion for these people," said Harmas, "but we cannot afford to take care of everyone who is sick. Furthermore, in our country, most of the money will go to treating injection drug users, who ought to know better than to get the disease in the first place. And for all of the poverty-stricken sick people in Africa and Asia, all I can say is 'I'm sorry, complain to your own government. We're broke.' " Do you agree or disagree with the congressperson's position?

## REFERENCES AND RECOMMENDED RESOURCES

### References

American College Health Association. (2008). National College Health Assessment. Available at: http://www.acha-ncha.org. Accessed September 26, 2008.

Dunne, E. F., et al. (2007). Prevalence of HPV infection among females in the United States. *Journal of the American Medical Association, 297,* 813–819.

Holmes, K. K., et al. (2007). *Sexually transmitted diseases, 4th ed.* New York: McGraw-Hill.

## Recommended Resources

Marr, L. (2007). *Sexually transmitted diseases: A physician tells you what you need to know.* Baltimore: Johns Hopkins University Press. Detailed information on all STDs.

United Nations. (2010). UNAIDS today. Available at: http://www.unaids.org. Basic information on the worldwide HIV/AIDS epidemic.

U.S. Centers for Disease Control and Prevention. (2010). Sexually transmitted diseases. Available at: http://www.cdc.gov/std. The most up-to-date information on sexually transmitted diseases.

World Health Organization. (2010). Sexually transmitted infections. Available at: http://www.who.int/topics/sexually_transmitted_infections/en. STDs from a global perspective.

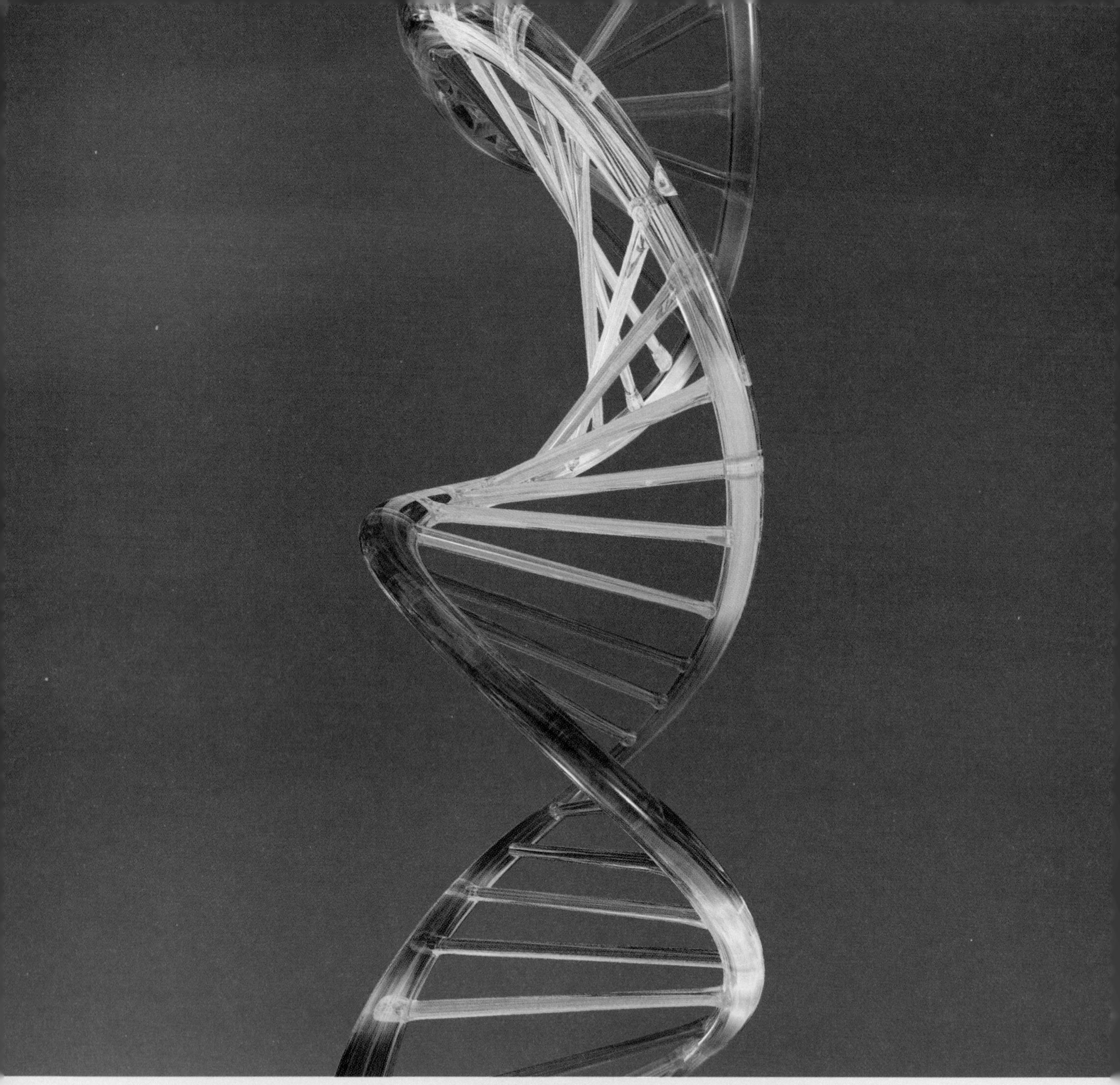

*"The finest inheritance you can give to a child is to allow it to make its own way, completely on its own feet."*

— Isadora Duncan

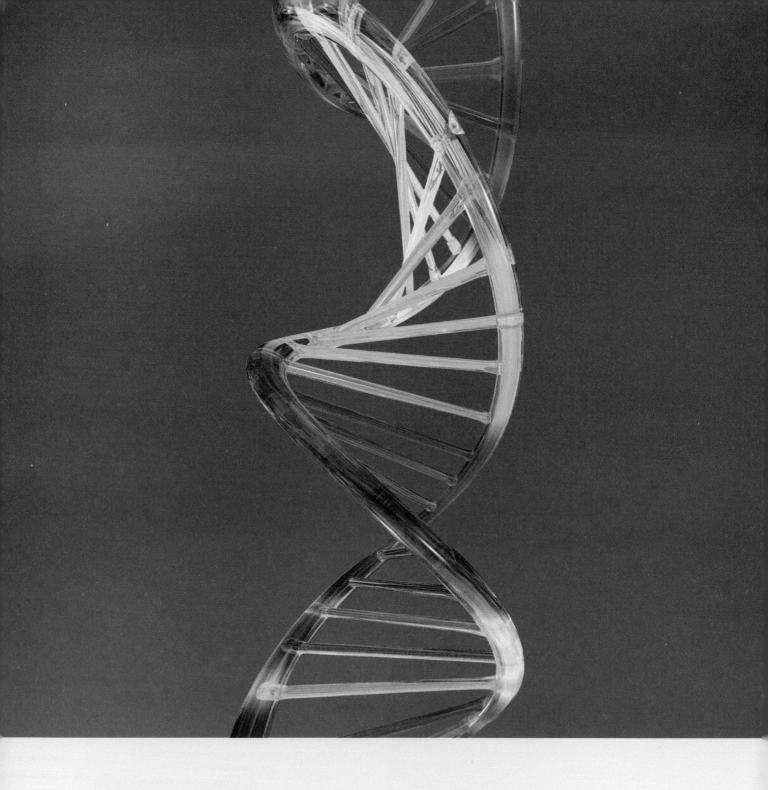

CHAPTER 7

# Genetics and Inheritance

## Student Learning Objectives

1. Know that almost every human cell contains about 20,000 genes carried in 23 pairs of chromosomes; one pair are sex chromosomes
2. Describe how genes affect development of the sex organs in the fetus
3. Give at least one example of abnormal fetal sex development caused by an abnormal chromosome and gene
4. Describe how genetic testing of a fetus is performed
5. Explain how genetic testing can be used to prevent genetic diseases and disorders
6. Explain why some forms of genetic testing of adults may be detrimental to health

genes chemical sequences in DNA that direct the synthesis of proteins in cells or which control other functions

deoxyribonucleic acid (DNA) large molecule in chromosomes that carries all the genetic information of an organism

chromosomes structures in the nuclei of cells that contain DNA and genes

Biological reproduction is the creation of new individuals that are unmistakably similar to the parent organisms from which they arise. Puppies always resemble adult dogs, and kittens always look like cats; puppies are never born to mother cats. This conservation of organic form occurs because offspring inherit genetic information from each parent that determines their biochemical, anatomical, physiological, and many behavioral characteristics. The inherited biological information consists of thousands of chemical factors called genes. The genes a child inherits determine the structure and function of the body, physical and mental abilities, susceptibility to illness and disease, and even how long he or she might live. The development and functioning of the human body is controlled by approximately 20,000 genes.

Each person's genes are derived from the parents. They are passed on when a male's sperm fertilizes a female's ovum. Genes are composed of a chemical called deoxyribonucleic acid (DNA). Every gene is a particular piece of DNA with a precise chemical structure. Each gene directs the manufacture of a specific biological substance, usually a protein, that plays a particular role in the development and maintenance of the body's cells. Genes are joined to one another in structures in the nuclei of cells called chromosomes.

At the moment of conception, an individual's genes begin to control her or his biological development, including the formation in the fetus of cells and organs, and in childhood and adulthood, their further growth and maintenance. A particular gene may act by itself to produce a specific trait, or more commonly, it may act as part of a team of many genes in controlling traits such as skin color, shape of the nose, height, and mental abilities. In this chapter we discuss human genes and chromosomes, genetic control of the development of the sex and reproductive organs, hereditary diseases and birth defects, and genetic tests that can help predict or prevent genetic diseases and disorders.

## Genes and Chromosomes

Nearly all of the genes a person inherits are contained in 23 pairs of chromosomes. One member of each pair of chromosomes is inherited from the mother, and the other is inherited from the father. Chromosomes extracted from cells can be

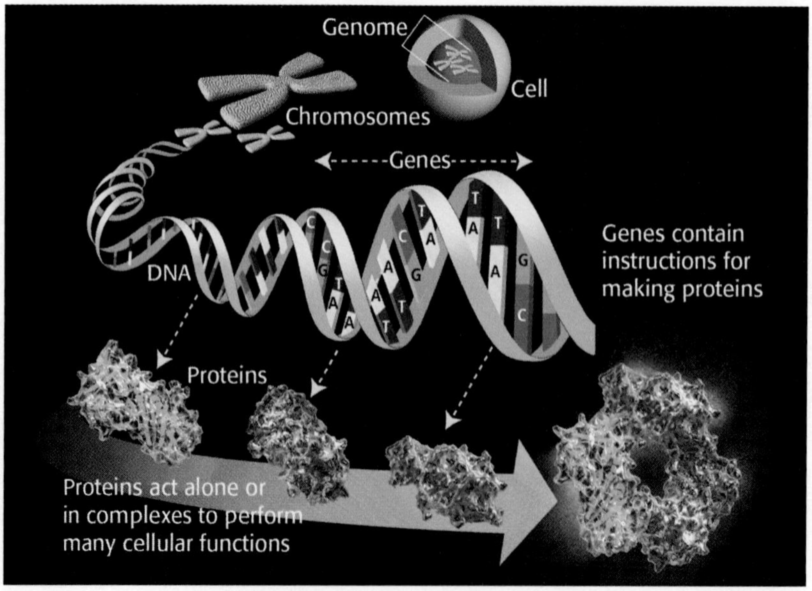

visualized under a microscope. Twenty-two of the chromosome pairs are classified according to size and shape and designated by numbers 1 to 22 (FIGURE 7.1). These 22 matched pairs of chromosomes are called autosomes. Both members of an autosomal pair appear identical when chromosomes are examined under a microscope. Although the chromosomes in each pair look alike, the actual genetic information they carry differs somewhat because they come from different parents who carry different genetic information in some of their genes. Many genes that govern the structure of substances in cells are identical in all people. For example, the gene for hemoglobin (the protein in red blood cells that transports oxygen throughout the body) is identical in everyone except for rare exceptions. These individuals carry mutations in the hemoglobin gene that produce inherited diseases such as *sickle cell anemia*.

**autosomes** the 22 pairs of human chromosomes except for the sex chromosomes

**sex chromosomes** the X and Y chromosomes in human cells; an XX constitution directs female development, and XY constitution directs male development

The 22 pairs of autosomes appear similar in size and shape. However, the twenty-third pair of chromosomes differs in appearance depending on the biological sex of the individual; hence, these chromosomes are called sex chromosomes. In females, the size and shape of the two sex chromosomes are identical; they are designated by the letter "X." (They are called X chromosomes because when they were first observed their functions were unknown.) In men, the two sex chromosomes are visibly dissimilar. One is an X chromosome identical in appearance to X chromosomes in females, and the other is much smaller in size; it is designated by the letter "Y." Thus, the complete chromosome set in females consists of 22 pairs of autosomes and one XX pair of sex chromosomes. The complete chromosome set in males consists of 22 pairs of autosomes, one X chromosome, and one Y chromosome.

A sperm and ovum originally contain 46 chromosomes, but they undergo a maturation process in which the number of chromosomes is reduced to 23, retaining one member of each pair. Then, when a sperm and ovum unite at fertilization, the normal number of 46 chromosomes (23 pairs) is restored. A human adult is composed of about 100 trillion cells of about 200 different types (e.g., lung cells, skin cells, brain cells), all of which are derived from the fertilized ovum. Thus, every one of an individual's cells contains exact copies of all the genes present in the original 46 chromosomes in the fertilized ovum. The different cell types that make up the body arise from activating and deactivating particular genes within them at specific times in development.

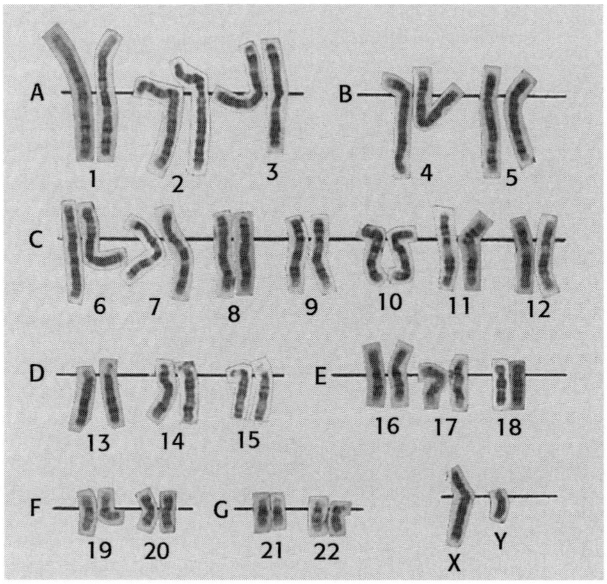


FIGURE 7.1 **Display of Human Chromosomes.** The chromosomes from a man's blood cell are dyed and photographed. The chromosomes are cut from the photograph, paired, and arranged by number. Note the large X and small Y chromosomes characteristic of a male.

## Inheritance of an Abnormal Number of Chromosomes

Errors in chromosome number occasionally occur during formation of sperm or ova, resulting in the birth of a child with an abnormal number of chromosomes. *Down syndrome*, for example, is characterized by anatomical abnormalities and mental retardation, is caused by inheritance of an extra chromosome 21; this results in every cell of the body having three copies of chromosome 21 instead of two (a condition called *trisomy 21*). Women over 35 years of age are at greater risk compared with younger women of conceiving a child with Down syndrome (FIGURE 7.2). For this reason, all pregnant women over age 35 are advised to undergo genetic testing of fetal cells (described later in the chapter) to determine if Down syndrome is present.

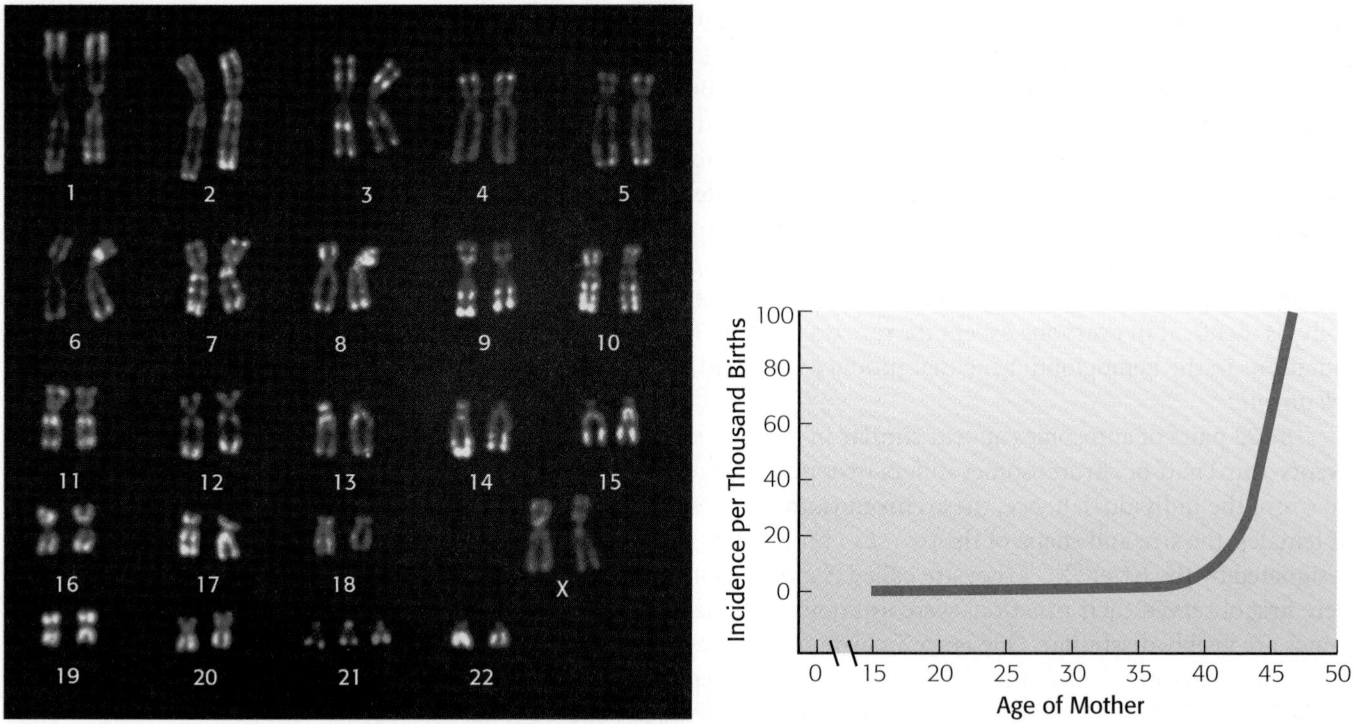


(a) (b)

FIGURE 7.2 **Chromosome Abnormality in Down Syndrome.** (a) Three copies of chromosome 21 characterize an individual with Down syndrome. (b) The frequency of children born with Down syndrome as a function of the age of the mother. Beyond age 35, the risk of a woman having a child with Down syndrome rises dramatically. All pregnant women in the United States over age 35 are advised to undergo amniocentesis in order to examine the chromosomes in fetal cells.

Individuals can also be born with an abnormal number of sex chromosomes. *Klinefelter syndrome*, for example, is associated with an XXY set of sex chromosomes, which can be produced either by the fusion of a normal Y-bearing sperm with an abnormal XX-bearing ovum, or by the fusion of an abnormal XY-bearing sperm and a normal X-bearing ovum. The presence of the Y chromosome gives a person with Kleinfelter syndrome many male characteristics, but because of the additional X chromosome, sexual development is abnormal. The testes are small and the seminiferous tubules are underdeveloped, and thus the individual is sterile. *Turner syndrome* is caused by the presence of only one X chromosome (designated XO). This condition is characterized by the absence of ovaries, sterility, underdeveloped breasts, and certain skeletal deformities.

About 20% of all conceptions have a chromosomal abnormality of some kind. Most fetuses with chromosomal abnormalities are lost spontaneously in the first weeks of a pregnancy (a condition called *spontaneous abortion* or *miscarriage*). Those that survive to term generally have severe developmental problems, as in Down syndrome. In contrast to a fetus with an abnormal number of autosomes, a fetus with an abnormal number of sex chromosomes has a good chance of surviving and will have less severe developmental problems.

## How Genes Work

Genes work by directing the manufacture of specific biological molecules that serve as one of the following:

1. *Building blocks of anatomical structures.* For example, *tubulin*, a protein that makes up the tailpiece of sperm, and *myelin*, a protein that makes up the sheath covering nerve fibers.
2. *Regulators of gene function.* For example, a gene in cells of the gastrointestinal tract controls the activity of the enzyme that digests the sugar lactose and allows all babies to thrive on breast milk (or milk obtained from animals such as cows). In almost all babies in the world, there is a control gene that switches on the production of the milk-digesting enzyme in infancy. At about age 2, however, when children usually stop breastfeeding, the control gene switches off the gene producing the lactose-digesting enzyme. But it turns out that it is not switched off in all populations. In Asians, most Africans, and many southern Europeans, the control gene *is* switched off. Generally, this is not a problem because at this age most babies are weaned and begin to eat semisolid or solid food. From this time on, however, if they ingest milk or lactose-containing milk products (cheese and yogurt are lactose free), they experience gastrointestinal distress or diarrhea and can even become sick. People who experience these symptoms after ingesting milk products are classified medically as *lactose intolerant*, a condition that can be tested for.

   Most people of northern European ancestry, however, are *lactose tolerant* and can drink milk throughout their lives. We now know that, about 10,000 years ago when Europeans began to domesticate cows, a change (*mutation*) occurred in a few individuals that weakened the lactose "control gene" and allowed people to continue to consume milk after infancy. Over time, this beneficial mutation allowing people to continue drinking milk spread throughout Europe and eventually overseas as people migrated.

## Genetic Control of Sexual Development

The pair of sex chromosomes inherited from parents at fertilization sets the stage for the development of an individual's sexual and reproductive organs during fetal development (FIGURE 7.3). By the fourth or fifth week after fertilization, even though many structures of the fetal body have developed, the sex organs have not. This is called the *indifferent stage* of sexual development. About the fifth week of development, under the direction of genes (many on the X or Y chromosomes), the fetal sex organs begin to develop in the following stages:

### Stage One: Gonadal (Testes/Ovary) Development

Very early in fetal development, specific genes on the pair of sex chromosomes (XX or XY) direct the formation of immature or *primordial* sperm or ova (that is, cells not yet capable of taking part in fertilization). During the fifth week of development, the primordial sperm or ova migrate to a pair of bulges in the fetal abdominal region, called the *gonadal ridges*, which are similar in every fetus regardless of genetic sex. If the cells are primordial ova, genes within them cause the gonadal ridges to develop into ovaries. In contrast, if the cells are primordial sperm, at about the seventh week of development, a gene on the Y chromosome, called the sex-determining region Y (SRY) gene, directs the production of a specific chemical called the *testis-determining factor*, or *TDF*, which directs the formation of testes. Embryonic testicular tissue quickly becomes capable of producing testosterone, which sets the stage for further male sexual development.

**sex-determining region Y (SRY) gene** a gene on the Y chromosome that controls development of a fetus as a male; in the absence of this gene, development proceeds as female

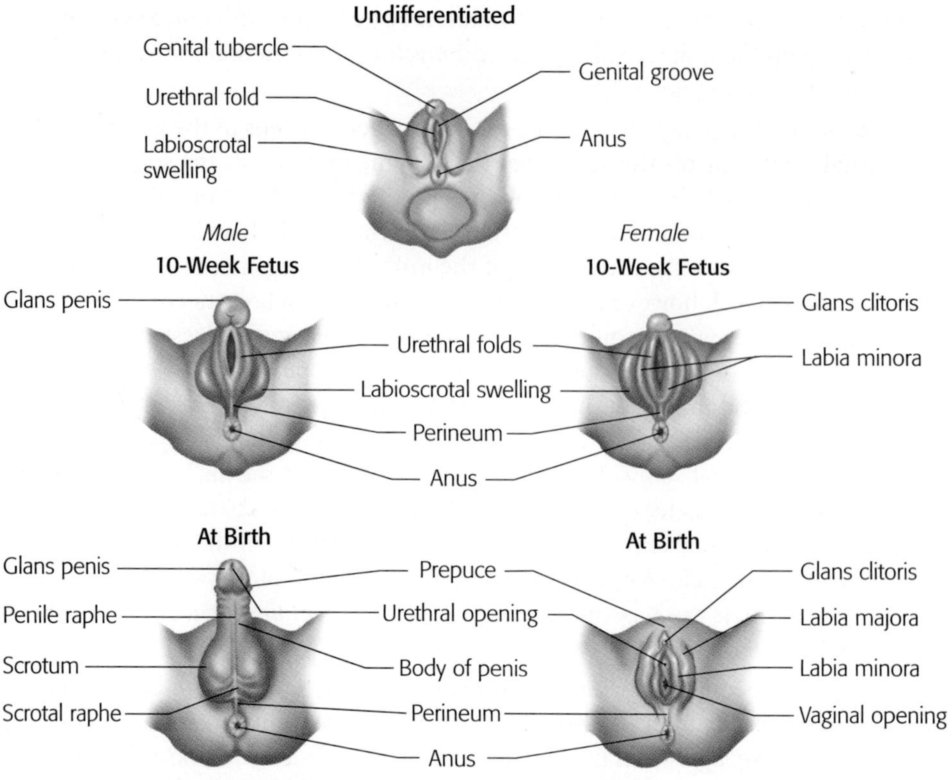


FIGURE 7.3 **Development of Male and Female Sex Organs.** The sex organs begin to develop about the fifth week of fetal life from tissue destined to become testes or ovaries and two sets of ducts (tubes) destined to become the internal and external sex organs. If the fetus is XY (male), testes develop and produce the hormone testosterone, which activates certain genes and deactivates others such that male sex organs develop and female organs do not. Without testosterone, the female pattern of development occurs.

Very rarely, a person is born with both testicular and ovarian tissue (*true hermaphroditism*) because an ovum was fertilized by a single sperm carrying both X and Y chromosomes. These rare sperm arise if sex chromosomes fail to separate properly when sperm are formed. (Ova also can carry abnormal numbers of chromosomes.) If a single X- and Y-bearing sperm fertilize an X-bearing ovum, one-half of that person's cells can have XY sex chromosomes and the other half will have XX sex chromosomes. In some instances, gonadal tissue is a combination of ovary and testis. In other instances, a testis develops on one side of the abdomen and an ovary on the other.

## Stage Two: Sex Duct and Gland Development

By about the seventh week of fetal life, fetuses of each sex possess two pairs of tubes (the *wolffian ducts* and the *mullerian ducts*) that lie next to each other in the abdominal region near the fetal kidneys. In genetic males, testosterone that is manufactured in each testis migrates to a nearby wolffian duct; the hormone activates genes that direct the development of the epididymis, vas deferens, seminal vesicle, and ejaculatory duct. The testes also manufacture a chemical substance called *mullerian inhibiting substance (MIS)*, which causes degradation of the mullerian ducts.

In genetic females, ovaries develop, and so testosterone is not produced to trigger the development of the male sex structures and no MIS is produced to trigger the degradation of the mullerian ducts. Instead, genes in cells of the mullerian ducts are activated, which directs mullerian duct cells to develop into fallopian tubes, uterus, and the upper one-third of the vagina. (The lower two-thirds of the vagina develop from tissue that also gives rise to the urinary bladder and the urethra.) Without testosterone, the wolffian ducts degenerate.

## Stage Three: External Genital Development

Before the seventh week of fetal development, all fetuses regardless of genetic sex possess three identical structures with the potential to become the external genitalia. These structures are called the *genital tubercle*, *urogenital folds*, and the *labioscrotal swelling*. The transformation of these structures into male or female reproductive organs is directed by many different genes. In male fetuses, at about the eighth week of development, a specific gene in certain cells in the testes directs the manufacture of an enzyme called *5-alpha reductase*, which converts testicular testosterone into a related hormone called *dihydrotestosterone (DHT)*. DHT switches on genes in the fetal genital tissues to direct the formation of the penis and scrotum. In female fetuses, genes that manufacture testosterone and DHT are not active, so these hormones are not available. This allows other activated genes to direct the transformation of the primordial genitalia into clitoris, labia minora, labia majora, and mons pubis.

The sex organs can develop abnormally if a fetus is exposed to large amounts of sex hormones or related substances. These can be produced by either the mother's body or drugs the mother ingests during pregnancy. Also, pollutants and chemicals in the environment that are ingested by a pregnant woman can affect the activities of genes responsible for fetal sexual development. These environmental chemicals mimic the actions of human sex hormones and are called **xenoestrogens**. They include many kinds of pesticides, polychlorinated biphenyls (substances formerly used in electrical transformers), and bisphenol-A, a chemical used in the manufacture of many kinds of plastics that are subsequently used to package and store food and beverages. Pregnant women are urged to avoid exposure to xenoestrogens in their food and environment if at all possible. Since development of the sex organs occurs during the first few months of pregnancy, women who are planning to become pregnant should live particularly healthfully prior to pregnancy.

**xenoestrogens** chemicals in the environment that mimic the actions of human hormones

## Sex Selection

Since biological sex is determined by sex chromosomes, it is possible for prospective parents to use reproductive technologies to select the sex of their child (*sex selection*). Using *preimplantation genetic diagnosis* (see a later section), the sex chromosomes of embryos developed in a laboratory dish can be analyzed. One or two embryos of the desired sex are then transferred into the prospective mother's uterus.

In an alternative method called *sperm sorting*, semen is collected from the prospective father, and X-bearing sperm are separated from Y-bearing sperm. After sorting, the prospective mother is artificially inseminated with only the sperm that will produce a child of the desired sex. Some parents use these procedures to balance their families with both boys and girls.

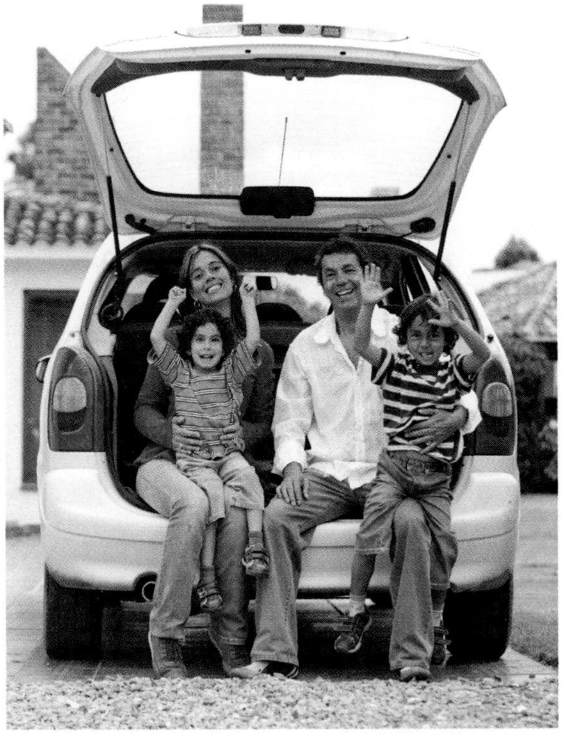

Reproductive technologies allow parents to choose the sex of their children.

Some people oppose sex selection because they fear that it will lead to selection of traits other than biological sex, so-called "designer babies." For example, a couple might select an embryo with genes that would help their child develop a particular body type or skill, such as being tall, athletic, musical, or exceptionally intelligent. The possibility of trait selection conjures up the specter of *eugenics* (selective breeding of people for particular traits), which was practiced by the Nazis in mid-twentieth-century Europe.

## Hereditary (Genetic) Disorders and Diseases

**hereditary (genetic) disorders and diseases** disorders or diseases that result from inheriting an abnormal chromosome or gene from one or both parents

**Hereditary (genetic) disorders and diseases** result from (1) a chromosome in a sperm or ovum that is abnormal in shape or number or (2) an abnormal gene passed from one or both parents in the chromosomes that are packaged into sperm or ova. Several thousand hereditary disorders and diseases caused by abnormalities in single genes have been identified (Table 7.1). Not all genetic abnormalities cause

**Table 7.1** Inherited Disorders and Diseases Caused By Single Gene Defects

The diseases and disorders listed here are all due to *mutations* (chemical changes in genes) that disrupt the activity of a single gene in human cells. Inherited diseases are described as *dominant*, *recessive*, or *X (sex)-linked*.

In cases of an inherited disease caused by a dominant defective gene, one parent will have a copy of the defective gene and will also have the disease or disorder; children have a 50% chance of inheriting the defective gene. Defective dominant genes cause serious diseases, but symptoms usually do not appear until adulthood.

In cases of an inherited disease caused by a defective recessive gene, each parent carries one copy of the defective gene. Parents are unaffected because the other copy of the gene that they carry functions normally. Children have a 50% chance of inheriting the defective gene from each parent and a 25% chance of being affected.

X (sex)-linked diseases are always passed on from the mother and only to male children. The defective gene is on one X chromosome; however, since the mother has two X chromosomes, she carries a functional gene on the other X chromosome. Male children have a 50% chance of inheriting the mother's X chromosome with the defective gene.

| Dominant Disease/Disorder | Symptoms |
|---|---|
| Achondroplasia (Dwarfism) | Short stature |
| Retinoblastoma | Blindness |
| Huntington Disease | Nervous system degeneration |
| Polydactyly | Extra fingers or toes |
| **Recessive Disease/Disorder** | **Symptoms** |
| Cystic Fibrosis | Respiratory disease |
| Albinism | Lack of pigment in skin and eyes |
| Phenylketonuria | Inability to digest the amino acid phenylalanine; mental retardation |
| Tay-Sachs Disease | Neurological deterioration |
| Sickle-Cell Disease | Anemia |
| **X (Sex)-Linked Disease/Disorder** | **Symptoms** |
| Hemophilia | Bleeding; failure of blood to clot after injury |
| Duchenne Muscular Dystrophy | Progressive muscular weakness |
| Lesch–Nyhan Disease | Mental retardation, self-mutilation |
| Agammaglobulinemia | Defective immune system; infections |

a disease; short stature ("dwarfism"), for example, is not a disease. Nor is *male-pattern baldness*, which is caused by a gene on the X chromosome. Sometimes, an inherited disorder or disease produces only minor symptoms; often, however, such disorders cause serious illness and premature death. In some cases, the symptoms occur before or just after birth; in other cases, disease symptoms do not appear until adulthood.

## Sexuality-Related Genetic Disorders

In 355 BC, Aristotle suggested that the difference between men and women was determined at the time of copulation. He thought that men produced hot or cold semen. Hot semen produced males; cold semen produced females. We now know that the sequence of events that determines male sexual development is due to presence of the SRY gene located on the Y chromosome—not to heat.

Occasionally, during sperm formation, the SRY gene moves from the Y chromosome to the X chromosome. If a child receives this X chromosome from its father, it will be genetically XX. But, since one of the X chromosomes has the SRY gene, the individual will develop male sex organs and be characterized as male at birth. However, because other genes on the Y chromosome are missing, the individual usually does not develop secondary male sex characteristics at puberty.

In a similar fashion, if a sperm carrying a Y chromosome that is lacking the SRY gene fertilizes an ovum, the resulting individual is genetically XY but, because the SRY gene is lacking, will develop female sex organs and be characterized as female at birth. Such a woman is sterile, however, and may not discover the male genetic legacy until she explores the reasons for her infertility.

Other genes also are essential for the normal development of male sex organs. For example, the development of male genital ducts, scrotum, penis, and secondary sex characteristics depends on the actions of the hormones *testosterone* or *dihydrotestosterone (DHT)* on hormone-sensitive cells in the fetus and also during puberty. For these hormones to work, they must attach to specific parts on the surface or inside a cell called *androgen receptors*. Occasionally, the gene that produces the androgen receptors (called the *AR* gene) is defective. A genetic male with a completely defective *AR* gene (located on the X chromosome inherited from his mother) will have an inherited disorder called **androgen insensitivity syndrome (AIS)** or **testicular feminization**. Persons with this disorder are genetically XY, but their physical anatomy varies from partly male to completely female, depending on the degree of androgen insensitivity.

**androgen insensitivity syndrome (AIS)** also called testicular feminization; an inherited disorder in which individuals are genetically XY males but, because their cells are insensitive to male hormones, develop female sexual anatomy

**Testicular feminization** also called androgen insensitivity syndrome; individuals with this inherited disorder are genetically XY but, because their cells do not respond to androgenic hormones, they often develop female-appearing anatomical structures

In AIS, the wolffian ducts cannot respond to testosterone and the genital tubercle cannot respond to DHT, resulting in the development of female external sex organs (clitoris, vaginal labia, and short vagina) rather than male organs. However, since affected individuals possess a Y chromosome with an active SRY gene, they will develop testes. Because of the presence of testes, the mullerian ducts disintegrate, and the fallopian tubes, uterus, and upper third of the vagina do not form. Because these individuals possess male and female sexual organs, they are referred to as *intersexed* or *pseudohermaphrodites*.

The lives of individuals with ambiguous sexual organs and altered sexual development can be difficult. Consider the case of Caster Semenya, a female track athlete from South Africa. In 2009 she won the 800-meter race for women at the world championship games in Berlin. She ran the race in a blistering time of 1:55:45, faster than most male athletes. After the race, her gender was questioned because of her muscular build and exceptionally fast time. The gold medal she won was taken away by the International Association of Athletics Federations. After almost a year of investigation, during which her career was in limbo, her female status was restored by the international organization. No details of her genetic sex or her physical sexual anatomy were officially revealed, but it was rumored in sports media that she lacks ovaries and a uterus. After a year of emotional turmoil, however, Caster Semenya was allowed to compete in women's events once again.

**congenital adrenal hyperplasia (CAH)** also called adrenogenital syndrome; an inherited disorder of sexual development in which an individual is born with ambiguous genitalia and cannot be classified as either male or female at birth

Another hereditary disorder of sexual development is congenital adrenal hyperplasia (CAH), also known as adrenogenital syndrome. This disorder is usually apparent at birth because the baby's genitalia do not appear distinctly male or female (a condition referred to as "ambiguous genitalia"). These infants are genetically female (XX), but because of a malfunction of the gene that manufactures an enzyme called *21-alpha-hydroxylase*, their adrenal glands overproduce testosterone-like hormones (androgens). This causes masculinization of the female external genitalia. The clitoris is greatly enlarged, and the labia fuse to give the appearance of a scrotum. Thus, at birth the female infant appears to have a penis. The developing brain of such infants also has been exposed to higher than normal amounts of androgens, which may have consequences for their sexual psychology (see Chapter 2).

## Congenital (Birth) Defects

**congenital (birth) defect** any abnormality in a newborn observable at birth

**teratogen** any environmental agent that causes abnormal fetal development and birth defects

Each newborn is examined immediately after birth for the presence of any physical abnormality; if one is found, it is called a congenital (birth) defect. A congenital defect can be caused by an abnormal gene, exposure to a harmful environmental agent during pregnancy, or a combination of both. Environmental agents that adversely affect normal fetal development and cause a birth defect are called teratogens (from the Greek meaning "to produce a monster"). Teratogens include

### Dear Penelope . . .

***A few weeks ago, my lover and I had a terrible fight, and we didn't see each other for a few days afterwards. That's all patched up now, and things are going all right again, except I feel terribly guilty. When things were so bad between us, I went to friend's party by myself and ended up getting drunk and "cheating" on my partner. It was just a one-time thing with someone from another college, but I still feel terribly ashamed and sorry. How do I tell my partner about this without dropping a bomb in the middle of my relationship?***

***—Case of the Guilts***

*Dear Guilts,*

Confession may be good for the soul, but it isn't always good for a relationship. If you have a specific contract with your partner to disclose situations like these, then you should make good on your promise. But if no such contract exists, then you have to weight the possible costs and benefits of revealing this incident. Unless you make it so, there is no rule that says that partners must tell each other everything. Very often the source of guilt is within our own minds, and it is we who have to forgive and accept ourselves for what we do. That's sometimes a lot harder than asking someone else for forgiveness, so we often turn outside of ourselves in such situations. Your guilt tells you that getting drunk and having sex with a stranger wasn't the best way to cope with your hurt feelings. That is a good thing to have learned. Now you know how your sexuality affects your well-being and self-esteem, and you can find better ways to cope with relationship stress.

Courtesy of the UC Davis *Aggie*

alcohol, chemicals in cigarette smoke, cocaine, certain industrial chemicals, several viruses, some prescription drugs, and heavy metals.

Most birth defects are caused by a complex interaction of genes and environmental factors. For example, some babies are born with *spina bifida*, in which a malformed spine exposes the spinal nerves to damage with resulting paralysis and increased risk for infection. The risk of spina bifida is related both to a fetus's genetic susceptibility and the mother's diet; the risk is reduced significantly if a woman consumes adequate amounts (about 400 micrograms per day) of the vitamin *folic acid* before and during the first weeks of pregnancy. For this reason, all grain products in the United States are fortified with folic acid.

Not all congenital defects are detected at birth. In some cases, a drug or toxic substance can alter fetal development and cause problems later in childhood. For example, children born to women whose food was contaminated with the heavy metal mercury (in the form of methylmercury) during pregnancy have a higher than average risk for mental retardation, speech and language delays, visual and hearing impairments, difficulties with balancing and walking, and emotional problems. Pregnant women are advised not to consume fish that are known to contain high levels of mercury and to limit overall fish consumption. A major source of mercury that contaminates the environment and food is coal-fired electricity-generating plants, which is a major reason for finding alternative ways to generate electricity.

## Testing Prospective Parents and Fetuses for Abnormal Genes

Most couples that want children understand that inherited disorders and diseases are a risk, especially if there is a family history of them. One of the major achievements of modern medicine is the ability to test prospective parents and a fetus for abnormal genes and chromosomes in order to prevent inherited disorders. This is called **genetic testing**. Based on the results of genetic tests, parents can decide if they want to risk conceiving a child or if they want to continue a pregnancy knowing that the child will be born with a genetic disease. Prospective parents who agree to genetic testing must also agree to *genetic counseling*, during which the risks and options are explained.

Genetic testing is recommended only for prospective parents who are at higher than average risk of having a child with an inherited disorder or disease (Table 7.2). If they decide to proceed with conceiving a child knowing that they carry abnormal genes, fetal cells can be tested to determine if the fetus has inherited any abnormal genes.

**genetic testing** testing for abnormal genes and chromosomes in cells taken from adults and fetuses

**amniocentesis** procedure for removing fetal cells from the uterus of a pregnant woman and examining the cells for inherited disorders or diseases

**chorionic villus sampling (CVS)** another procedure for testing fetal cells during pregnancy for inherited defects

**preimplantation genetic diagnosis (PGD)** used during in vitro fertilization to screen for the presence of genetic (inherited) diseases before an embryo is transferred into the uterus

### Testing a Fetus for Genetic Abnormalities

Genetic testing of a fetus requires analyzing fetal cells for the presence of abnormal genes and/or chromosomes. The commonly used medical procedures for genetic testing of fetal cells are **amniocentesis**, **chorionic villus sampling (CVS)**, and **preimplantation genetic diagnosis (PGD)**.

Amniocentesis involves analyzing fetal cells taken from the amnion, the fluid-filled sac in which the fetus develops inside the uterus (FIGURE 7.4). About the fifteenth week of pregnancy, a few fetal cells present in the amniotic fluid are extracted and grown in laboratory dishes to amplify their number. The cells are then tested for genetic, chromosomal, or biochemical abnormalities.

## Table 7.2 Risks for Having a Child with an Inherited Disorder

| |
|---|
| Prenatal testing and genetic counseling are advised if a person falls into any one of the following risk categories: |
| High or low levels of alphafetoprotein during pregnancy (risk of neural tube defect) |
| Woman had a previous child with a chromosomal abnormality or neural tube defect |
| Woman had a previous stillbirth or neonatal death |
| Woman or mate carries a previously diagnosed chromosomal or genetic abnormality |
| Woman carries a previously diagnosed defective gene |
| Woman and mate carry the same previously diagnosed defective gene |
| Close relatives have a child with an inherited disorder |
| Woman has been exposed to a teratogenic agent during pregnancy |
| Woman has recently been infected by rubella (measles) virus or cytomegalovirus |

**ultrasound scanning** use of sound energy to obtain an image of a fetus in the womb of a pregnant woman, as well as determine the presence of multiple fetuses, the orientation of the fetus, and the location of the placenta

When amniocentesis is performed, the fetus is also visualized by **ultrasound scanning** so that the fetus's position in the uterus is known and it is not harmed when amniotic fluid is removed. Ultrasound scans are also used to determine the presence of multiple fetuses, the orientation of the fetus, and the location of the placenta, and to measure the size of the fetal head, which helps estimate fetal age (FIGURE 7.5). An ultrasound image can also show the sex of the fetus.

Chorionic villus sampling, performed around the eighth week of pregnancy, involves retrieving tissue that is destined to become the placenta. These cells are fetal in origin, so analysis of their genes and chromosomes provides the same information that is obtained through amniocentesis. One advantage of CVS is that information regarding the genetic status of the fetus is obtained earlier than with amniocentesis; the procedure is also slightly less risky than amniocentesis, although both procedures are extremely safe.

Preimplantation genetic diagnosis (PGD) is used during in vitro fertilization (IVF) to screen for the presence of genetic (inherited) diseases before an embryo is transferred into the uterus. IVF involves creating embryos in a laboratory dish by fertilizing several ova with sperm. When embryos have developed to the eight-cell stage, one cell is removed. The genes and chromosomes taken from this cell

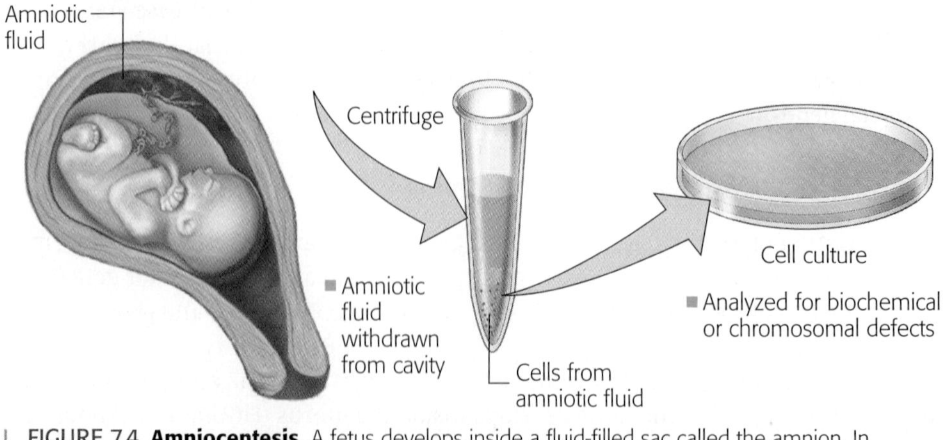


FIGURE 7.4 **Amniocentesis.** A fetus develops inside a fluid-filled sac called the amnion. In amniocentesis, a small amount of amniotic fluid is collected. This fluid contains some fetal cells that have sloughed off of the fetal body. After collection, the fluid and the fetal cells are analyzed for biochemical, genetic, or chromosome defects.

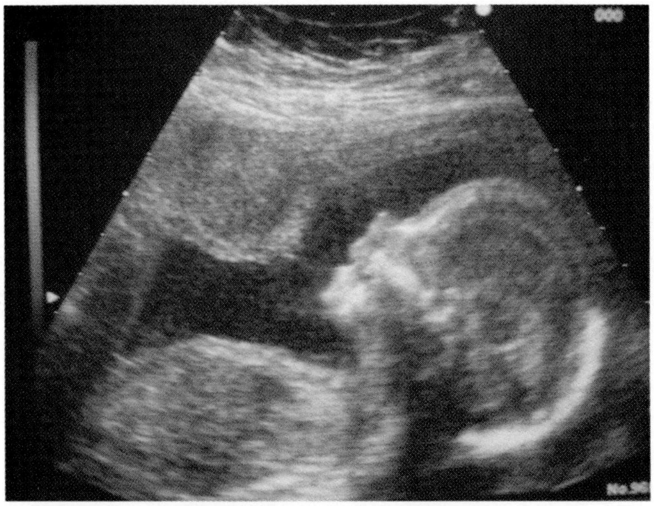

FIGURE 7.5 **Ultrasound Scans.** Ultrasound scans are used during pregnancy to reveal the position of the fetus in the uterus, the sex of the fetus, and certain physical abnormalities. Ultrasound scans are required only for those pregnancies in which a problem is suspected. Ultrasound scans are used during amniocentesis to locate the fetus and prevent injury during removal of amniotic fluid.

are examined for any genetic abnormalities. Embryos found to be free of genetic anomalies are selected for transfer to a woman's uterus. (The woman has been prepared for pregnancy by previous hormone treatment.) Remarkably, an eight-cell embryo can lose one of its cells for this test and still develop normally.

## Genetic Testing: Risks and Benefits

Genetic testing is an enormous help in having a healthy child. Genetic tests of fetuses and prospective parents are a great medical advance but a mixed blessing in situations that are not related to having a healthy baby. Genetic tests are now available for finding genes that make a person more susceptible than average to a wide range of health problems, including heart disease, cancer, alcoholism, depression, diabetes, Alzheimer's disease, and many others.

Any person thinking about getting a genetic test for these conditions or others should consult a trained genetic counselor before providing blood samples for testing. Simply knowing your inherited risks for a disease can change your life in ways you may not predict. Testing positive for a gene that is *associated* with alcoholism or depression is not the same as testing positive for a gene known to *cause* a serious disease. However, being told one has a higher than average risk of acquiring a disease or condition can cause unnecessary worry, which itself may cause health problems.

## Widespread Genetic Testing of Adults

There are many situations in which genetic testing is not appropriate, and there are valid reasons for deciding not to know what deleterious genes you may, or may not, carry. Some general problems with currently marketed genetic tests are:

1. Most inherited disorders or diseases cannot be cured or even treated effectively, so finding out that you might be affected by a genetic disease in the future may, in itself, be unhealthy due to the added stress and worry.

HEALTHY SEXUALITY

### Is There a Gay Gene?

In modern society, the word *gay* is used to refer to a homosexual male. Historically, the word meant "mirthful, high spirited;" later, it began to be associated with sexual conduct, as in "gay blade." But how the term *gay* became associated with male homosexuals is still uncertain. In 1993, a scientific research team claimed to have discovered the biological basis of male homosexuality by identifying a "gay gene." However, their methods involved statistical associations, and no actual gene was ever identified. Furthermore, genetic studies by other researchers failed to confirm the original observations or analysis. Although researchers presume that homosexuality has a basis in biology and genes, there is still no convincing evidence to support this presumption. Perhaps the best evidence is that many gay persons report that they were aware at a very early age of their attraction to other males—but this is not scientific evidence for a gay gene.

Should future research uncover specific genetic influences on sexual orientation, and given its complex nature, it seems highly unlikely that a single gene (or even a few genes) can account for homosexuality. Sexual orientation is most likely determined by hundreds of genes and numerous environmental factors that affect brain development in utero as well as after birth. The factors underlying sexual orientation are probably at least as complex as the ones that affect intelligence.

Research on the genetic basis of homosexuality is extremely controversial for many reasons. In the past, and even now, most homosexual men would have chosen to hide their sexual orientation because of the dire consequences of "coming out." In the United States prior to the 1970s, homosexuality was medically classified as a disease, and homosexual men often were forced to undergo painful psychological or physical treatments to "cure" their homosexuality. Until recently in China, shock therapy was used to "treat" homosexuals. Although gay men are well integrated in most aspects of American society today, strong prejudice still exists in many areas of the United States and in other countries around the world (read "Brokeback Mountain" by Annie Proulx or watch the movie based on it). Extreme prejudice or hatred of homosexuals is called *homophobia* and is still a problem in the United States and elsewhere in the world.

Anthropological evidence indicates that homosexuality has existed in all human cultures past and present and that, in general, male homosexuals constitute between 2% to 4% of any human population. Thus, homosexuality is a typical variation among people, just like genetic variation in height or intelligence. For example, only a small percentage of people are over 7 feet tall or have the minds of geniuses, but they are not stigmatized. If one or several genes are eventually found that make an individual more likely to have a same-sex orientation, it is not hard to imagine many people wanting to undergo genetic testing for such genes. A positive test for homosexuality susceptibility genes could be used to determine the suitability of a marriage partner or to abort a fetus. The hypothetical possibility of a genetic test for homosexuality is disturbing and could create significant social problems.

2. Effects of genes vary widely from one individual to another depending on a person's overall genetic makeup. In one person a particular defective gene might produce symptoms; in another person the same defective gene may have no effect whatsoever. Simply knowing that you have a particular defective gene does not tell you how it will be expressed in your body.
3. Genetic tests are like other biological tests in that they generate a certain number of false positives and false negatives. That is, the test might indicate that you have a particular defective gene when in fact you do not. Or, it might indicate that you do not have the gene when in fact you do have it. All tests have some small percentage of error.
4. Genetic testing is not regulated, and there is no governmental oversight of quality, as there is for prescription drugs, for example. Companies that sell genetic tests may make claims about accuracy, but there is no way to know if such claims are true. For example, a company marketed a blood-based test to determine the sex of a fetus based on a sample of the pregnant woman's blood. The company claims that its test is the gold standard of gender tests and has a 99.9% accuracy rate. However, more than 100 women who took the test filed a class action lawsuit against the company for false results. Until companies marketing genetic tests face the same degree of scrutiny and regulation by the federal government as drug companies do, it will be difficult for consumers to trust the results.

Despite the many pitfalls of some genetic tests, there are situations in which people can benefit from them. However, ordering tests online or obtaining them from unregulated sources is risky. Genetic testing should be done only with supervision by trained health professionals. Your genes are your most valuable personal resource; do not let others obtain your genetic information without your full knowledge and understanding of the consequences.

## SEXUALITY IN REVIEW

- Human traits and sexual characteristics are determined by each person's genetic information that was inherited from parents.
- Human genes are packaged into 23 pairs of chromosomes; each individual inherits half of her or his genes from the mother and half from the father.
- Anatomical, physiological, and many behavioral characteristics result from the actions of one or more genes and environmental factors.
- Many genes control the development of the sex organs in male and female fetuses.
- Abnormal chromosomes and genes can cause a variety of abnormalities in sexual development that give rise to individuals whose sex is ambiguous.
- Inheritance of single abnormal genes can cause genetic disorders, genetic diseases, birth defects, and abnormal sexual development.
- Genetic testing can detect abnormal genes and chromosomes in fetuses, children, and adults, thereby helping to prevent inheritance of abnormal genes.

## CRITICAL THINKING ABOUT SEXUALITY

1. A few years ago, the U.S. military ordered all service personnel to provide a sample of their DNA, which was to be analyzed and placed on file in order to identify remains from future combat. A soldier refused to provide his DNA, arguing that he had no assurance that his DNA profile would be kept private and not used for purposes of discrimination or to his detriment in other ways. Some lawmakers want to have the DNA profile of every person in the United States on file to help in solving crimes. Discuss the benefits and drawbacks of having the DNA profiles of everyone in the United States on file in a federal agency so that anyone could be identified by law enforcement, government agencies, hospitals, or other agencies.
2. A growing number of parents in the United States are choosing the sex of their children. In some instances, the choice is simply one of preference, often to "balance the family" by having equal numbers of female and male children. In other instances, sex selection is based on medical issues. However, with identification of more and more genes that control specific traits, there is growing concern about "designer babies." The techniques for sperm sorting and preimplantation testing were explained in this chapter. What are the benefits and drawbacks of sex selection? Do you approve of some forms of sex or trait selection but not others? Do you think any kind of sex selection is immoral? Discuss your views regarding sex selection and/or trait selection by prospective parents.
3. What is your opinion of the following (fictitious) television interview with Donald Trumpet, the renowned real estate mogul and reality show host? Do you think there are "money genes" or "political orientation" genes?

   Q: Mr. Trumpet, I want to thank you for coming in to discuss genes and money with us.

DT: No problem. I'm glad to share my wisdom with your audience.

Q: You claim to have inherited a money gene. Is that correct?

DT: Certainly. I'm very rich, my parents were rich, and their parents were rich. It's obvious that I inherited my family's money gene.

Q: Isn't it true that even though something "runs in a family," it does not necessarily mean it is inherited? For example, political party affiliation runs in families, but we don't say there are genes for Republicanism.

DT: I'm not sure about political genes, but I do know about the money gene. The Rockefellers have it and so do the Rothchilds. The Bushes certainly have a money gene, and I might have the same one they do. I haven't traced it back yet.

Q: Assuming you do have a money gene, Mr. Trumpet, do you know the pattern of inheritance?

DT: Oh, I'm pretty sure it's sex linked and that the gene is on the X chromosome. I got the gene from my mother, and she got it from her father, who was filthy rich. It's always transmitted from mother to son, which is why really rich people are almost always men. Most women get their money from their ex-husbands, of course.

Q: With all this talk about genetic tests for this and that these days, do you think there should be a genetic test for the money gene?

DT: I've already offered my DNA so they can identify the gene. Other rich people might have some kind of money gene, but I think mine is the best one. I want to share it with others.

Q: That's very generous of you. To give it away I mean.

DT: My money gene is the Rolls Royce of genes. My lawyers have already patented my gene. People who want it will have to pay. What a terrible world it would be if everyone had a money gene like mine.

Q: I see what you mean. Thank you very much for speaking with us today. Time is money, as they say.

DT: Sure, no problem. My lawyers will bill you later.

## REFERENCES AND RECOMMENDED RESOURCES

### References

Barry, P. (2009, July 4). Seeking genetic fate. *Science News*, 16–21.

Hartl, D. L. (2011). *Essential genetics: A genomics perspective, 5th ed.* Sudbury, MA: Jones & Bartlett Learning.

Hvistendahl, M. (2009). Making every baby count. *Science*, 323, 1164–1166.

Sadler, T. W. (2009). *Langman's medical embryology, 11th ed.* Philadelphia: Lippincott Williams & Wilkins.

### Recommended Resources

Feero, W. G., Guttmacher, A. E., & Collins, F. S. (2010). Genomic medicine—an updated primer. *New England Journal of Medicine, 362*, 2001–2029.

MedlinePlus. (2010). Available at: http://www.nlm.nih.gov/medlineplus/genetictesting.html. Information on genetic testing from the U.S. National Library of Medicine.

Online Mendelian inheritance in man. (2010). Available at: http://www.ncbi.nlm.nih.gov/omim. A list of every known single gene defect and the disease or disorder it causes.

U.S. Department of Energy. (2010). Available at: http://www.ornl.gov/sci/techresources/Human_Genome/medicine/medicine.shtml. Information about the Human Genome Project.

U.S. National Institutes of Health. (2010). Stem cell information. Available at: http://stemcells.nih.gov. Stem cell information. Provides current news on stem cell research.

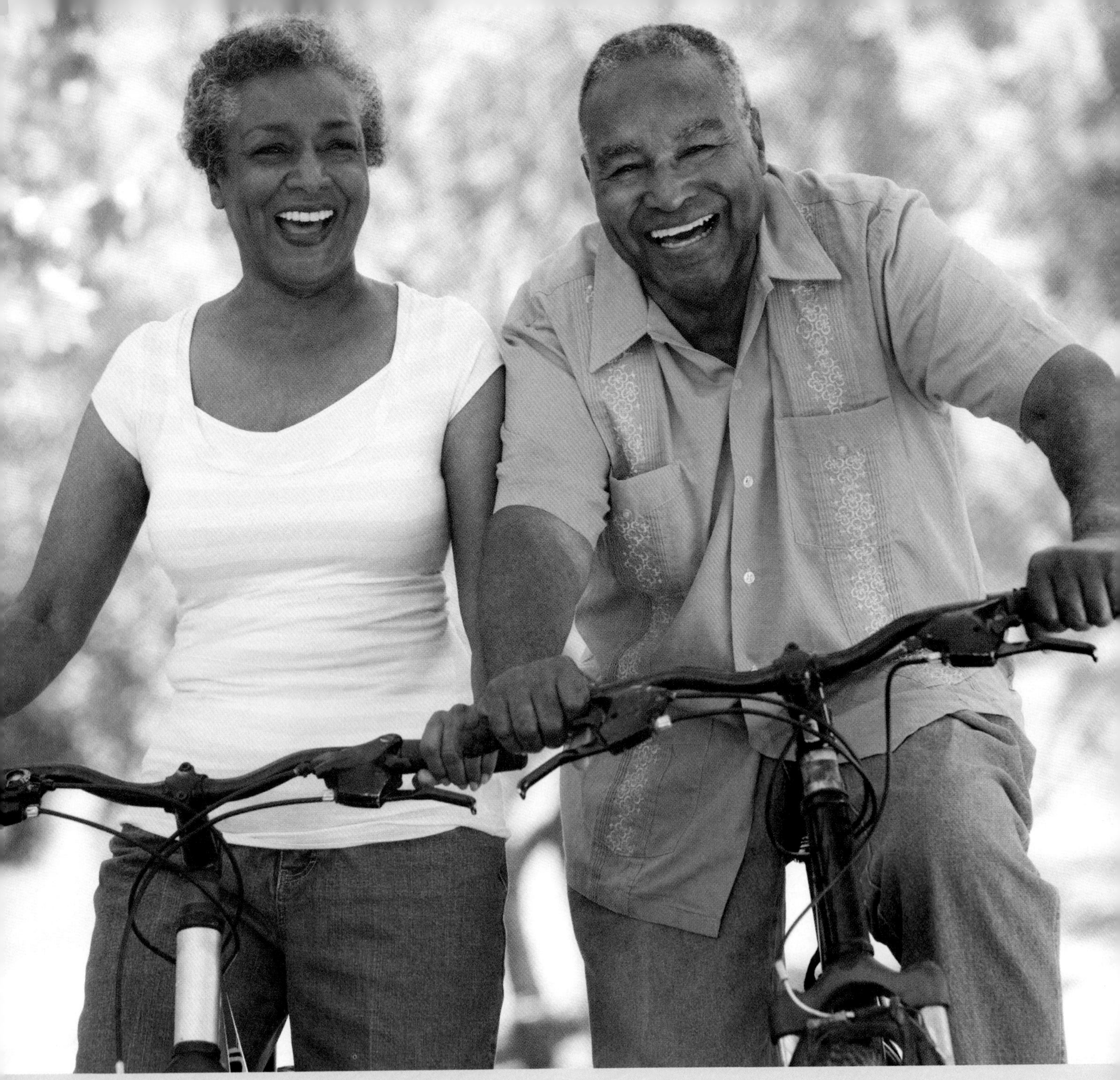

*“Sex is a lifetime career.”*

— Jack Annon

CHAPTER 8

# Sexuality Development Across the Lifespan

## Student Learning Objectives

1. Describe the five categories of sexual learning characteristic of childhood: gender, body, emotions, appropriate sexual behavior, and attachment patterns
2. Distinguish between adolescence and puberty
3. List the major pubertal changes in males and females
4. Describe the characteristics of adolescent sexual behavior
5. Describe the predominant patterns of sexual relating in early to middle adulthood
6. Describe factors affecting sexual expression in late-life adults

It is common to think that how you experience your sexuality now is how you will experience it in the future. However, looking back on your own life, you know that a person's sexuality can change significantly. Recall, for example, when you changed from a child to adolescent.

With regard to sexuality development, it is useful to divide the lifespan into the following stages:

- Fetal life, during which the sex and reproductive organs develop and hormones affect brain development.
- Childhood, during which individuals learn about themselves and appropriate social behaviors.
- Puberty and adolescence, during which the body changes from the child to the adult form, individuals begin to experience sexual (erotic) sensations, thoughts, fantasies, and desires, and they begin to explore acting on their sexual feelings.
- Early and middle adulthood, during which sexual identity and sexual experience become important aspects of one's life and one's emotionally close, personal relationships.
- Late adulthood, during which sexual experience may continue or diminish due to lack of a partner or changes in health.

In Chapter 2 we discussed hormonal influences on the developing brain, and in Chapter 7 we discussed fetal development of the sexual and reproductive organs. In this chapter we discuss the developmental changes in sexuality during childhood, adolescence, early and middle adulthood, and late adulthood.

## Sexuality in Childhood

As discussed in Chapter 7, the biological foundations of a person's sexuality are established at fertilization with the inheritance of the sex chromosomes (XX for females and XY for males). During fetal life, the sex chromosomes influence the formation of the gonads (ovaries or testes), which in turn produce hormones and other substances that influence the formation of the internal and external sex and reproductive organs and certain regions of the brain. By the time a child is born, the sex and reproductive organs, while reproductively nonfunctional, are formed anatomically.

During the first decade after birth, other than growth in proportion to the rest of the body, an individual's sexual biology changes little. However, considerable sexual development occurs in the form of establishing the psychological and social foundations of adult sexuality. About a century ago, Sigmund Freud postulated that much of the adult personality is the result of sexual development in childhood, specifically the interplay of instinctual sexual drives (hypothesized to be derived from patterned neurological activity in the brain) and pleasurable/erotic sensations in the genital and anal regions (**Table 8.1**). Contrary to Freud's view, many modern psychologists interpret sexual development in childhood as part of a broader developmental pattern centered on learning about gender, one's body, emotions, sexual values, attachment-based relationship patterns, and relationship management skills.

### Learning About Gender

**gender identity** the sense of oneself as being biologically male or female

One of the most significant features of sexuality development in childhood is the establishment, by about age three, of **gender identity**—the integration into one's sense of self and self-concept which biological sex, either male or female, one is. Although

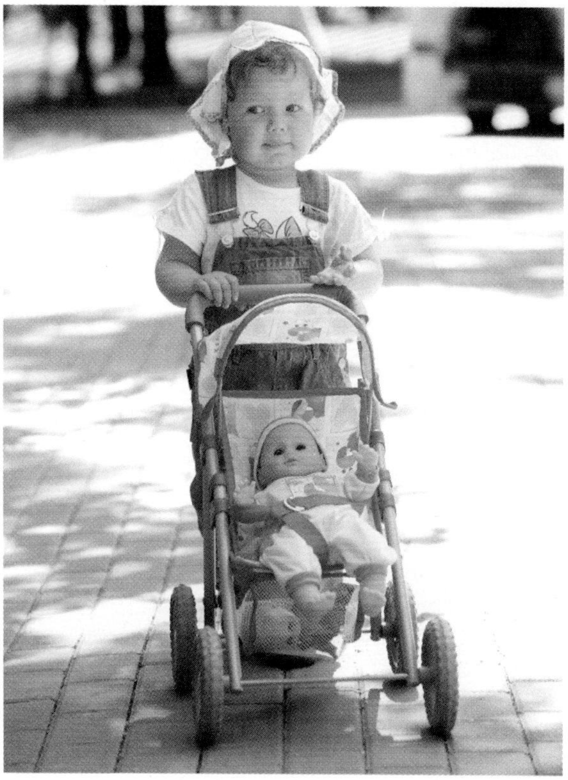

Sexuality in childhood consists of establishing the psychological and social foundations of adult sexuality.

neurobiological factors may play a role, the major influence on the establishment of gender identity is believed to be sex typing (sex assignment), which occurs at birth (or prior to birth if parents are informed of the results of ultrasound scans or prenatal chromosomal analysis; see Chapter 7) when parents and other adults, noting the appearance of the child's genitalia, proclaim a child to be a boy or a girl. From that time onward, parents and others reinforce sex assignment by treating the child in terms of their own gender stereotypes (e.g., the color blue and short hair for boys, the color pink and long hair for girls) and socializing the child into what they believe are appropriate gender-based attitudes and behaviors. Also, in time, children become aware of the sex-specific nature of their own genitalia, which, most of the time, leads to self-identification with the corresponding biological sex.

**sex typing (sex assignment)** the assigning of a gender to newborns, generally based on the appearance of genitals

**Table 8.1** Freud's Stages of Psychosexual Development

| Stage | Age | Description |
|---|---|---|
| Oral | 0–1 | Erotic pleasure is derived from sucking, chewing, and biting. |
| Anal | 1–3 | Erotic pleasure is derived from expelling or retaining feces. |
| Phallic | 3–5 | Erotic pleasure is derived from genital sensations. Boys develop erotic feelings for their mothers and girls fall in love with their fathers. Children eventually give up their erotic longings for the other-sex parent and instead identify with the same-sex parent. |
| Latency | 5–12 | Sexual urges are minimal; children focus on learning to control and find non-sexual outlets for their drives. |
| Genital | Puberty | Erotic drives are genital in focus as individuals look to peers as sexual partners. |

Freud proposed that some of the energy for life was derived from biological sexual urges that are present at birth. As children develop, sexual energy (called *libido*) is centered on different body regions, and if development proceeds healthfully, children pass through the stages and become healthy sexual adults. However, if circumstances (including parenting practices) are not optimal, individuals may not move from stage to stage, resulting in various kinds of personality and behavioral problems.

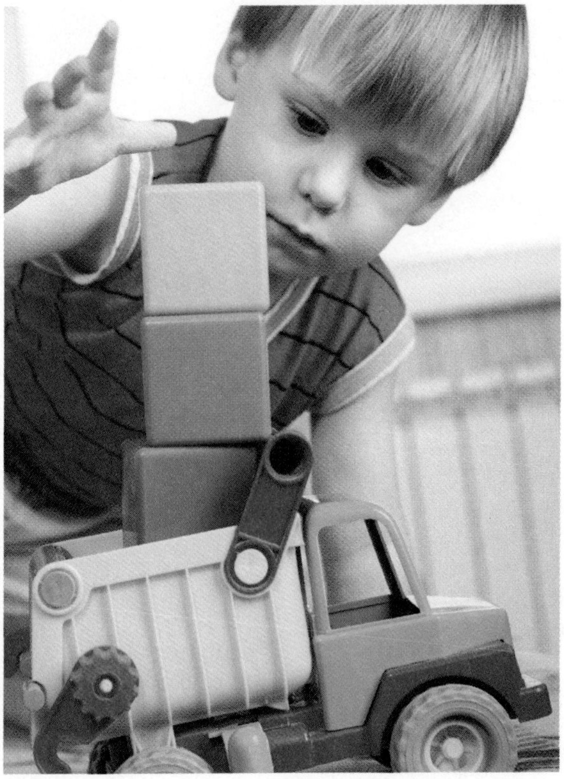

By age three, children can cite behaviors stereotypically appropriate for each sex.

As they develop, children use their gender identity to help them know which gender stereotypes and gender role behaviors apply to them. Children as young as three years old can cite long lists of behaviors expected of one sex or the other. Adults—particularly parents—influence the development of a child's sex-based attitudes and behaviors by rewarding what is considered proper, discouraging improper sex-based behavior, and modeling appropriate sex-based behaviors. Siblings, peers, school, religion, and the media also affect gender identity. Temperament, which is considered inborn and biologically based, may also influence gender-specific attitudes and behaviors. For example, boys and girls tend to differ in activity level and social behavior. Many boys tend to seek playmates who prefer movement and rough-and-tumble play, and are competitive. Many girls, in contrast, tend to prefer less-active, cooperative play. These tendencies lead adults to provide toys and play opportunities that fit a child's temperament, thus reinforcing what appear to be gender stereotypes (e.g., males as active and competitive, females as passive and cooperative).

## Learning About the Body

Children are naturally curious and playful. They will explore themselves and their surroundings, notice what others say and do, ask questions, react to how others respond to their inquisitiveness and behaviors, and do in their play what is fun and/or that they see adults and older children doing. In their explorations, children will touch their genitals and may even acknowledge pleasurable—although not necessarily erotic—sensations stemming from this kind of activity. They may mention or inquire about others' genitals and sex-specific body parts (e.g., dad's penis, mom's breasts, sister's absence of a penis). They may engage in "bathroom talk" (e.g., pee, poo, fart) or repeat acceptable sex words or "dirty words" they've heard at home, at school, or in media to establish their meaning, to feel grown up, or to see how their parents will react. They may ask "how babies are made" in anticipation of their own parenting, or perhaps because mom is pregnant with a sibling. Curiosity and the desire to play "grown-up" may lead to games such as "doctor," "house," and "I'll show you mine if you show me yours" or to experiment with kissing or genital touching.

By about age six, children become more private about their bodies. They may close the bathroom door and be more circumspect about who is permitted to see them naked or in their underwear. They may resist another's touch or, conversely, use inappropriate touching as an expression of dominance.

## Emotional Learning

Emotions are at the core of sexual experience, sexual intimacy, and close relationships. Although children do not experience *the sexual* as adults do, childhood is nevertheless when individuals can learn to identify and manage their own emotions and to express emotions to accomplish personal goals and to foster personally rewarding relationships. Emotions generally arise from mental assessments of the state of one's being and the need to alter that state in some way. A hungry infant will cry, an angry toddler will grab another child's toy, a frightened child will seek comfort, and a joyful middle schooler will jump, spin, smile, and shout. Barring some neurological incapacity or psychological trauma, as development progresses children learn that certain experiences within them are called feelings, they learn to distinguish one feeling sensation from another, and they learn to label specific feelings ("I am happy," "I feel angry"). Children also learn to appraise their own emotional experiences within the social contexts in which they arise ("I am mad at Mom because she yelled at me"), and they learn to regulate their emotional experiences, perhaps by diverting attention to another experience, toning down their intensity (*self-soothing*), or choosing the circumstances for expressing them.

Throughout childhood, individuals develop competencies with regard to emotional expression. They learn which emotions to express and how to express them in order to obtain their goals and to facilitate harmonious social interaction—for example, by expressing anger through words rather than by hitting or throwing something. They also learn the ways emotional expression can affect relationships—for example, by saying "I like you" to a friend or hugging a parent. Children who are adept at sending emotional messages (particularly positive ones) tend to have successful relationships with peers. Children also learn to assess when it is personally beneficial *not* to express a particular emotion. For example, a child might feel lonely, frightened, or upset, but she knows that seeking comfort from a stranger is inappropriate or possibly dangerous.

## Learning Appropriate and Inappropriate Sexual Behavior

Parents, religion, peers, and other elements of society transmit to children a variety of values and behavioral norms intended to make them cooperative members of their social group. Some of these values and norms pertain to sexuality. For example, children learn that certain words and behaviors are "appropriate" and others are not.

Being sexually curious and engaging in play that adults may perceive as sexual are normal aspects of childhood. And so is learning society's rules about sexual conduct. A child who is punished for expressing her or his sexual curiosity can experience self-doubt or confusion and develop sex-negative attitudes. Accepting children's natural sexuality and helping them to express it properly can help them develop a much more balanced attitude toward sexuality and more responsible sexual conduct.

In North America, parents are expected to be the primary sex educators of children, but many parents are reluctant to discuss sexuality with their children. This is so for a variety of reasons. For example, parents may have limited sexual knowledge and be embarrassed to admit this to their children, believe that sex is dirty or sinful, or fear that educating children about sex encourages them to be sexual.

When parents do not educate their children about sex, peers and the media become a child's most influential sex educators. Unfortunately, peers and the media are often misinformed, and, unlike parents, neither peers nor the media have a young person's best interests in mind when they impart information and suggest sexual values. Without parental guidance, many young people are forced to learn about sex and sexuality on their own. Also, parents who do not discuss sexuality with their children impart the message that sex is taboo or bad, which can establish negative attitudes about sex that carry into adulthood and often are perpetuated in succeeding generations.

### Development of Attachment Patterns

During infancy and childhood children experience intense emotional attachments to their parents (or other emotionally significant adults). These early attachment relationships establish expectations and beliefs about trust, intimacy, and emotional bonding, which may affect a person's behavior in emotionally close relationships later in life. Individuals whose childhood attachments are trusting, secure, supportive, and pleasant grow up believing that others are likely to be caring, responsive, and fun and that they themselves are worthy of another's trust, love, support, and playful interaction. In contrast, individuals whose early attachment relationships are characterized by neglect, abuse, instability, and abandonment tend to expect relationships to be unpleasant and to see themselves as not worthy of another's caring, love, and support.

## Sexuality in Adolescence

**Adolescence** is the time of life when individuals transition from childhood to their society's definition of adulthood. In some societies, adolescence might involve little more than a few weeks or months of instruction in the ways of adulthood and a ceremony marking the transition to adulthood. In other societies, adolescence might involve considerable learning and rehearsal beginning at around age 10 and extending well past age 20 with no particular ceremony or event to mark the attainment of adult status (i.e., graduating from high school or college, getting a job, having a child, or getting married).

**adolescence** the stage of life when individuals transition from childhood to adulthood
**puberty** specific biological changes that transform a child's body into a sexually and reproductively capable adult's

In all societies, the central feature of adolescence is **puberty**, a set of specific biological changes that transform a child's body to that of a sexually and reproductively capable adult (**FIGURE 8.1**). Individuals get taller, heavier, and hairier (*puberty* is derived from the Latin word *pubes*, meaning "to become hairy"). Males become more muscular and females deposit body fat on the hips, buttocks, and breasts. In additional to anatomical changes is the hormonally driven emergence of erotic capacity in the form of heightened erotic feelings and the desire to act on them.

Besides profound changes in the body, adolescence is characterized by the opportunity to develop and attain a fuller sense of personal identity. In the mid- to late teens, changes in the brain endow greater degrees of abstract thought,

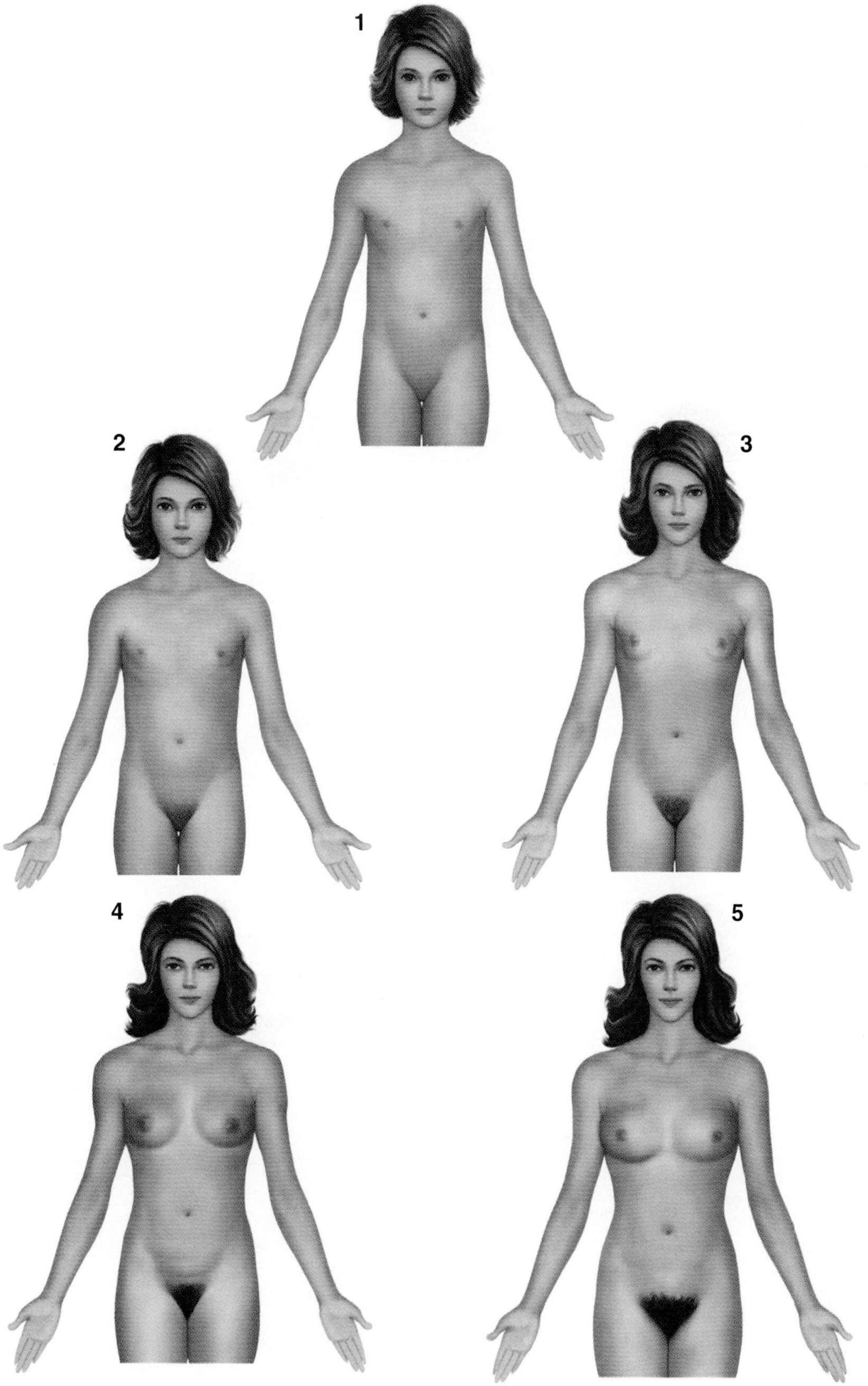


FIGURE 8.1 **Changes in Sexual Anatomy at Puberty.** Puberty is characterized scientifically into five stages, called *Tanner Stages* or the *Sexual Maturity Rating. (Continues)*

Adapted from Marshall, W. A., & Tanner, J. M. (1969 June). Variations in pattern of pubertal changes in girls. *Archives of Disease in Childhood, 44*, 235, 291–303; and Marshall, W. A., & Tanner, J. M. (1970 February). Variations in the pattern of pubertal changes in boys. *Archives of Disease in Childhood, 45*, 239, 13–23.

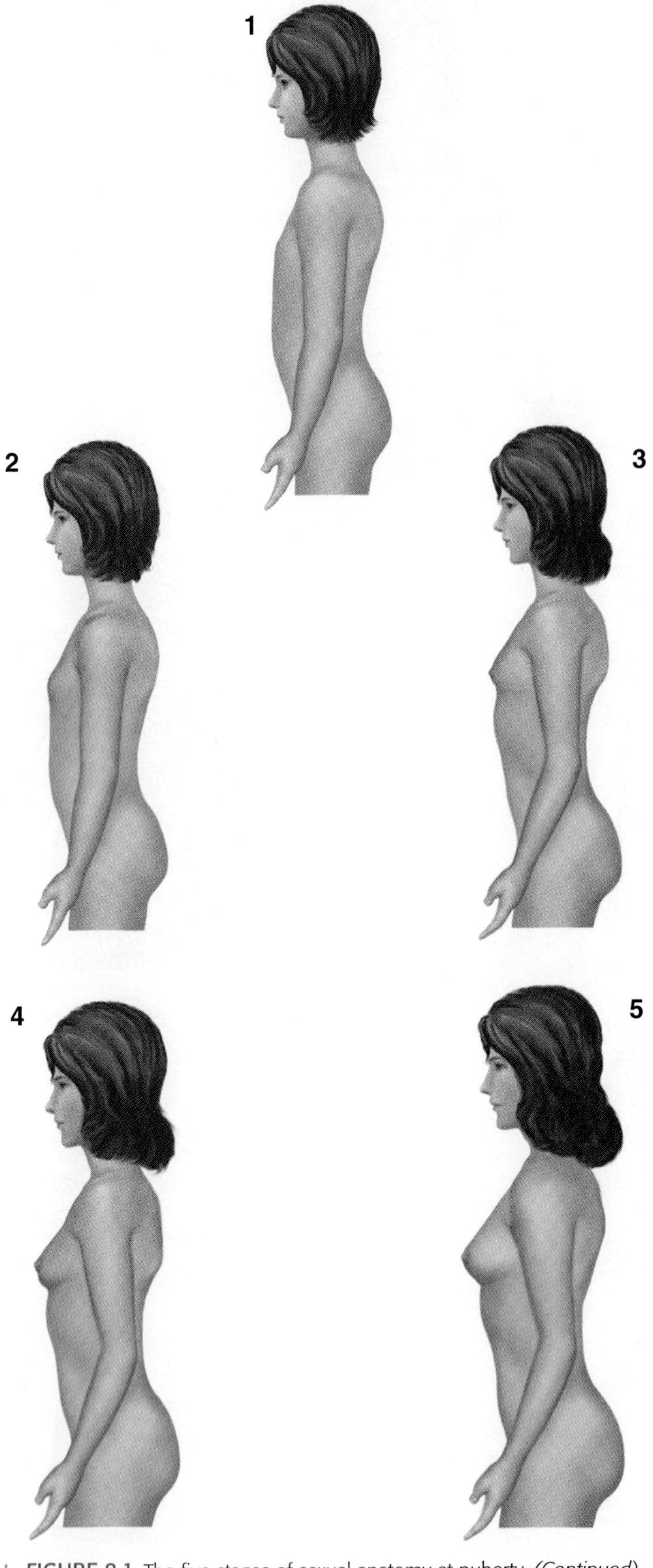


FIGURE 8.1 The five stages of sexual anatomy at puberty. *(Continued)*

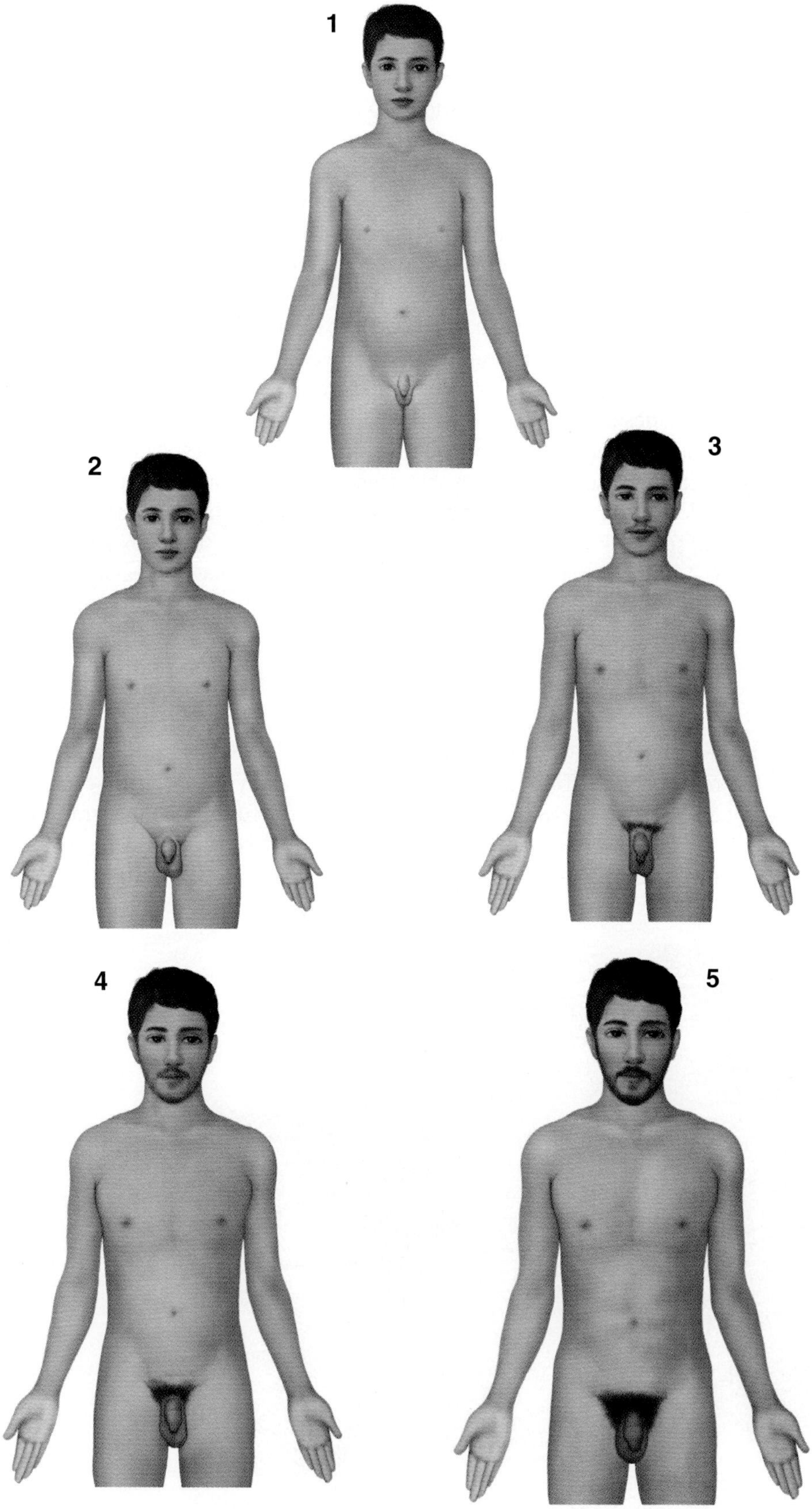


FIGURE 8.1 The five stages of sexual anatomy at puberty. *(Continued)*

advanced planning, the application of critical thinking and judgment, and greater regulation of emotions. These neuropsychological capacities combine with social expectations to provide an opportunity to commit to beliefs and values that are experienced as one's own rather than adopting those of others. Not only does one commit to a set of self-chosen beliefs, but also one experiences oneself as a *chooser.* Without much life experience to guide choices, however, adolescence is generally a time of developing and committing to hopes, dreams, and goals rather than undertaking specific activities to manifest them (other than going to college).

Adolescence is also a time of developing more complex strategies for relating to people outside of one's family. For along with development of a more profound sense of identity is the desire to turn to peers more often than family for self-expression, companionship, emotional support, love, and intimacy. Thus, one key social skill in adolescence is learning to balance being oneself and fitting in socially. This includes developing healthy attitudes about one's body (*body image*) and the expression of one's gender-based attitudes and behaviors. And, because adolescence is the first time in life they experience intense erotic feelings intermingled with desires for peer-to-peer emotional bonding, individuals also must develop a set of social skills to help them meet their needs for sexual expression and intimacy. Adolescents accomplish this by drawing on what was learned in childhood about values, appropriate social behaviors, emotional expression, and emotional closeness.

## Puberty

Puberty is the time of life when an individual develops the biological capacity to take part in reproduction. Thus, puberty is characterized by rapid increases in body height and weight (the *adolescent growth spurt*), the functional maturation of the sexual and reproductive organs, the development of secondary sex characteristics (see Chapters 2 and 3), and specific sex-related changes in the brain.

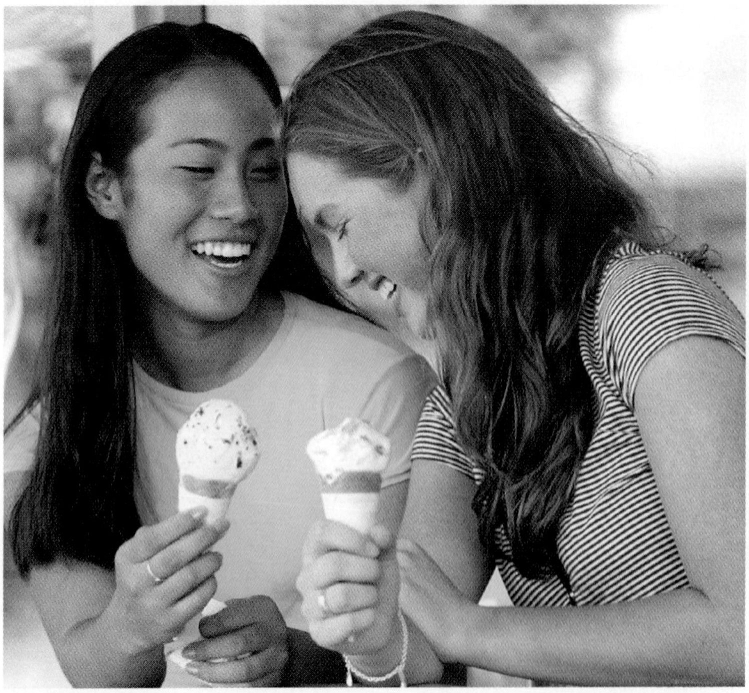

Adolescents rely on peers for self-expression, companionship, and emotional support.

The onset of puberty is triggered by the actions of brain and pituitary hormones, which cause the ovaries and testes to grow and release sex hormones, principally estrogen in the female and testosterone in the male. The onset of puberty also brings an increase in secretion of the androgenic hormone *dehydroepiandrostenedione sulfate (DHEAS)* from the adrenal glands. In females, DHEAS stimulates growth of the long bones, underarm and pubic hair, and sebaceous glands in the skin. In males, analogous changes are brought about by testosterone, which is a more powerful androgen than DHEAS. The actions of skin bacteria on exudate from the sebaceous glands are responsible for underarm odor, musky scents in the genital region, and acne.

Among North American females, puberty generally begins between the ages of 9 and 12, and the period of change lasts about three years. The first sign of puberty is either the beginning of breast growth or the appearance of pubic hair. Within a year or two after the onset of puberty, the ovaries, fallopian tubes, uterus, vagina, and external genital structures grow and become functional. As puberty continues, the breasts develop the adult form; the hips become wide in comparison to the waist; subcutaneous fat accumulates on the hips, thighs, and buttocks; and the young woman experiences her first menstrual period, called the menarche. After menarche, even though menstrual cycles occur, a young women may not be immediately fertile because the ovaries are not yet producing fertilizable eggs and the uterus is not yet capable of carrying a pregnancy. Most of the time, these capacities are attained within the first year after menarche. Late in puberty, estrogen produced by the ovaries arrests bone growth and the adult height is attained.

**menarche** first menstrual period
**endocrine disruptors** industrial chemicals that disrupt the functions of sex hormones

In North American males, puberty generally begins between the ages of 12 and 14 and lasts about five years. The first sign of puberty in boys is growth of the testes and scrotum. About a year after the onset of testicular growth, the growth spurt begins, the penis grows, the shoulders broaden, the larynx enlarges (causing the voice to "crack" before it attains its deep pitch), and facial hair becomes prominent. Also at this time, the seminal vesicles and prostate begin to grow, becoming functional and producing seminal fluid. This permits a male's first ejaculations, some of which occur via masturbation and others spontaneously during sleep ("wet dreams").

The timing of the onset of puberty varies by age of the child and is thought to depend on inheritance and the following factors:

- *Physical factors.* The age of first menstruation has been declining among young women in industrialized countries for over a century: In 1880 menarche occurred around age 17; in 1930, age 15; from 1980 to the present, age 12.5. This trend has been attributed to improvements in nutrition and physical health. The amount of body fat may also influence the onset of puberty, perhaps signaling a girl's biological capability to reproduce.
- *Psychosocial factors.* Girls in father-absent families or who live in the presence of non–biologically related males tend to enter puberty earlier than do girls who live with their biological fathers. Girls who live in stressful environments (as in situations of extreme poverty, war, or abuse) tend to enter puberty later than average.
- *Environmental factors.* Certain industrial and agricultural chemicals that are present in water, food, clothes, and household items (e.g., polychlorinated biphenyls, phthalate esters, furans) may be endocrine disruptors, which alter the actions of natural estrogen and testosterone in the body. Specific endocrine disruptors, called *xenoestrogens,* alter the actions of natural estrogen and are suspected to cause early, or precocious, puberty in girls. In

one case, an 8-year-old boy experienced precocious puberty from exposure to testosterone on his father's skin (the boy's father used a testosterone-containing skin cream). Chemicals called phthalates, which are widely used as plasticizers in the manufacture of thousands of kinds of packaging, plastic toys, and plastic pipes, are xenoestrogens that also may trigger early onset of puberty in girls.

## Adolescent Sexual Behavior

Although they prepare the body for reproduction, the biological changes at puberty do not endow human children with knowledge of how to behave sexually. Appropriate expression of sexual and romantic feelings and desires must be learned from family, peers, and other agents of socialization within a young person's culture, and, perhaps more importantly, from personal exploration and experience.

In some cultures, adolescent sexual learning and experience are carefully directed by adults according to long-standing traditions and rituals. Young people may receive instruction in sexual relating and marriage roles, and their interactions with peers are likely to be closely scrutinized and chaperoned by adults. Premarital sex, especially for females, may be considered a severe violation of cultural or religious norms and punished by ostracism, physical abuse bordering on torture, and even death. In contrast, in other societies, older children and adolescents are permitted to explore sexuality with some adult guidance in sexual and marital skills and few behavioral restrictions other than the expectation that young females not become pregnant.

Currently, in the United States, most adolescents receive contradicting messages about sexual behavior. On the one hand, adults permit (and in some instances encourage) adolescents to dress provocatively and to consume sex-related media such as teen magazines, music videos, advertising, television, and films. Adults also accept the fact that young people will form emotionally close relationships with peers, although such relationships are often referred to as "puppy love" to distinguish them as nonadult—that is less meaningful and not sexual. On the other hand, even though certain adult modes of dress, exposure to sexual imagery in media, and falling in love are permitted, adults discourage adolescent sexual activity to limit the risk of unintended pregnancy, acquiring an STD, or experiencing emotional hurt and loss of self-esteem and self-confidence that can result from

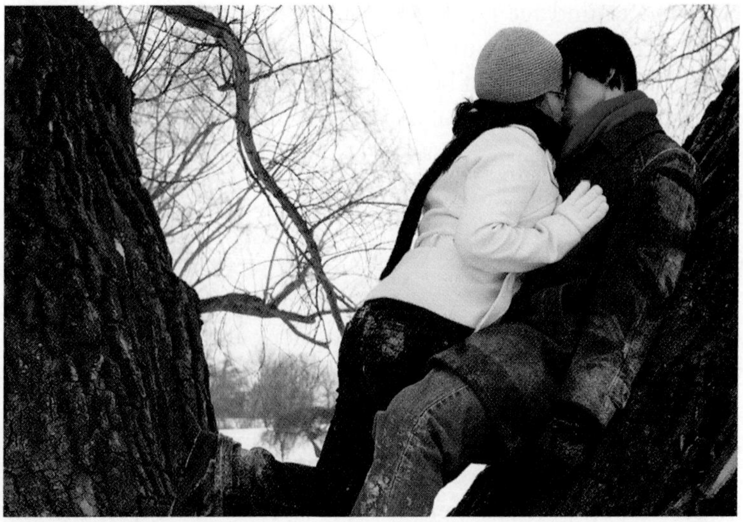

a breakup of a "love" relationship. Adults also may discourage adolescent sexual activity because they wish not to accept a child's emerging adulthood and its associated emotional independence from the family.

Even though there are strong cultural taboos against adolescent sexual activity and a lack of mentoring in being a sexual adult, young Americans, nevertheless, explore their emerging sexual interest though a stepwise pattern of ever-deepening erotic experience. For many individuals, sexual exploration begins around age 10–12 as an interest in and curiosity about sex and love increase. Young adolescents may experiment with hugging and kissing and become interested in sex/love-related media. By age 12, nearly 50% of American young people have experienced an "in love" or "like" relationship with a peer. In these early relationships, partners may engage in hugging and kissing and may talk about sex.

Around age 13, as sex hormone levels rise, adolescents begin to experience more intense erotic feelings. Touching one's genitals no longer occurs simply because it feels good; when it occurs (generally more frequently in males than in females), it is authentic sexual masturbation for the purpose of erotic experience. Young people experiment with flirtation and explore ways to become attractive to potential relationship partners. And as adolescence progresses, the likelihood of being in a romantic or "like" relationship increases. By age 15, because of love, curiosity, and sexual desire, sexual activity among partners expands to include embracing, kissing, touching breasts first over and then under clothes, and manual and oral stimulation of the genitals. Avoiding AIDS/STDs, pregnancy,

## Dear Penelope . . .

***I'm really mixed up! I'm in love with two very different people. Comparing the two is like looking at purple and green. I could see myself spending the rest of my life with either person. It's almost like I have a split personality and they come out depending on the one I am with. I know I'm supposed to choose, but how? (This sounds so totally high school, and I'm a senior in college!)***

***— So Confused***

*Dear So Confused,*

Matters of the heart can definitely be confusing. Perhaps your head can help your heart.

Start by identifying what each of these attachments tells you about yourself. Instead of focusing on having to make a choice, look inside yourself and ask what needs each relationship meets, and with which aspects of your personality each person resonates.

It's likely you'll find that one or both of these attachments is related to some "new" aspect of your own psychological growth. This is why you feel you have a split personality. In some ways you do.

Also, as a senior in college you are in transition from the familiar and somewhat sheltered to the new and unknown. It's possible that your openness to these attachments is related to this period of transition.

The choice for you now is *not* to force yourself to choose either of these persons, but instead to allow the growth to take place and your life to settle down. A signal from your psyche like this one means it isn't time to make decisions for "the rest of your life."

Before choosing a life partner, you'll do yourself a favor if you wait until you have a more solid life-concept. Give yourself a chance to find out who you are. Moreover, you'll want to make the decision on more than love. You'll want to consider how your beloved's values, plans, and dreams fit with yours.

Courtesy of the UC Davis *Aggie*

and parents' anger, as well as feeling "not ready," are reasons not to have sexual intercourse.

Adolescents also engage in sexual, romantic, and erotic/romantic fantasy. In the fantasies of younger teens, the identity and characteristics of the partner(s) and behaviors tend to be vague. However, as adolescence progresses, fantasy partners and behaviors become more specific and detailed. Romantic and sexual fantasizing (which may be accompanied by masturbation) provides pleasure, opportunities to learn about one's own sexual and romantic needs and preferences, mental experiencing of situations that are unattainable in real life, and rehearsing sexual and romantic experiences in preparation for actual activity.

In the United States, the average age of first intercourse for both sexes is about 16.5 years. Although first sexual intercourse may be an isolated episode with a friend or stranger, in the vast majority of instances, first intercourse is voluntary and takes place in a serious, emotionally close love relationship that has persisted at least three months and tends to continue after first intercourse. First intercourse tends to be spontaneous rather than planned, although it may not be unexpected, and without the influence of alcohol. The reasons for first intercourse include curiosity; to express mutual affection, closeness, and love; to meet physical urges and desires for sex; to be like—or more mature than—one's friends; to feel like an adult; and to "get it over with" (losing virginity).

Adolescents' reactions to first intercourse generally depend on the circumstances. When planned, or at least not unexpected or undesired, first intercourse can be a positive experience for the individuals and regarded as a profound positive change in their relationship. When forced or pressured "to go all the way," alcohol-related, or otherwise undesired, even if anticipated at some future time, first intercourse can be a negative experience characterized by shock, regret for not waiting, anger, guilt at behaving contrary to one's own and one's parents' values and society's norms, and anxiety regarding becoming pregnant or acquiring an STD.

By age 20, about 80% of American youth have experienced sexual intercourse. To a considerable degree, sexual intercourse among older adolescents takes place in romantic relationships. However, many adolescents have sexual relations with strangers or individuals known only casually (e.g., friend of a friend, seen around before), referred to as "casual sex" or "one-night stands." Meetings-for-sex, or "hook-ups," often occur at parties, bars, and school events. They tend to be spontaneous, impulsive, based on physical sexual attraction, emotionally superficial, and, about two-thirds of the time, involve alcohol or drugs to lower the natural inclination to be sexually/emotionally cautious and to increase the perceived desirability of potential partners ("beer goggles"). Occasionally, participants expect the encounter to be more than "a one-time thing"; however, some expect it to evolve into a regular casual sexual relationship or a serious love relationship. Nonromantic sexual encounters also occur among friends ("friends with benefits"), whose sexual behaviors tend to involve more affection (holding hands, hugging, kissing, and massage) than those of individuals engaging in one-time casual sexual encounters.

## Sexuality in Early and Middle Adulthood

In a variety of ways, much of childhood and adolescence are given over to preparing young people to assume the responsibilities of adulthood, and to some extent this holds for sexuality. During childhood, individuals develop self-concepts and learn values, rules of social behavior, and social skills that serve as foundations for sexual and intimate experiences later in life. During adolescence, individuals begin to explore the scope and significance of their sexual/erotic feelings and capacities and develop skills for peer-to-peer sexual and intimate interaction. Then, during the 40–50 year span of adulthood, the learning and experiences of the first 18–20 years of life can be realized in full.

A survey of over 27,000 adults in 29 countries, including the United States and Canada, showed that most men and women believe sex to be important to their overall lives. Worldwide, about 83% of men and 66% of women report having had sexual intercourse in the previous year; the majority of those having sex do so about 50 times a year. Societies generally encourage and/or condone sexual activity only between individuals engaged in that society's definition of marriage, whether a legal contract or regularized by custom and/or religious ceremony. In the United States, marriage is the only legally sanctioned social context for sexual activity. Over 90% of Americans marry at some point in their lives; about 72% have married by age 34.

Although Americans tend to value marriage as the primary context for adult sexual activity, they tend not to limit their sexual activity to marriage. For example, even though the average age of first marriage for women is about 25 years, and for men, 27 years, the average age of first intercourse for young Americans is about 17. Among those aged 18–24, 34% are in ongoing, nonmarital sexual relationships, referred to by social scientists as *dating*, and another 10% live together in sexual relationships, an arrangement called *cohabitation*. Only 20% of Americans age 18–24 are married. About 40% of Americans believe that sex before marriage is always or almost always wrong.

About 50% of American marriages end in divorce. Among the divorced aged 18–60 who are not remarried, a majority are either in sexual dating relationships or cohabiting. Thus, though a marriage may end, sexual activity may continue in other relational contexts.

Over 90% of Americans believe that sex with someone other than a marital partner is always or nearly always wrong. Nevertheless, extramarital sexual relations occur with some frequency. Not being sexually exclusive is generally taken to symbolize a lack of emotional investment in a relationship with a primary sexual partner due to to dissatisfaction, disharmony, conflict, or loss of interest in the primary relationship. For example, of Americans admitting to having had sexual relations with someone other than the spouse during the prior 12 months, 7% report they are happy or pretty happy with their marriages, but 14% report they are not too happy.

## Sexuality in Old Age

To be old is a new dimension in human history. In ancient Rome the average life expectancy was 20 years; in the middle ages, it was 35 years; in 1900, the average American's life expectancy was about 50 years. Today, most North Americans in their 20s and 30s can expect to live into their 80s and 90s.

The increase in life expectancy has created a new social phenomenon, the "graying America." By 2030, one American in five will be over 65 years of age and one in 10 will be over 80. Scientists are only beginning to determine the biological aspects of aging, and as of yet there is no way to stop or reverse it. Everyone can expect to have gray hair, a gradual decline in physical endurance, a decline in or loss of some bodily functions, and a variety of wrinkles, bulges, and sags.

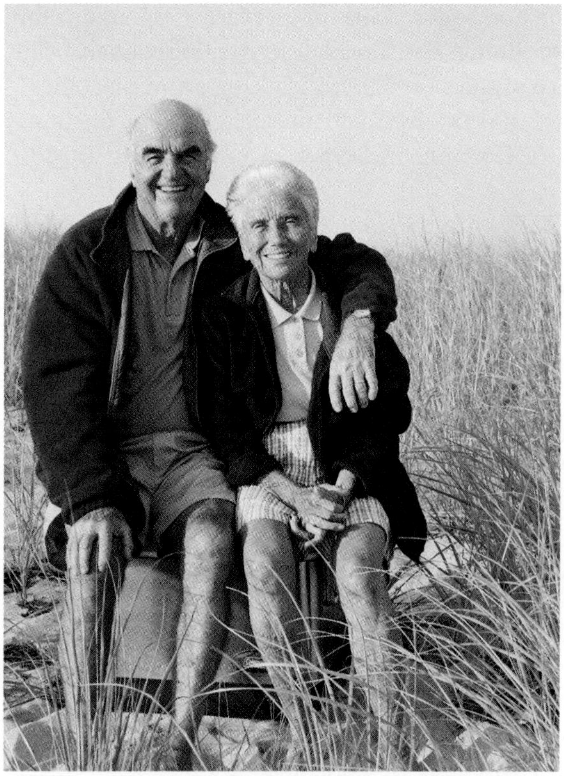

As people become 50 and 60 years old, biological, psychological, and lifestyle changes may occur that diminish sexual interest and the ability to engage in sexual activity as one did when younger. Menopause in women and lower levels of testosterone or prostate and urinary problems in men may usher in changes in sexual needs and performance. A chronic illness, such as diabetes, high blood pressure, or heart disease, can reduce sexual desire in both the ill person and a sex partner. And, an older person may become widowed and be unable to find another intimate partner. This is particularly true for women, who far outnumber men as age advances. Nevertheless, many older people find sex to be a vital part of their lives and continue to enjoy sex well into their 70s and 80s.

## Female Sexuality in the Later Years

Although American women tend to be sexually active in the later years, particularly if they are healthy and involved in an intimate relationship, they may be less interested in sex and less sexually active than their male age peers. Many women seem less concerned about their own age-related diminished sexual capabilities and desires than the quality of their intimate relationship.

## Menopause

**menopause** the cessation of ovulation and menstrual periods

A major factor affecting sexuality in middle-aged women is the menopause, the gradual cessation of ovulation, sex hormone production, and menstruation. For most American women, menopause occurs between age 50 and 52; however, it can occur as early as age 35 and as late as age 55. The age at which menopause occurs may be affected by hereditary, social, and nutritional factors. There is no relation between the age at which menopause occurs and the age at which a woman begins to menstruate.

Biologically, menopause occurs because a woman's ovaries stop producing eggs and sex hormones. Beginning at puberty and continuing until menopause, a woman has near-monthly menstrual cycles, driven by estrogen and progesterone, hormones made in the ovaries (see Chapter 3). At menopause, the ovaries stop producing eggs, estrogen and progesterone production decline, and menstrual cycles stop.

Low levels of estrogen in the body may reduce vaginal tone and the ability to produce adequate lubrication during sexual intercourse. Using new sexual techniques and alternate lubricants can help women adjust to these changes. Some women choose to take estrogen pills or use estrogen-containing vaginal suppositories to replace the lost hormone.

Although menopause brings biological changes, some of which may be uncomfortable for a while, it is not a disease. The tendency among women and their healthcare providers to medicalize menopause led to more than 30 years of drug treatment for menopause (called *hormone replacement therapy [HRT]*), which originally was thought to be safe but ultimately was shown to increase somewhat the risk of heart disease and cancer. Now, HRT is recommended only for women with specific symptoms related to menopause or for other conditions in which benefits outweigh risks.

The menopause often is called "the change," not only because a woman's body is changing, but also because it comes at a time when a number of nonbiological changes are occurring. A woman's grown children may be leaving home, her husband may be coping with his midlife issues, and her aged parents may need care. Coping with any of these occurrences may demand time and energy, which may lessen a woman's interest in sexual activity. On the other hand, coping with difficult life issues may increase the desire for emotional (and practical) support, which may manifest as wanting more emotional closeness with a partner even if it is not sexual.

Because menopause signifies the end of a woman's reproductive capacity, some people believe that it necessarily means the end of her sexual interest and ability. Whereas this belief is not supported by biological fact, menopause can have a powerful effect on a woman and her partner and alter their sexual relations. However, women who accept menopause as a normal life transition can continue to be sexually active.

## Male Sexuality in the Later Years

Do men have a menopause? Not really, despite the attempt of drug sellers to suggest otherwise in order to sell testosterone-like drugs and growth hormone. There is a decline in androgen as men age, but the experience of change is gradual over many years. Because androgen supports the sex drive in males (and females; see Chapter 2) and the functionality of the sex organs, over time the lessening of androgen production with age can reduce sexual desire and activity. Erections may come slower and less often, they may be less hard, and the intensity of ejaculation and the volume of ejaculate may decrease. After sexual activity, a man may not feel ready to have sex again for a while.

Changes other than a decline in testosterone may be more significant for an older man's sexuality. Men facing retirement may become concerned about what they are going to do with their lives without having a job to go to. They may feel depressed by the realization that the career goals they set for themselves as young men have not been met. A marriage may have ended in divorce. Serious health problems such as overweight, diabetes, heart disease, prostate disease, and other

## HEALTHY SEXUALITY

### Anti-Aging Hormones

In recent years, the centuries-long, unfruitful search for the "fountain of youth" has focused on pharmaceutical-grade hormones. Among the most studied of possible anti-aging hormones are human growth hormone (hGH), estrogen, and testosterone and similar-acting substances such as dehydroepiandrosterone (DHEA). To date, none of these hormones has been shown to slow the aging process in healthy individuals; the hormones may have minimal beneficial effect in some individuals with a clinically evident hormone deficiency. In all cases, anti-aging hormones have been shown to be dangerous. Apparently, the best way to remain healthy in old age—including sexually healthy—is to adopt and maintain a healthy lifestyle.

That no anti-aging substances exist has not stopped unscrupulous individuals from proffering worthless, and in some cases dangerous, substances to people seeking a youthful state. Experts in medical quackery caution consumers to be wary of these signs of fraud:

- Claims that are publicized directly to the media without evidence of unbiased scientific analysis.
- Claims that the purveyor's work or message is being suppressed by the scientific establishment.
- Use of phrases such as "scientific breakthrough," "exclusive product," "secret ingredient," "ancient remedy," or "natural."
- Testimonials and anecdotes unsupported by scientific data.
- Claims that centuries-old remedies are credible because they have withstood the test of time.
- Attempts to convey credibility with doctors' coats or the use of the words "MD," "academies," or "institutes," and testimonials by celebrities and "media" doctors.
- Absence of adverse reactions and the making of claims that sound too good to be true.
- Misleading interpretations of studies or outright false claims that something works.
- Use of disclaimers, money-back guarantees, and the phrase "We are on your side."

Should scientists ever find a safe, credible way to slow or reverse the aging process, we all will learn about it in short order. Until then . . .

chronic health problems of old age may affect an older man's sexuality and ability to get an erection or to maintain one sufficiently long during sexual intercourse to satisfy himself or a partner.

## SEXUALITY IN REVIEW

- As with other personal qualities and capabilities, sexuality develops after birth throughout the lifespan stages of childhood, adolescence, early and middle adulthood, and late adulthood.
- Sexuality development in childhood is characterized principally by learning about gender, the sexual body, emotional experience and expression, and social skills.
- Adolescence is characterized as transformation of the child's body into that of a reproductively capable adult, experiencing of sexual/erotic feelings, and exploring personally and socially appropriate ways to meet those feelings.
- Sexuality in early and middle adulthood tends to occur within the context of relatively stable pair-bonded sexual/romantic relationships, such as marriage.
- In late life, people may maintain significant interest in sexual expression, although sexual interest and activity may decline with declining health and the absence of a suitable sex partner.

## CRITICAL THINKING ABOUT SEXUALITY

1. How do the messages about sex and sexuality that you received as a child affect your sexuality today and how you relate to intimate partners?
2. Interview someone over 55 years old regarding their sexual development in middle adulthood. Obtain information about sexual values, gender role expectations, agents of socialization, attitudes about affection and intimacy, and any other factors that you think are important.

3. Write a personal essay using the following as a topic sentence: "When I was growing up, talking about sexual matters with my parents . . . because . . . Now the situation is . . ."
4. Imagine that you are a parent. How would you respond to these situations?
   a. Your preschool child asks you, "How does the baby get inside the mother's tummy?"
   b. Your 6-year-old child comes into the bedroom while you and your partner are having sex.
   c. By accident you discover several extremely pornographic magazines in your 14-year-old son's room.

## REFERENCES AND RECOMMENDED RESOURCES

### References


Abma, J. C., et al. (2010). Teenagers in the United States: Sexual activity, contraceptive use, and childbearing, 2006–2008, *Vital and Health Statistics, 23*, 30.

Berk, L. E. (2009). *Development through the lifespan, 5th ed.* Boston: Allyn & Bacon.

Bleakley, A., et al. (2008). It works both ways: The relationship between exposure to sexual content in the media and adolescent sexual behavior. *Media Psychology, 11*, 443–461.

Halberstadt, A. G., Denham, S. A., & Dunsmore, J. C. (2005). Affective social competence. In: C. Lewis & J. G. Bremmer (Eds.), *Developmental Psychology II, vol. 5.* Thousand Oaks, CA: Sage.

Moore, S., & Rosenthal, D. (2006). *Sexuality in adolescence.* London: Routledge.

Schoeters, G., et al. (2008). Endocrine disruptors and abnormalities of pubertal development. *Basic Clinical Pharmacology and Toxicology, 102*, 168–175.

Smith, T. W. (2006, March). *American sexual behavior: Trends, socio-demographic differences, and risk behavior.* General Social Survey Topical Report No. 25, Version 6. Available at: http://www.norc.org/NR/rdonlyres/2663F09F-2E74-436E-AC81-6FFBF288E183/0/AmericanSexualBehavior2006.pdf. Accessed November 1, 2007.

Waite, L. J., et al. (2009). Sexuality: Measures of partnerships, practices, attitudes, and problems in the National Social Life, Health, and Aging Study. *Journals of Gerontology (Series B), 64*, 56–66.

Zani, B., & Cicognani, E. (2006). Sexuality and intimate relationships in adolescents. In S. Jacobson & L. Goossens (Eds.), *Handbook of adolescent development.* New York: Psychology Press.


### Recommended Resources


Grello, C. C., Welsh, D. P., & Harper, M. S. (2006). No strings attached: The nature of casual sex in college students. *Journal of Sex Research, 43*, 255–267. Discusses "hooking up" and other types of sexual encounters.

Laumann, E. O., et al. (2006). A cross-national study of subjective well-being among older women and men. *Archives of Sexual Behavior, 35*, 145–161. Describes sexual behavior among the elderly.

World Health Organization. (2006). Sexual and reproductive health. Available at: https://www.who.int/reproductive-health/gender/sexualhealth.html. A definition of sexual health and goals for attaining it.

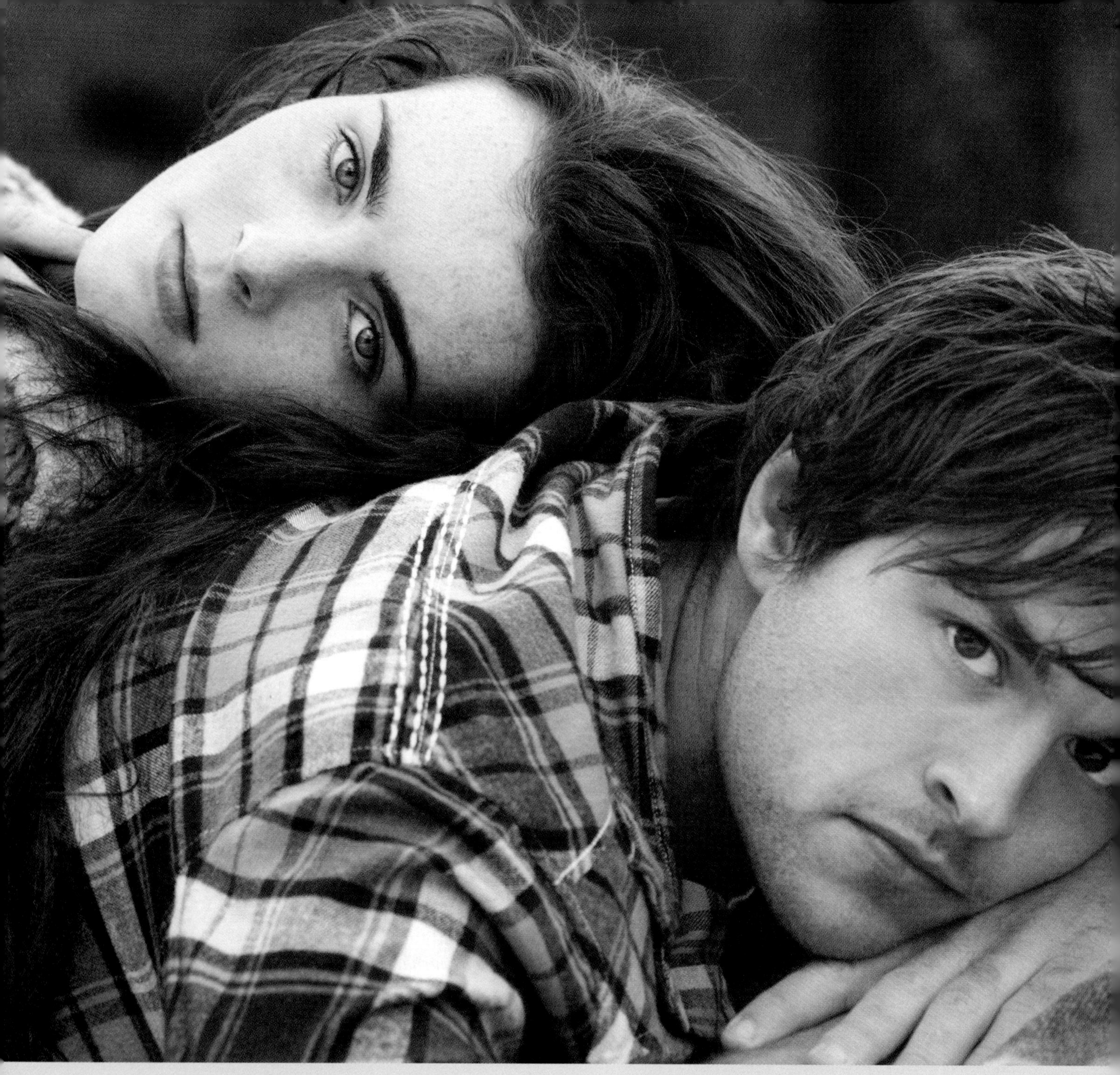

*❝And, in the end, the love you take is equal to the love you make.❞*

— John Lennon and Paul McCartney

CHAPTER 9

# The Sexual Self

## Student Learning Objectives

1. Describe and give an example of each of the three categories of beliefs
2. List and describe the characteristics of values
3. Explain and give examples of the relationship of beliefs and values to behavioral norms
4. Define and give examples of three kinds of sexual scripts
5. List and describe the three aspects of gender
6. Define sexual orientation

A basic aspect of personhood is a sense of self, which we experience as both our subjective, inner, generally moment-to-moment thoughts and feelings, and what we and others experience as our objective personal traits and patterns of interaction with the social and physical environments (*personality*). Furthermore, most of us believe that we are physically and psychologically unique in that our experiences, thoughts, feelings, ideas, and personal history—even if shared by others—are uniquely and unquestionably our own.

**sexual self** a sense of oneself as a sexual being

A significant part of your sense of self is your **sexual self**, which includes not only your awareness of your sexual biology and your sexual desires and feelings but also the beliefs and values that guide your sexual behavior, your sense of yourself as male or female and the ways you express that part of yourself, and your disposition regarding the sexuality of potential sex and intimate partners. In this chapter we examine these aspects of the sexual self.

## Beliefs

*Do you believe that men and women think differently?*

*Do you believe that being in love makes a person happy?*

*Do you believe that a special someone could be attracted to you?*

*Do you believe that sexual activity is OK only if the partners are married?*

**beliefs** thoughts and ideas you assume to be true
**conscious beliefs** thoughts one is aware of
**unconscious beliefs** thoughts one is unaware of
**attitudes** beliefs that are associated with a positive or negative judgment or evaluation of an idea, person, object, or group

**Beliefs** are thoughts and ideas that are assumed to be true. Beliefs can be taken on faith, or they can originate from having been tested against reality. We use beliefs to make sense of our experiences and to guide behaviors that are intended to satisfy our wants and needs and avoid suffering and pain. **Conscious beliefs** are ones you are aware of, which means you could describe them, and depending on your degree of self-knowledge, perhaps even describe how they affect your inner experience and your behavior. **Unconscious beliefs** are tucked away out of everyday conscious awareness, which means you cannot readily describe them or easily identify how they affect your inner experience or behavior. Unconscious beliefs are sometimes accessible through hypnosis, fantasies, dreams, and various forms of creative experience. And, they are sometimes evident to others from your behavior, even if you are not aware of them.

**Attitudes** are beliefs that are associated with a positive or negative judgment or evaluation of an idea, person, object, or group. For example, you might believe that men are by nature competitive, but your attitude about male competitiveness could be either positive or negative. Or, you may believe that sexual activity is pleasurable, but your attitude about sexual pleasure could be positive or negative.

In general, you have beliefs about (1) yourself as a unique physical and psychological entity, (2) how the social and physical/biological environments work, and (3) the consequences of particular *interactions* with the social and physical environments.

*Self-beliefs* refer to your view of yourself as a unique and separate physical and psychological entity. Kinds of self-beliefs include the following:

- *Self-image:* beliefs about your character or nature (I am generous; I am ambitious)
- *Self-esteem:* attitudes about yourself (I am good; I am flawed)
- *Body image:* beliefs about the appearance of your body (I am tall; Others find me attractive)
- *Body esteem:* attitudes about the appearance of your body (I like my body; I hate my body)

- *Agency:* believing that you can set goals and carry out strategies for accomplishing them rather than having your fate determined by people and circumstances not in your control (I can accomplish things; I am timid and need a lot of luck and others' help to get by)
- *Self-efficacy:* beliefs about how effectively you accomplish goals you set for yourself (I'm pretty good at starting up conversations with strangers I find attractive)

*How-the-environment-works beliefs* are about the nature of the physical and social environments, which you experience as outside of you. These beliefs include scientific or "natural" laws—for example, males make sperm, females bear children, or certain kinds of touching produce erotic arousal. They also include beliefs about aspects of human behavior that seem fundamental or "natural" ("human nature") whether or not they really are—for example the beliefs that men only want sex, women are more emotional than men are, and true love lasts forever.

*Self-in-world beliefs* are about the nature of your interrelatedness and interactions with the social and physical environments. Examples of these kinds of beliefs include the following:

- Strategies for getting your wants and needs met (If I get hammered when I party, I'll score some sex)
- Whether your personal attributes can lead to success in developing and maintaining a sexual or intimate relationship (When I am affectionate, my partner likes me)
- The kinds of sexual behaviors that are considered "proper" (Sexual intercourse is OK, but oral sex is not)
- Who may have sex with whom (Sex is OK for partners who love each other)

Self-in-world beliefs often include a sense of identification or belonging to something larger than oneself, such as a pair-bonded love relationship, a family, a clan, a religious group, a society, all of humanity, or some universal force or deity. Identification with a larger group brings a sense of safety and security, and the expectation of benefiting in various ways from interactions with other members in the group.

## Emotions

Beliefs are associated with emotions (**FIGURE 9.1**). **Emotions** are patterns of brain activity that can arise spontaneously or in response to what a person experiences, has experienced, or believes he or she may experience. Emotions generate a sense of pleasantness or unpleasantness, which helps someone evaluate as positive or negative an actual or anticipated experience and the outcome of a planned or actual behavior. The subjective experiencing of an emotion is a feeling.

**emotions** patterns of brain activity that generate a sense of pleasantness or unpleasantness, which leads to evaluations of anticipated or actual experience and the outcome of a planned or actual behavior

Besides providing an evaluation of an experience, emotions provide the energy or motivation for behavior. In general, pleasant emotions (e.g., joy, interest, contentment, love) motivate the pursuit of novel, creative, enjoyable activities, whereas unpleasant emotions (e.g., anger, fear, anxiety, disgust, guilt, shame) motivate aversion or avoidance to perceived threats to one's sense of well-being, physical safety, or survival.

One characteristic of mental health is having beliefs and emotions that are congruent with reality. This increases the likelihood of choosing behaviors that facilitate getting needs met and avoiding harm. Sometimes a belief is not congruent with reality because a person misperceives or misinterprets reality. Sometimes

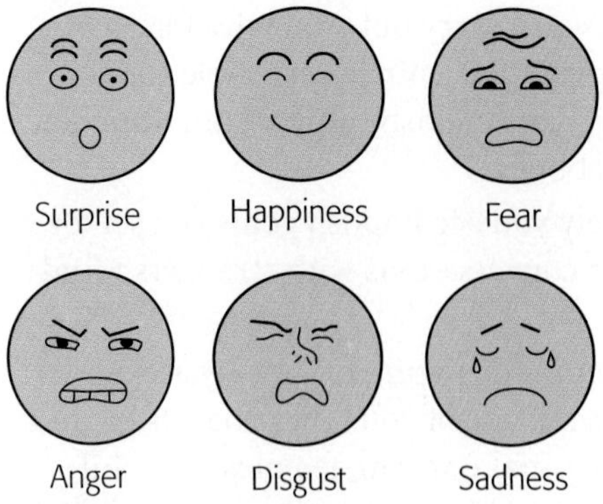


FIGURE 9.1 **Human Emotions.** Human emotions include interest, enjoyment, surprise, sadness, anger, disgust, fear, shyness, shame, and guilt. Forty-three muscles in the face automatically express six of the basic emotions: surprise, happiness, fear, anger, disgust, and sadness.
Adapted from Harrison, R. P. (1974). *Beyond words: An introduction to nonverbal communication*. Prentice-Hall, 120.

a person distorts the perception and interpretation of reality in order to avoid experiencing unpleasant thoughts, memories, emotions, and situations. These distortions are called *psychological defense mechanisms*. For example, *denial* is the defense of not believing a truth or believing a nontruth. An example of denial is not using a condom with a new sex partner even though one knows that this behavior risks getting an STD.

## Sexual Values

**values** beliefs pertaining to concepts of right and wrong, good and bad, moral and immoral

**Values** are a category of beliefs pertaining to concepts of right and wrong, good and bad, moral and immoral. Examples of values are "human life is precious," "all people are created equal," and "erotic pleasure is natural and therefore good." Values represent what are considered basic, universal truths derived from "natural law," "the universe," or a deity. Furthermore, values are believed to endure over time and transcend specific situations and an individual's unique attitudes. For example, the value that sex before marriage is wrong cannot be held in some situations and not others (*situation ethics*). Values are among people's most important beliefs (which is why they are called values and not something else). Values can be so important that people will fight and even die to defend them.

Sexual values can be represented through language. For example, the value "sex is wrong because it is of the flesh" gives rise to permissible ("clean") and nonpermissible ("dirty") sex-related vocabularies (Table 9.1). Permissible vocabularies include medical/scientific language (e.g., "penis," "breasts"), child euphemisms ("pee pee," "doo doo"), and personal sex-related vocabularies ("Mr. Jones," "cupcakes"). These represent ways to identify and describe sex-related body parts, reproduction, and sexual activities and experiences without engendering guilt or feeling immoral. Nonpermissible sex-related vocabularies include slang or "dirty" words, which generally are considered offensive but are often used.

All major religions provide guidance to adherents regarding sexual values, attitudes, and behaviors. For the most part, religions advocate that sexual activity occur only among heterosexual couples in permanent, marital-type relationships, claiming that same-sex and nonmarital sexual unions are sinful and contrary to God's intentions. Some religions also teach that the purpose of sexual activity is reproduction, and hence fertility control is disapproved of. American youth report that religion is one of the least influential factors in their sexual learning.

**Table 9.1** Sexual Vocabularies

| Vocabulary | Description | Examples |
|---|---|---|
| Medical/Scientific | These are "proper" words used when talking to adults, which are used sparingly to avoid being judged as impolite, vulgar, or immoral. One feature of medical/scientific sex-related vocabulary is that it is often too difficult to spell and pronounce to use in everyday discourse. | Penis, vagina, breasts |
| Child Euphemisms | Euphemisms are indirect words or expressions that substitute for terms that are considered improper or offensive. Sex-related euphemisms often are used when referring to sex or reproductive body parts in order to "protect" children from "adult" words that presumably would destroy a child's innocence. | Pee pee, wee wee, privates |
| Personal | These are unique words and expressions that families, friends, or intimate partners use for fun and/or because other words are difficult to pronounce or using them makes one feel guilty. | "Snoopy," "Mr. Jones," "cupcakes" |
| Slang/Dirty | These words must not be uttered, especially in front of children. Many parents try to prevent children from hearing and saying them. Warnings are provided to potential viewers that certain films and other media that may contain "adult language." It is a violation of federal law to air "obscene" programming at any time and "indecent" programming or "profane" language during certain hours. | Tits, cock |

## Sexual Norms

A group's shared beliefs, values, and attitudes give rise to rules of appropriate behavior (for that group) called **norms**. For example, the value that sexual activity is wrong except for producing children and maintaining marriage gives rise to norms permitting sexual intercourse only among individuals married to each other and prohibiting sexual intercourse with non-spouses, among all non-married adults, and between adults and children. A group can consist of many millions of individuals who share a set of religious beliefs, such as the people who adhere to traditional Judeo-Christian philosophy. Or, the group can consist of individuals in a particular society, a subcultural or ethnic group within a larger society, or a small number of students in a particular social clique in a particular school.

**norms** rules of appropriate behavior for a specific group based on that group's shared beliefs and values

**social role** a position or status within a group

Some norms are written into law—for example, our society's prohibition of prostitution. Some take the form of religious edicts or avowed expectations, such as the Sixth and Tenth Commandments ("Thou shalt not commit adultery;" "Thou shalt not covet thy neighbor's wife") and the Catholic Church's proscription against using fertility control methods. And some can be informal, which are understood but usually not codified, such as the expectation that men initiate sexual activity with women sex partners.

Norms apply to individuals within social roles. A **social role** is a position or status within a group. For example, in a college classroom, the person lecturing is in the role of teacher; those listening and taking notes are in the role of students. When the lecturer sits in a class and listens to another person lecturing, that person is in the role of student. A social role is analogous to a theatrical role in that it specifies appropriate (and inappropriate) behaviors for individuals in particular social roles instead of actors in theatrical ones. Most adults fill several roles simultaneously, such as student, employee, friend, boyfriend/girlfriend, spouse, parent, caretaker of a parent, and so on. They also fill sexual/relationship roles—for example, initiator and/or choreographer of a couple's sexual activities or being responsible for birth control.

Norms enable individuals to meet their basic biological and psychosocial needs in ways that sustain social harmony and cohesion and promote social continuity. When behavior is guided by norms, individuals know how to behave and what to expect. This lowers uncertainty, increases security, and sets the opportunity for collective action. If people behaved in any ways they pleased in order to meet their individual wants, needs, and goals, the result would be social chaos.

Sexual norms can vary tremendously among human societies and subgroups within a particular society. For example, when anthropologists first observed the Mangaians, who inhabit one of the Cook Islands in the South Pacific, they found that the culture placed a high value on erotic experience and encouraged all its adult members, whether or not they were married, to partake of this experience often.

In contrast to the Mangaians, anthropologists found that the inhabitants of the island of Inis Beag in Ireland did not value sexual experience. On the contrary, these people considered sex dirty and evil. Parents did not teach their children about sex or reproduction, principally because they were ignorant about such matters themselves. Young women were not prepared by their mothers (or other women) for their first menstrual periods, and many women went through life not knowing the significance of that biological occurrence. The people of Inis Beag lacked knowledge of French kissing, oral breast stimulation, female manipulation of the male genitals, oral sex, anal intercourse, and premarital and extramarital

## Dear Penelope . . .

***I'm 20 years old and have been heterosexual since I can remember, including beginning sexual activity with the opposite sex three years ago. Now I find myself strongly attracted to someone of my own sex, and that person is attracted to me, too.***

***If you told me a year ago this would happen to me, I would have said you were crazy. But now that it's happening it feels OK. I still like the opposite sex. Does this mean I'm bisexual? What will it mean for my future if I am?***

***— Bi-ding My Time***

*Dear Bi-ding My Time,*

Being attracted to individuals of both sexes is exceedingly common. And during their years of sexual emergence, many individuals experience same-sex as well as other-sex relationships. But attraction and the behavior or lifestyle you follow are separate issues. Whether you eventually develop the capacity to form strong sexual and emotional attachments to both sexes or orient to one remains to be seen.

Seeking to label your attractions (bisexual? Not bisexual?) is confusing. Instead, think in terms of what is actually happening right now: "I'm attracted to this person and that's how it is for now." Then think about what you want to do about this situation at this particular time in your life and what the consequences of the various choices might be.

The most important things are to accept yourself as you are and to be the best person you can be. It makes little difference whom you love—the key to fulfillment is how you love.

Courtesy of the UC Davis *Aggie*

sex. Female orgasm was completely unknown. Men believed sexual intercourse to be debilitating, and they refrained from sex if they anticipated having to do difficult work. Marital sex consisted primarily of a brief episode of sexual intercourse, with the man-on-top position the only one ever used. Since nudity was abhorred (the islanders bathed only once a week and in complete privacy), sexual interaction occurred while wearing underclothes.

## Sexual Values and Norms in North America

Common sexual value systems in North America include the following:

1. *Procreational*, which is based on the value that sexual activity is morally right only for reproduction. It establishes the following norms:
   - Sexual activity is limited to vaginal intercourse between male and female spouses.
   - Sexual activity is permissible only if conception is possible, which means sexual activity is not permitted during menstruation, pregnancy, or after menopause.
   - Sexual activity is prohibited prior to marriage, after marriage has ended through death of a spouse or divorce, with a person other than one's spouse, with children, and through masturbation.
2. *Relational*, which is based on the value that sexual activity is morally right in adult–adult, emotionally close relationships. It establishes the following norms:
   - Appropriate sex partners are adults regardless of marital status.
   - Close family members and persons married to others are not permissible sex partners.
   - Casual (nonemotional) sexual activity is wrong.
   - The main purpose of sexual activity is enhancing emotional closeness, not necessarily producing orgasms or pregnancy.
   - Any behavior is sexually permissible if the partners agree to it.
3. *Recreational* (hedonistic), which is based on the value that erotic pleasure is "natural" and can be experienced for its own sake. It establishes the following norms:
   - Sexual behavior is appropriate with any consenting adult(s).
   - An emotional or social relationship among the sexual partners is not required.
   - The goal of sexual activity is personal pleasure.
   - Any mutually agreed on activity that enhances sexual pleasure is permissible.

## Socialization

Beliefs, values, and norms are acquired through **socialization**, the process by which individuals learn the behavioral rules of the social group(s) to which they belong, and thereby learn how to get along with others. They also learn the penalties for not conforming to their group's expectations. Individuals acquire their beliefs, values, and behavioral expectations from a variety of influences, called **agents of socialization**, including the family, school, peer group, religion, employment settings, organizations to which individuals belong (e.g., fraternities, sports teams), and the mass media.

**socialization** the process by which individuals learn the behavioral rules of the social group(s) to which they belong

**agents of socialization** social and cultural groupings that instill in members group-specific beliefs, values, attitudes, and rules of behavior

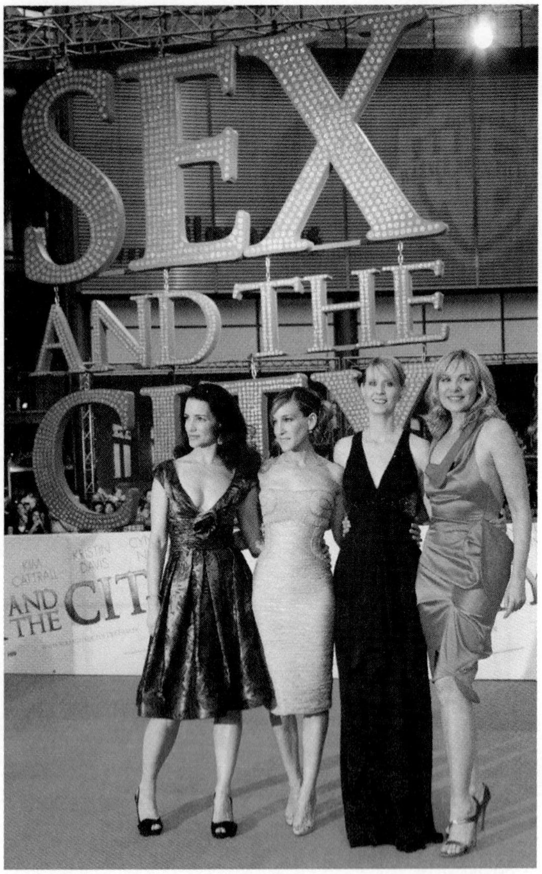


Mass media (such as television, magazines, and the Internet) are major influences on sexual socialization.

In North America, *sexual socialization* is primarily influenced by peers and media. Both other- and same-sex peers share information about sex (although not always correct, such as "You can't get pregnant the first time you have intercourse"), and they model sexual behavior. Peers provide an opportunity to talk openly about sex, to shape gender and sexual attitudes, and influence behavior through discussion, questioning, teasing, daring, and shaming. Most important, peers provide the relational contexts for experimenting with sex and developing one's sexual identity.

Mass media (television, magazines, popular music, film, and the Internet) have a major influence on sexual socialization. For example, more than half of adolescents cite television as an important source of information about preventing unintended pregnancy. Most scripted television programming for adolescents contains sexual content, including talking about sex and to a significant degree precursory sexual behaviors such as flirting and passionate kissing; some programs present implied or actual sexual intercourse. About half of the content of popular music is sex related. Some is playful and romantic, and some is hostile and degrading.

It might be assumed that parents are major influences on their children's sexual socialization. In some instances, parents are effective guides and role models, enabling their children to learn the facts of their sexual biology, clarify their sexual values, manage their emerging sexual identity and feelings, and adopt appropriate sexual behaviors. However, in many instances, parental influence on children's sexual development is problematic. Parents may be sexually uninformed and hence refrain from discussing sex with their children for fear of embarrassment or losing status. They may harbor sex-negative attitudes and experience sexual communication with children or anyone else as distasteful and difficult. Typically, parent–child communication about sex is infrequent, and when it occurs, it tends to be conducted by mothers. In general, communicative parents talk about biological development (e.g., bodily functions, menstruation, biological changes) and sexual safety (e.g., contraception, STD, HIV/AIDS prevention) but not about sex in relationships, sex and love, or sexual pleasure. Apparently this is all right with many preteen and adolescent children, who find discussions with parents intrusive, less informative than with peers, more controlling, more likely to involve unwanted topics, and more likely to avoid issues important to them.

## Sexual Scripts

**sexual scripts** norms of preferred sexual behavior

Norms of preferred sexual behavior are called **sexual scripts**. These include contextual scripts, behavioral scripts, and motivational scripts.

*Contextual scripts* specify the social context for permissible sexual activities—for example, who may be sexual with whom based on the sexual partners' role relationships. An example of a contextual sexual script is according marital partners the right—and in some societies the duty—to be sexual with each other. When individuals enter their society's definition of marriage, and hence adopt the social role of spouse, they receive their society's permission to be sexual with each other, and in about half of human societies, to be sexual with no one else. In contrast, in many human cultures, sexual relations with a non-spouse are permitted in certain circumstances or contexts. For example, among Eskimos, a male visitor to a household is permitted to have sex with the woman of the host couple. Contextual scripts can have names, such as "marriage," "having an affair," or "casual sex," which help the participants know how to behave and what to expect.

*Behavioral scripts* specify which activities are deemed "proper" for creating sexual experiences and also the sequence of such activities ("sexual choreography"). Examples of behavioral sexual scripts include that heterosexual intercourse always take place in the man-on-top position, that heterosexual activity almost always begin with breast stimulation, or that one partner be active and the other passive during sex.

An example of sexual choreography is the script that calls for erotic pleasure to be created in a specified sequence of acts—for example, first kissing, then touching of the female breasts, then mutual touching of the genitals, then oral–genital stimulation, and finally sexual intercourse. A different script would call for only some fondling prior to intercourse, or perhaps engaging in intercourse soon after partners agree to have sex, and nonintercourse sexual arousal ("foreplay") occurs subsequent to the initial episode of sexual intercourse and as a prelude to a second.

*Motivational scripts* specify the "appropriate" reasons for sexual activities. People can have sex for a variety of reasons: to create children, to experience sexual pleasure for its own sake, to create and enhance intimacy and feelings of emotional bonding, and for a variety of nonsexual reasons, such as earning money, accomplishment, giving/getting comfort, relieving loneliness, escaping boredom, duty, confirming one's social desirability, or proving one's masculinity or femininity (see Chapter 2).

Motivational scripts also include the internal and environmental cues that can permissibly be interpreted as *sexual cues* or *sexual signals* (see Chapter 10). They include a person's feelings of sexual desire, the behavior of a potential sex partner, interacting with certain objects that suggest sex, seeing regions of another's body such as the genitalia or breasts, and being touched in certain ways.

*Individual scripts* are personally designed modifications (or even replacements) of a group's acceptable sexual scripts intended to meet the designers' individual needs. For example, a group's norm might call for men to initiate social activity, but a woman in that group may find it necessary or more in keeping with her personality to ask men for dates. Trying to meet one's needs by behaving in accordance with an individual sexual script may pose problems. If others consider the behaviors "unnatural" or dangerous, the individual may be punished, castigated, or exiled from the group. Another potential problem with individual scripts is that a sexual partner who does not know the script may not know what to expect or how to behave, leading to confusion and hurt feelings. For example, one partner may be behaving in accordance with a "sex-for-fun" script and another a "sex-for-getting-emotionally-involved" script.

## Maleness/Femaleness (Gender)

A fundamental aspect of the sexual self is **gender** (derived from the Latin *genus*, meaning type, kind, or sort), which refers to the tendency for individuals to classify themselves—and be classified by their social group—socially, psychologically, behaviorally, and even morally according to their biological sex. Gender is a complex attribute encompassing beliefs about the basic nature of each sex (*gender*

**gender** classifying individuals socially, psychologically, behaviorally, and even morally according to their biological sex *stereotypes*), social expectations based on biological sex (*gender role*), and a fundamental part of one's sense of self (*gender identity*).

## Gender Stereotypes

**gender stereotypes** beliefs about the "natural" or "typical" characteristics of men and women
**gender role** socially desirable behavioral expectations of men and women

A stereotype is an exaggerated image of the characteristics of a particular group. **Gender stereotypes** are beliefs about the "natural" or "typical" characteristics of men and women. For example, men, as compared with women, might be believed to be aggressive, logical, independent, and unemotional, whereas women, as compared with men, might be believed to be cooperative, intuitive, dependent, and emotional. Nearly all social groups possess gender stereotypes.

Many individuals do not conform to a gender stereotype even if they endorse one for others and wish they could be more like a stereotype (*gender ideal*). Some males are cooperative and some females are competitive. Some males are competitive but not aggressive. Some women are aggressive and emotionally expressive. *Androgyny* (*andro* refers to male and *gyn* refers to female) is the tendency to express characteristics typical of both gender stereotypes.

Gender stereotypes often are enforced by negative attitudes about and consequent shaming of individuals who do not conform to the accepted stereotype. For example, a boy who plays with dolls may be derided as a sissy. A girl who plays football and climbs trees may be called a tomboy. Women who are aggressive and competitive (for example, a female corporate CEO or national leader) might be considered by some to be, at the least, unfeminine and possibly even masculine (a "ball buster").

## Gender Role

The **gender role** consists of socially desirable behavioral expectations of men and women (e.g., men are lumberjacks, women clean the house, men take the lead in sex). For example, the traditional gender role for American males calls for them to

### HEALTHY SEXUALITY

### Civil Unions and Same-Sex Marriage

Marriage is a social custom that is thousands of years old. Although varying in detail depending on the society, marriage is fundamentally a system of rules, the purposes of which are to control reproduction (who procreates with whom), manage property rights, identify lineage, and form stable, parental, social, and economic units (families). For almost all of recorded history, marriage was entered into by interpersonal agreement. Although marriage can still be entered into by interpersonal agreement ("common law" marriage), many cultures now codify marriage as a legal institution requiring a civil marriage license and adherence to a variety of laws relating to the rights and responsibilities of spouses. Besides a legal institution, in some cultures marriage is also a religious entity.

One aspect of marital law is codifying who may marry whom. The defining criterion can be age, religion, social class, income, race, prior and current marital status, and/or sexual orientation. For many centuries, a variety of societies have prohibited interracial marriage and interracial sexual relationships (referred to by the pejorative *miscegenation*, meaning to "mix races"). In the United States, anti-miscegenation laws came into being during colonial times and persisted in many jurisdictions for hundreds of years despite the fact that the U.S. population has always been a mixture of different races and ethnic groups. The last U.S. anti-miscegenation law (in Virginia) was struck down by the U.S. Supreme Court in 1967. Today, one in 15 American marriages is interracial. Clearly, American society has changed its views on interracial marriages, but it took a long time.

Currently, many countries, including the United States, are considering extending *legal* marital status—and the rights, benefits, and responsibilities that accompany it—to same-sex couples. To separate legal status from religious and other cultural definitions of marriage, in many countries same-sex relationships are called *civil unions* and not marriages. In 2003 Massachusetts became the first state to grant same-sex couples the status of legally *married*, acknowledging that denying this right is a form of discrimination similar to anti-miscegenation laws. Same-sex marriage is now under consideration in many states, especially since in 2010 a U.S. court ruled that the Defense of Marriage Act (DOMA), passed in 1996, is discriminatory in that it deprives same-sex couples many rights enjoyed by legally married couples; for example, filing joint tax returns, adding a partner to a health policy, or leaving an inheritance to a longtime partner.

compete for economic resources and to share what they acquire with a chosen mate and any children they have. Men also are expected to defend themselves, their families, and their social group with acts of violence. The traditional gender role for women calls for them to marry, see to the emotional and physical needs of spouses and children, and maintain the household. This is true even if a woman also works outside the home in the paid workforce.

It has been suggested that the traditional American gender roles—the male as provider and protector and the woman as child caretaker and homemaker—are vestiges of a division of labor based on biological sex that might have existed thousands of years ago among the first human groups. Back then, as the theory goes, people were nomadic hunters and gatherers that roamed the countryside looking for food. By virtue of their physical strength and agility, males in these groups fought and hunted, whereas the females, their mobility hindered by the needs of small children to be breastfed and otherwise cared for, benefitted from the hunting and fighting skills of a male.

Whereas such sex-specific behaviors may have been necessary for the survival of early humans, they no longer strictly apply in modern, technologically based societies. In some families, a complete gender-role reversal occurs, with the female assuming the provider role and the male serving as the caretaker of children and the home.

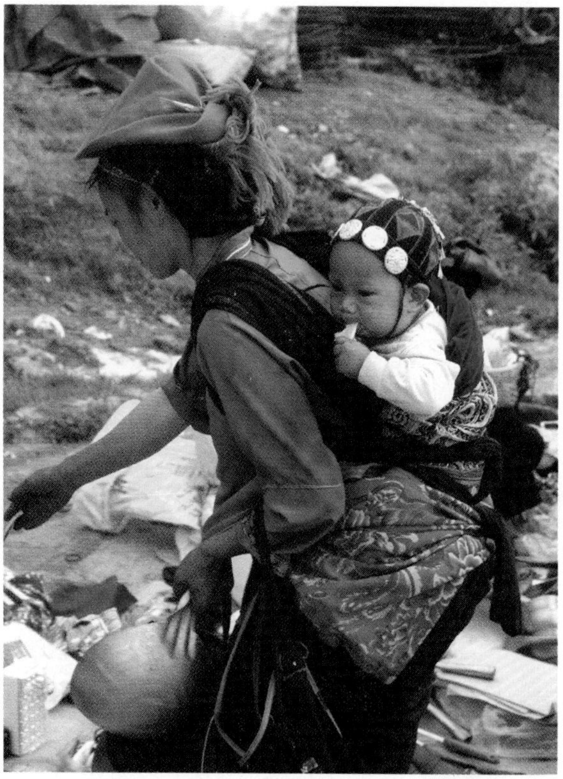

In many cultures, gender role behaviors represent a division of labor based on biological sex.

## Gender Identity

**gender identity** self-identification as a biological and social male or female

**transgenderism** gender identity not congruent with the biological sex

**Gender identity** is the personal sense of one's maleness or femaleness. Individuals use their gender identity to classify themselves as members of either the male, female, or nongendered social group and to adopt beliefs, attitudes, and behaviors they believe to be characteristic and appropriate for members of their group (e.g., "boys don't cry," "girls play with dolls") and avoid attributes believed to be characteristic of the other groups. Gender identity is a core belief, which means that it is deeply integrated into one's sense of self. Gender identity develops in most individuals by the age of two, and it tends not to change, although occasionally some individuals may "role play" as the other gender from time to time for amusement.

Most of the time, one's gender identity is consistent with one's anatomical sex—that is, the presence of male biology goes with an inner sense of maleness and the presence of female biology goes with an inner sense of femaleness. However, in a very few individuals, the gender identity is not consistent with the biological sex, a situation referred to as **transgenderism**. These individuals fundamentally and sincerely believe themselves to be women or men "trapped" in the body of the other sex. As children they insist they are the other biological sex. They often dress like, play with toys characteristic of, and prefer playmates of the other sex. As teenagers and adults, they may reject their own biological sexuality and dress and behave as the other biological sex. They may take hormones or undergo surgery to attain a body that is congruent with their gender identity. A biological male who feels like a female and is attracted to men probably would not consider himself homosexual, although some others might.

People often confuse transgenderism, transvestism, and homosexuality.

- Transgenderism refers strictly to gender identity, and whether this sense of oneself is congruent with one's sexual anatomy.
- Transvestism is adopting the appearance of the other sex. Societies tend to dictate how men and women should dress; whether or not to wear jewelry, or which kind; the type of body art; and the length of the hair. It is possible to adorn oneself as a member of the other sex so thoroughly that hardly anyone can discern the ruse. For example, a human sexuality instructor may wear a man's business suit, have short hair, speak in a baritone voice, and insist on being addressed as Mr. So-and-so, and may even tell personal stories suggesting a typical male life history, but none of this can assure students that their instructor is a biological male.
- Homosexuality is the propensity to be sexually attracted to and generally desirous of emotional attachment to members of one's own biological sex. Nearly always, a homosexual individual's gender identity is consistent with her or his biological sex. Homosexual men and women do not consider themselves to be members of the other sex, and they do not wish to be so.

## Sexual Orientation

**sexual orientation** the propensity to be sexually attracted to and generally desirous of emotional attachment to members of a particular biological sex

**Sexual orientation** is the propensity to be sexually attracted to and generally desirous of emotional attachment to members of a particular biological sex (**Table 9.2**). In some individuals, sexual orientation is exclusive for members of their own biological sex (called *homosexuality*) or the other biological sex (called *heterosexuality*). In others, sexual orientation is not particularly exclusive; sexual and romantic attraction can be for men and women, although attraction for one sex may predominate. This type of sexual orientation is called *bisexual*. For some, a particular sexual orientation is lifelong, whereas for others it may change—more than once.

Many people have some same-sex sexual experience, often occurring in childhood and adolescence when sexual experimentation is common. About 10% of American adults say they are occasionally erotically aroused by same-sex individuals, although they do not wish to act on those feelings. An additional 5% of American men and 3% of American women are exclusively attracted to mem-

**Table 9.2** Factors Associated with Sexual Orientation

| Factor | Description |
|---|---|
| Orientation Identity | The self-identification of one's orientation as same sex, other sex, any sex, or none. |
| Sexual Attraction | The biological sex of persons found sexually attractive and arousing. Attraction can be exclusively to same- or other-sex individuals, or both. |
| Sexual Behavior | The sex of partners with whom one engages in sexual activity. |
| Sexual Fantasies | The biological sex of partners in sexual fantasy. |
| Emotional Bonding | The sex of individuals with whom one "falls in love." |
| Social Preference | The orientation of people with whom one socializes ("hangs out"; parties). |
| Lifestyle | The social/political/community subculture in which one participates (gay, lesbian, bi, queer, straight). |

Adapted from Klein, F., Sepekoff, B., & Wolf, T. J. (1985). Sexual orientation: A multi-variate dynamic process. *Journal of Homosexuality, 11*, 35–49.

bers of their own sex. These people tend to call themselves and are labeled by others as *homosexuals*, *gays*, and if women, *lesbians*. The prevalence of sexual orientation among American and Canadian college students follows a similar pattern: approximately 3% of males and 2% of females identify themselves as homosexual, 80% to 85% are heterosexual, and others are bisexual.

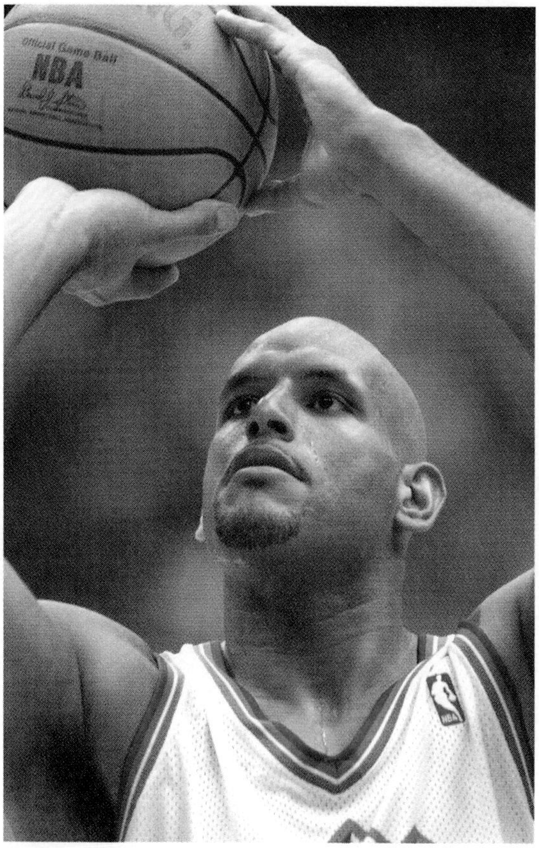

Former NBA star John Amaechi is gay.

Almost from the beginning of the scientific study of human sexuality about 150 years ago, with some exceptions, researchers have generally assumed that heterosexual orientation is fundamental to human sexuality because it facilitates reproduction. If there were no mechanisms to orient adults into other-sex sexual unions, it is argued, people might have sex with anyone. In this circumstance, many sexual encounters would be reproductively fruitless, and hence biologically maladaptive.

Within this line of thought, homosexual orientation is considered aberrant because it does not produce children (although many gay and lesbian individuals and couples adopt children and are excellent parents). Indeed, for many years homosexuality was referred to scientifically as "sexual deviation" or "sexual inversion" to denote its seeming opposition to the biological norm. This kind of thinking supported the myth—now completely rejected—that homosexual men were "feminized" males and homosexual women were "masculinized" females. Ample scientific evidence, however, has shown that there is no relationship between sexual orientation and either sexual anatomy, gender identity, or gender role beliefs and behaviors.

Because of the reproduction bias, much research has been—and continues to be—focused on finding explanations for how the presumed "normal" developmental path to heterosexual orientation is diverted to a homosexual one. So far, however, scientific studies have failed to uncover any social, developmental, genetic, hormonal, or metabolic explanation for homosexual orientation, although there are many theories (Table 9.3). The neuropsychological mechanisms underlying the development and patterning of sexual orientation—whether exclusively same-sex, other-sex, or either sex—are unknown. A vast majority of male homosexuals and lesbians believe that genetics (meaning biology and not necessarily heredity; see Chapter 7), as opposed to family environment, parenting style, or positive or negative influences with same- or other-sex individuals, has a great impact on the development of sexual orientation in anyone.

Traditionally, American culture has strongly forbidden same-sex intimate and sexual relationships, asserting that they are wrong, immoral, unnatural, or indicative of psychological illness. Thus, those whose sexual orientation is homosexual and who choose to live in accordance with their orientation—that is, by "being out"—often face prejudice, social ostracism, and even physical danger and death. Such prejudice and ostracism make it very difficult for people to live an openly homosexual lifestyle, and for young people to accept, assert, and openly display their sexual orientation ("come out") if it is not heterosexual (Table 9.4). Neither the American Psychological Association nor the American Psychiatric Association considers same-sex orientation to be a mental illness, nor is it associated with an increased risk of any kind of abnormal behavior, including child molestation. In 2010, the U.S. military stopped its practice of banning homosexual and bisexual persons from military service.

**Table 9.3** Causative Hypotheses of Same-Sex Orientation

Note that no hypothesis has yet to explain the "causes" of sexual orientation.

| Hypothesis | Description |
|---|---|
| Birth Order | Pregnancy with a male fetus produces an anti-androgen immune response, which lowers androgen levels in subsequent male fetuses, thus explaining the observation that gay men tend to have older brothers. |
| Prenatal Hormonal Environment | Exposure of the brain to low levels of androgen in fetal life fosters same-sex orientation in males, and exposure to high androgen and low estrogen fosters same-sex orientation in females. |
| Hormonal | Homosexual men have less testosterone or other androgens, and lesbians have more estrogen, than heterosexual peers |
| Genetic | Among twins, the probability of both individuals having same-sex orientation is greater (but *not* absolute) if the twins are identical rather than fraternal. Some variants of particular genes on the X chromosome are found more often in male homosexual twins. |
| Freudian Psychoanalytic | Failure to psychologically identify with the same-sex parent results in stunted sexual development, including rejection of other-sex individuals as potential sex partners. |
| Parental Dynamics | Homosexual males have a dominant, overprotective mother and a passive, distant father with whom a son could not identify. Lesbians have rejecting or indifferent mothers. |
| Learning/Conditioning | Early-life experiences condition an individual to dislike members of the other sex (intended or inadvertent fondling of the genitals by a same-sex individual, negative messages about heterosexual orientation, inadequate heterosexual social skills). |
| Gender | Fearing rejection by same-sex peers, boys exhibiting traditionally feminine characteristics and girls exhibiting traditional male characteristics may label the arousal from that fear as sexual attraction for others experienced as different and intriguing. |

**Table 9.4** Features Associated with "Coming Out"*

| Feature | Description |
|---|---|
| Personal Confusion/Fear | Awareness (often since childhood) of same-sex attractions and awareness that such attractions are different and perhaps wrong |
| Self-Identification | Considering or actually acknowledging one's same-sex orientation to oneself |
| Exploration | Reading about, talking to others about, and possibly experimenting with same-sex identity, activities, relationships, and lifestyle to investigate the personal and social meanings of same-sex orientation |
| Personal Integration | Willingness to integrate same-sex orientation into one's personality and, when appropriate, to share that aspect of oneself with others |
| The "First Telling" | Speaking or writing to a trusted other (friend, family member, teacher, counselor, support group), or messaging someone online, about one's orientation |
| Unsupportive Reactions | Understanding and preparing for others to be shocked, frightened, disappointed, or angry to learn of one's orientation |
| Rejection | Being prepared to accept another's rejection with the knowledge that one's self-esteem and personhood need not be subject to another's fears and prejudices, and with the hope that education and a prior healthy relationship may lead to eventual understanding and acceptance |

*Coming out is acknowledging and accepting one's sexual orientation as lesbian or gay and generally sharing that aspect of oneself with others.

Sexual orientation does not, in itself, affect the desire to love and be loved and to be involved in a committed, caring relationship. Many people believe same-sex couples should be legally permitted to marry and thereby gain the same rights and social status that other-sex couples have. With the possible exception that they involve far fewer gender-stereotypical behaviors, by and large, same-sex intimate relationships are similar to other-sex ones:

- Same-sex-oriented individuals tend to meet potential dating, sexual, and romantic partners through work, school, friends, and recreational activities. More frequently than in other-sex romantic relationships, same-sex relationships tend to develop from the partners' friendship.
- Relationship satisfaction and stability are related to similarity in partners' values and backgrounds, perceptions of equity, experiencing togetherness, intimacy, commitment, and sexual exclusivity, and being embedded in a supportive family and community environment.
- Relationship dissolution occurs at the same frequency as that of other-sex, cohabiting pairs. Individuals from "broken" same-sex relationships tend to remain friends more often than those from other-sex relationships do.
- Sexual satisfaction is related to overall relationship satisfaction. Sexual relating among lesbians can include considerable hugging, cuddling, and fondling without emphasis on orgasm; in some lesbian relationships sexual contact, although not expressions of emotional closeness, is infrequent. Male same-sex relationships may or may not include sexual exclusivity even if the partners have a long-term emotional commitment.
- Relationship violence occurs for the same reasons as it does in other-sex relationships: dependency, jealousy, money, power, and substance abuse.

## SEXUALITY IN REVIEW

- Fundamental to personhood is the sense of oneself as a sexual being, involving sexually related beliefs, attitudes, feelings, behavioral tendencies, and preferences for potential sexual and intimate partners.
- Beliefs are thoughts that are assumed to be true. There are beliefs about oneself, how the world works, and interaction with the physical and social environments.
- Values are beliefs pertaining to concepts of right and wrong, good and bad, moral and immoral. Values have the quality of coming from nature, a deity, or the universe and persisting over time.
- Beliefs and values give rise to rules of social behavior called norms.
- Beliefs, values, and behavioral norms are acquired by the process of socialization.
- Sexual orientation is the propensity to desire sexual and intimate interaction with individuals of one's same biological sex (homosexual), the other sex (heterosexual), or both sexes (bisexual).

## CRITICAL THINKING ABOUT SEXUALITY

1. Agents of socialization are elements in society that influence the adoption of values, beliefs, attitudes, and rules of appropriate behavior by society's members. Agents of *sexual socialization* influence the adoption of *sexual*

values, beliefs, attitudes, and behaviors. Examples of socializing agents are family, peers, media, school, and religion. Consider yourself a sociologist who is interested in determining the relative strength of the various possible agents of sexual socialization on college students. Regardless of the method you use to carry out your research, you must first choose what you think are the most influential agents of sexual socialization to consider. Make a list of the most influential agents of sexual socialization on college students. Rank your choices from most to least influential. Write a paragraph or two justifying each choice, using your own life experience and observations of your peers. What kind of study would you use (see Chapter 1) to test the validity of your list?

2. Imagine that you are a parent of a 15-year-old who has recently become involved in a very intense "first love" relationship with a 16-year-old schoolmate. What advice, if any, would you offer your child about the role of sex in life and relationships? What criteria would you want your child to use to guide her or his sexual life?
3. Describe three social expectations of you as a member of your biological sex. How do these expectations affect you personally? Are these expectations fair?
4. Respond to this letter as if you were Penelope, the advice columnist:

***Dear Penelope,***

***One of my friends is gay and so far has been hiding it from almost everyone (including parents) except a few of us close friends. Now that we're in college my friend doesn't want to hide any longer and wants to "come out." This is a scary prospect for my friend. What can I do to support my friend's courageous move?***

***— Wants to Be a Good Friend***

## REFERENCES AND RECOMMENDED RESOURCES

### References

Brannon, L. (2008). *Gender: Psychological perspectives, 5th ed.* Upper Saddle River, NJ: Prentice-Hall.

Diamond, L. M. (2003). What does sexual orientation orient? *Psychological Review, 110*, 173–192.

Ellis, R., Robb, B., & Burke, D. (2005). Sexual orientation in United States and Canadian college students. *Archives of Sexual Behavior, 34*, 569–581.

Gavin, L. E., et al. (2010). A review of positive youth development programs that promote adolescent sexual and reproductive health. *Journal of Adolescent Health, 46*, S75–S91.

Kinnish, K. K., Strassberg, D. S., & Turner, C. W. (2005). Sex differences in the flexibility of sexual orientation: A multidimensional retrospective assessment. *Archives of Sexual Behavior, 34*, 173–183.

Otis, M. D., & Skinner, W. F. (2004). An exploratory study of differences in view for factors affecting sexual orientation for a sample of lesbians and gay men. *Psychological Reports, 94*, 1173–1179.

Sax, L. (2006). *Why gender matters.* New York: Broadway.

Seidman, S. (2009). *The social construction of sexuality, 2nd ed.* New York: W. W. Norton.

## Recommended Resources

Cloud, J. (2008, January 17). Are gay relationships different? *Time*. A first-person account of a love relationship between two men.

Connell, R. W. (2005). *Masculinities*. Berkeley: University of California Press. Argues that there are many concepts for masculinity and shows how males strive to achieve their masculine identities.

Gagnon, J. H., & Simon, W. (1973). *Sexual conduct: The social sources of human sexuality*. Piscataway, NJ: Aldine. Discusses how sexual activities of all kinds may be understood in terms of sexual scripts, the ways in which sexuality is learned and expressed as different modes of behavior.

Ghosh, S. (2009). Sexuality, gender identity. Available at: http://emedicine.medscape.com/article/917990-overview. A professor of pediatrics explains the development of gender, gender identity, and gender role.

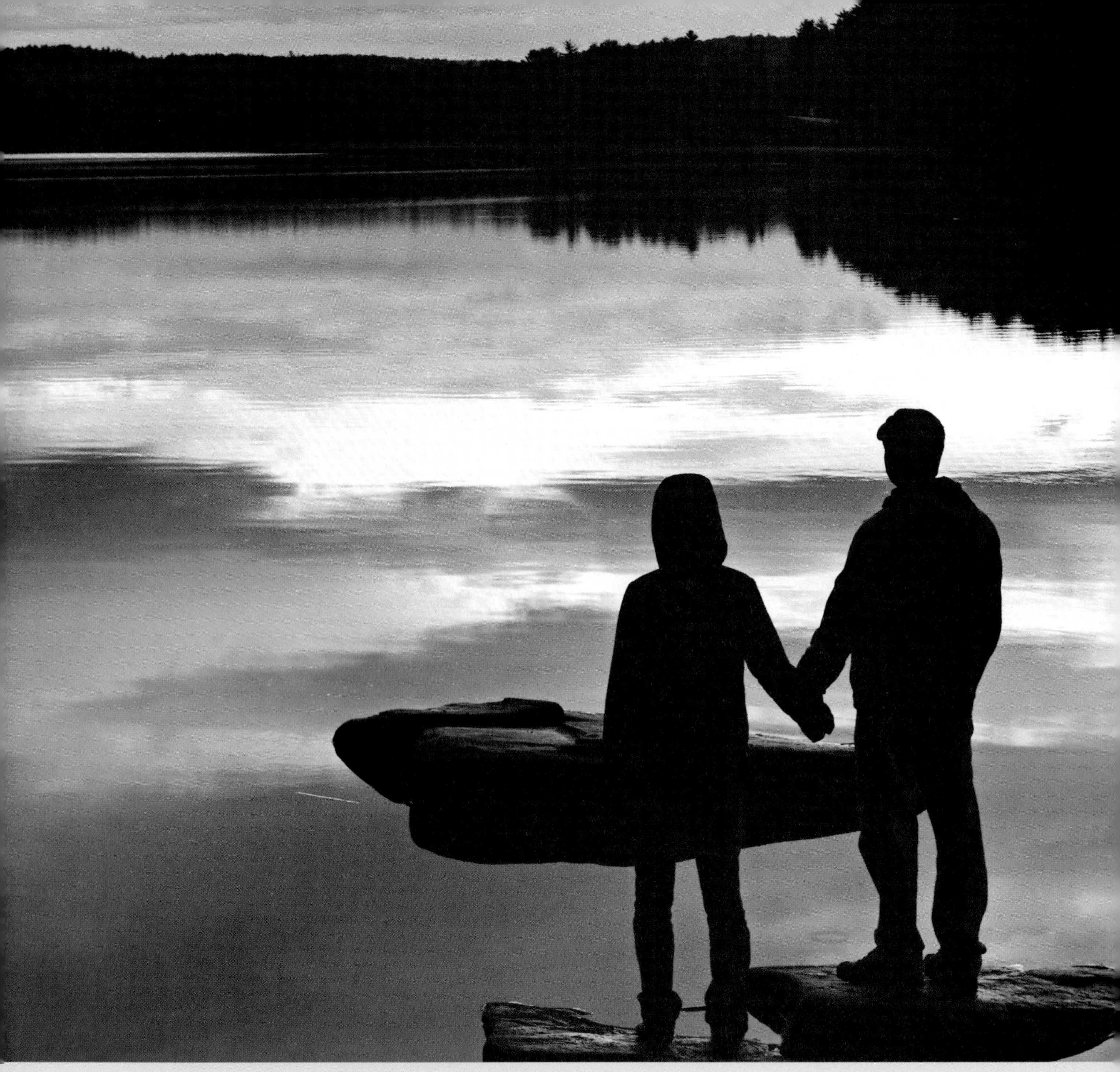

*"Sex and beauty are inseparable, like life and consciousness."*

— D. H. Lawrence

CHAPTER 10

# Sexual Arousal and Response

## Student Learning Objectives

1. Describe sexual interest and desire
2. Define transitioning to an erotic experience
3. Define and list factors that produce sexual arousal
4. Describe the characteristics of human sexual response
5. List and describe common sexual difficulties and their management
6. Provide examples of effective sexual communication
7. Describe the effects of drugs and alcohol on sexual experience
8. Explain masturbation and sexual abstinence

Sexual experiences are often thought of in terms of genital stimulation, genital responses, and orgasm. However, sex is a whole-person experience involving the body, mind, emotions, and spirit. The body dimension is one of sensations and physiological responses. The mental dimension consists of meaning-making: what is the significance of this experience to my life? The emotional dimension is one of feelings, such as joy, excitement, pleasure, and often also love and affection. The spiritual dimension is a state of consciousness that carries the sense of being part of something greater than oneself.

Sexual experience generally involves a change from an everyday, task-oriented, nonerotic state of being to an erotic one characterized by sexual arousal, erotic adventure, and/or sexual intimacy. The erotic state of being generally includes the following elements:

- *Sexual interest:* an openness or willingness to being erotically aroused
- *Sexual desire:* having an urge for erotic experience
- *Decision:* offering or accepting invitations for sex
- *Participation:* engaging in behaviors that produce erotic arousal
- *Evaluation:* interpreting and judging erotic experience

In this chapter we discuss these elements of sexual experience as well as sexual fantasy, drugs and sexual experience, masturbation, and sexual abstinence.

## Sexual Interest

Sexual interest is a willingness to have sexual experiences. Sexual interest is characterized by the awareness in oneself of sexual feelings, the presence of sexual thoughts and/or sexual fantasies, and a psychological openness to experiencing erotic sensations and pleasure. Every human society ever studied acknowledges that most of its adult members are interested in sex. Fifty percent of adult American men and 20% of adult American women report thinking about sex daily.

Although interest in sex is prevalent, it is neither universal nor constant among individuals. A few individuals claim never to have been interested in sexual experience. Many adults are aware of times in their lives when sexual interest was low or seemingly absent (FIGURE 10.1). For example, some women report a transient loss of sexual interest during pregnancy and for a time after childbirth. Both women and men may experience loss of sexual interest due to stress, overwork, fatigue, illness, fear of emotional closeness, and prior sexual trauma.

### Hormones and Sexual Interest

In both men and women, sexual interest is influenced very strongly by androgenic hormones, which are manufactured in the testes, ovaries, and adrenal glands (see Chapters 2 and 3). That sexual interest increases dramatically during the surge of androgenic hormones in both sexes at puberty suggests this relationship. By contrast, men with very low levels of androgens usually report little or no interest in sex. However, testosterone replacement in such individuals frequently increases the level of sexual interest, as measured by the frequency of erotic thoughts, erotic fantasies, sex-seeking behaviors, and sexual activity.

Similarly, women who have had their ovaries and adrenal glands surgically removed for treatment of cervical or breast cancer (to prevent secretion of bodily hormones that might facilitate cancer growth) often report a loss of interest in sex; however, interest in sex can be restored by treatment with testosterone but not with estrogen or progesterone.

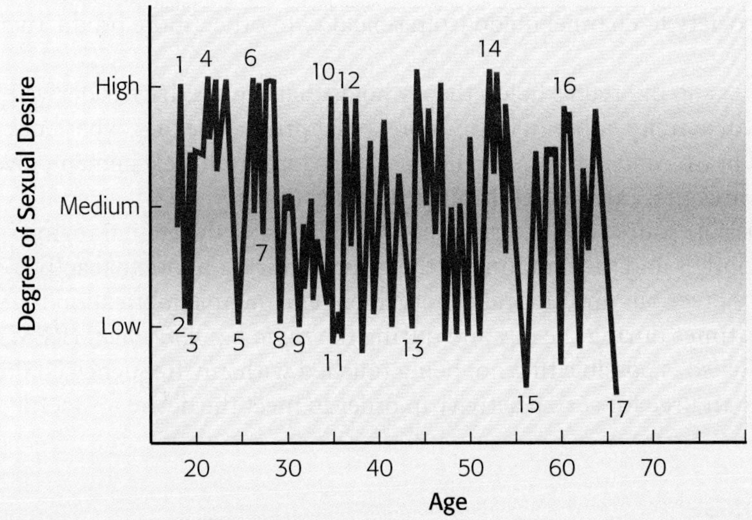


1. First serious love relationship
2. Breakup of first serious love relationship
3. College final exams
4. Love relationship with future spouse
5. Pre-wedding jitters
6. Honeymoon
7. Relocation to new community
8. Pregnancy, birth, and care of first child
9. Pregnancy, birth, and care of second child (and first child)
10. Two-week vacation in Hawaii without children
11. Job Loss
12. Start new family business
13. Business setbacks, marital stress, first child school problems
14. Both children in college in another state
15. Intense caretaking of sick parent
16. Retirement travel
17. Loss of spouse to death

FIGURE 10.1 **Variations in the Degree of Sexual Interest Across the Lifespan.** The cultural stereotype holds that sexual desire increases at puberty, remains high throughout early adulthood, and then wanes with increasing age. The reality is that sexual interest varies over time, often influenced by life events.

## Sexual Desire

**sexual desire** an urge to experience sexual pleasure and/or sexual intimacy

Sexual desire is an urge that motivates a person to experience sexual pleasure and/or sexual intimacy. Unlike sexual interest, which tends to be relatively stable over time, sexual desire, similar to hunger for food, is periodic.

Sexual desire can manifest as focused thinking about sex, seeking or being receptive to participating in sexual activity, or heightened states of sexual arousal *during* sexual activity. Whereas the media and popular myth espouse the expectation that one should be highly desirous of sex almost all the time, in reality, both the frequency and intensity of sexual desire vary from person to person and from day to day in the same person (FIGURE 10.2). Sexual desire often is affected by nonsexual aspects of one's life. For example, a high degree of sexual desire/passion is common at the beginning of an emotionally close relationship. In contrast, sexual desire may lessen due to illness or stress and the effects of certain medications.

### The Sex Drive

Sexual desire can be experienced as occurring spontaneously within oneself, producing a state of biological or psychological hunger, tension, or need, called the *sex drive*. The hunger created by the sex drive (referred to as sexual passion, lust, "being horny") is usually genitally focused and motivates seeking sexual pleasure or release to reduce sexual tension or need.

Sigmund Freud referred to the sex drive as *libido*, which means "pleasure seeking." Freud postulated that libido was instinctual—that is, a product of human biology. Freud further

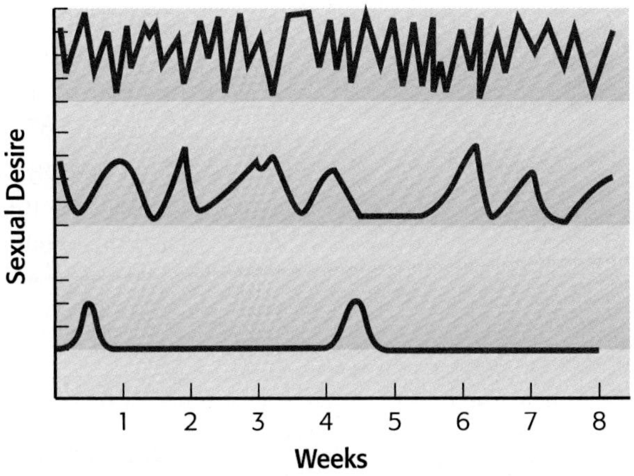


FIGURE 10.2 **Patterns of Sexual Desire Among Married Couples.** Researchers asked married couples to keep diaries of their sexual desire over a 56-day period. Analysis of the data suggested patterns. No pattern was associated with a greater or lesser degree of marital and emotional satisfaction. In other words, each pattern is "normal" and satisfactory for each couple.

Adapted from Ridley, C. A., et al. (2006). The ebb and flow of marital lust: A relational approach. *Journal of Sex Research, 43*, 144–153.

postulated that libido provided the force or energy for all human motivation. It was the role of society to channel libido from sexuality to other, more productive pursuits.

A modern version of Freud's libido theory holds that the sex drive is derived from neurological activity either in brain centers that produce sexual experience or in nonsexual brain centers that underlie the drives for novelty, excitement, love, or security—desires that can be met through sexual activity.

Another possible source of the sex drive is stimulation of the genital region by the rubbing of clothes and the handling of the genitals during nonsexual activities, and spontaneous erections and clitoral engorgement and vaginal lubrication that occur at various times during the day and during the *rapid eye movement* (REM) phase of sleep. It also is possible that not being touched with any frequency could create indirectly an urge for sexual activity in order to meet the desire for tactile contact.

## Sexual Incentives

Besides seeming to emanate spontaneously from within oneself, sexual desire can arise from a particular environmental cue, event, or situation (called a *sexual incentive*, *sexual stimulus*, or *sex releaser*) (**Table 10.1**). For example, someone may be in the library studying for an exam and not be particularly desirous of a sexual experience. However, that person might see someone whose posture and countenance trigger thoughts of a former lover, which may engender feelings of sexual desire. Perhaps the most potent sexual incentives are cues that suggest another's sexual availability and desire to be sexually involved with you.

Positive expectations about the outcome of a sexual experience increase sexual desire. Negative expectations can diminish sexual desire. Sexual disincentives include not feeling emotionally ready for sex; not liking the partner; fear of pregnancy or contracting an STD; being uncomfortable with nudity, touching, and contact with the genitals; and believing that sex is disgusting, sinful, dirty, or dangerous. Sometimes a person will have negative and positive expectations simultaneously. For example, some unmarried persons may desire sex and at the same time avoid it for moral and social reasons.

Relationship factors can affect sexual desire. Some people require that they be in a committed, emotionally close relationship to be sexually desirous at all. At the beginning of a love relationship, sexual desire may be high because partners anticipate creating exciting, new experiences. In a mature love relationship, sexual desire is often less intense than at the beginning. Also, sexual desire often is affected by the nonsexual aspects of a relationship, such as how well conflict is resolved.

**Table 10.1** Types of Sexual Invitations

| Direct Invitations | Indirect Invitations |
|---|---|
| Press against your partner | Make yourself attractive to your partner |
| Return a kiss passionately | Wear (or not wear) certain clothes |
| Let your hands wander over your partner's body | Tell your partner you are about to take a bath or shower |
| Touch more than usual | Change the usual routine |
| Prolong a touch | Suggest taking a bath together |

## Sexual Decision-Making

Being sexually interested and desirous does not necessarily mean that a person will behave sexually. Instead, being sexual is the result of a decision (except in instances of sexual coercion and assault) that is based on one's willingness to have sex when a sexual invitation occurs, feelings and fantasies about the sexual partner, and expectations about the outcome of a sexual episode. Also, the decision to accept a sexual invitation depends on the context in which sexual activity takes place. Social norms and laws govern who may have sex with whom and where sexual activity can take place.

Even if one is in a situation or relationship in which periodic sexual activity is expected and permitted, every sexual opportunity is unique, and one can decide "yes," "no," or "maybe" to each one. The decision is affected by how one feels physically and emotionally at the time, one's personal criteria for being sexual within the presenting situation, and one's expectation of how being sexual at that time will affect one's self-esteem and the relationship.

## Sexual Participation

In the day-to-day world of exams, work, and doing tasks, a person may have fleeting thoughts of sex and even sexual sensations in various places in the body. But, because the mind is focused on everyday matters, sexual thoughts generally pass out of conscious awareness. On some occasions, however, in response to one's

### Dear Penelope . . .

***I'm 20 years old and haven't had sex yet. I'm beginning to think that's weird. I've rejected a few invitations I've gotten because casual sex isn't for me. Or at least it hasn't been. Now I'm wondering: should you have sex to satisfy your curiosity? Is this an OK reason for losing your virginity?***

***— Losing Patience***

*Dear Losing Patience,*

Being a virgin at 20 isn't as unusual as you may think. Based on what we hear in popular music, see in the movies, and what our friends brag about, it seems that everybody is having the time of their lives hooking up as often as possible. Don't you believe it. While it can be fun and pleasurable, sex is also serious because it involves emotions and self-esteem. There are many valid reasons for saying "no" or "not yet" to sex, whether or not you are a virgin.

It's difficult to feel different. But it's more difficult to act contrary to your personal values and psychological needs. Trust your intuition. Since you say "casual sex isn't for me," you probably should wait for someone you know well, care for, and trust enough that you can surrender to the experience. Many people who have their first sexual intercourse in a casual encounter report that it was much less enjoyable that they expected.

If you decide to "satisfy your curiosity," make the experience meaningful by incorporating as much caring and sexual responsibility (no unintended pregnancy, no sexual infections, no hurt feelings) as possible.

Courtesy of the UC Davis *Aggie*

own sexual thoughts and feelings, another's sexual invitation, or a variety of other motivations for sex (see Chapter 1), individuals will decide to turn their attention from everyday concerns to having sex.

## Sexual Transition

**transitioning** a progressive mental and physical "letting go" of the everyday so that a full sexual experience can occur

Shifting from everyday to erotic experience generally requires **transitioning**—a progressive mental and physical setting aside of everyday concerns so that a nearly total mental focus on erotic experience can occur. Transitioning from everyday reality is common. For example, in athletics or the theater, participants change into special clothes and do "warmup" activities to focus the mind and body on the forthcoming performance and to distance themselves from everyday concerns. Going to sleep can also be facilitated by transitional or "winding down" activities.

With sexual transitioning, individuals and partners may seek a private location that facilitates creating a pleasurable sexual experience without fear of discovery or interruption. Once in a sexually facilitative environment, individuals and partners may undertake "transitioning activities"—for example, talking about shared interests, listening to music, taking a shower (alone or together), massaging, or being together quietly. They may partially or completely undress and kiss or touch each other. Partners may mentally transition long before the physical transition occurs (called *simmering*), awaiting the appropriate time and circumstances to proceed sexually.

As the transition from the everyday to the sexual continues, the mind increasingly imbues with sexual meaning sights, bodily sensations, and feelings that, in the everyday world, may have little or no sexual significance. Time may become distorted because sexual experience progresses not in minutes but in stages of increasing sexual intensity involving the pleasures of the moment, increasing desire for different and more intense sensations in forthcoming moments, and complete focus on the sexual experience.

Transitions to sexual experience can be halting or smooth. Individuals new to sexual experience may not yet know which sexual transitioning activities work for them. Also, an individual's personal motivations and conditions for sex must be appropriate to prevent worry and judgment, which can inhibit the free flow of sexual experience. In new sexual relationships, individuals may become distracted from sexual experience by worries about "looking good" or "doing it right," as determined by what is occurring in their own and the partner's body. Partners in established sexual relationships generally have fewer worries, and a sexual experience is likely to progress without distracting thoughts.

## Sexual Arousal

Sexual arousal involves feelings of excitement, joy, and erotic pleasure brought about by activation of specific nerve networks in the brain. These nerve networks can become activated by thoughts, fantasies, daydreams, or night dreams, and the interpretation of nerve signals from the body's sense organs as erotic stimuli.

Many years ago, research on possible treatments for epilepsy showed that the *septal region* of the human brain is involved in producing sexual feelings. In one case, a male patient was given a device that would deliver small electrical impulses to various brain regions in the hope of controlling seizures. During three-hour test sessions, the man delivered hundreds of pulses to the septal region of the brain and very few to any others. According to the researchers, such stimulation produced feelings of pleasure and sexual arousal with a desire for sexual release.

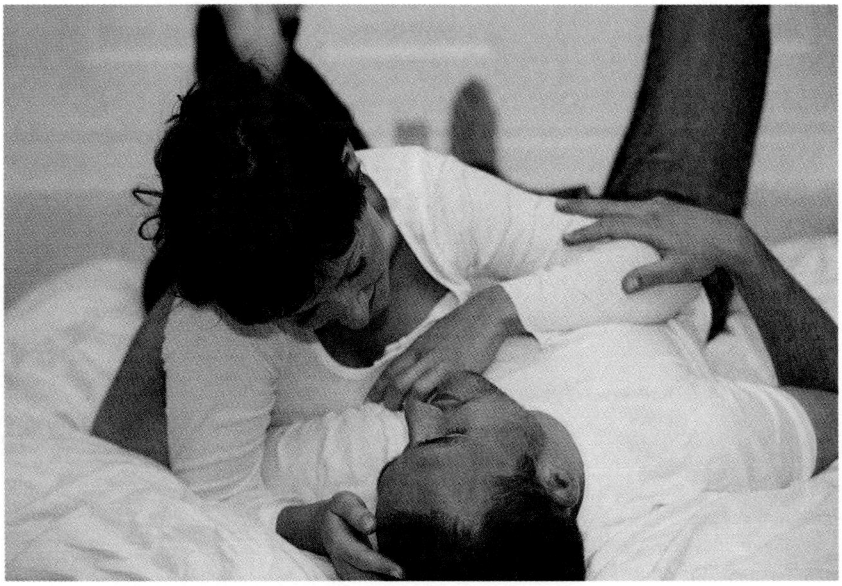

In a different experiment, microscopic tubes were implanted in various regions of a woman's brain to permit the introduction of the neurotransmitter acetylcholine. Activation of the septal region produced positive emotions, an increased level of awareness, and a desire for sex that culminated in repeated orgasms both reported by the woman and confirmed by the researchers who observed her movements.

Sophisticated modern methods such as positron emission tomography (PET) and functional magnetic resonance imagery (fMRI) can produce images of the brain as it functions. Using these methods, scientists have identified regions of the brain that become activated when subjects are presented with erotic stimuli. Although the brain possesses neurological networks or regions that produce sexual feelings, pleasure, and responses, one must always remember that to become sexually aroused a person must first deem a potential sexual situation appropriate and safe.

## Sexual Stimulation

Sexual stimulation is the process of producing sexual arousal by activating nerves that produce sensations of sight, taste, smell, hearing, and touch. Certain regions of the body, called **erogenous zones**, are highly sensitive to tactile stimulation when one's personal conditions for becoming sexually aroused are met. These regions include the mouth, glans penis, glans clitoris, the outer third of the vagina, the nipples, and the anal region. During sexual excitement, erogenous zones also can be less sensitive to discomfort from rubbing, pinching, or biting. For example, when a man is sexually excited, his erect penis is much less sensitive to pain and heat than when he is not sexually aroused, thus reducing discomfort from friction associated with intercourse. When a woman is sexually excited, she may not feel the discomfort that usually accompanies pressure on the breasts and nipples when she is not sexually excited.

**erogenous zones** body regions that are highly sexually sensitive, including the lips, glans penis, glans clitoris, the outer third of the vagina, the nipples, and the anal region

Besides the well-known erogenous zones, with repeated experience just about any region of the body can generate sexual sensations. For example, many people with spinal cord injury report eroticizing parts of the body that are still neurologically capable of sending signals to the brain, such as elbows, fingers, and eyelids.

## Sexual Fantasy

Besides physical activities, sexual stimulation can occur by means of thoughts, fantasies, and images. Sexual fantasies can be fleeting thoughts or elaborate stories. They can involve realistic or bizarre imagery of romantic or sexual experiences. They can be completely novel images, sometimes surprising even to the imaginer, or memories of past occurrences, perhaps mentally edited or altered to enhance their erotic potential. Sexual fantasies can occur spontaneously or intentionally or they can be triggered by other thoughts, feelings, or external circumstances. When

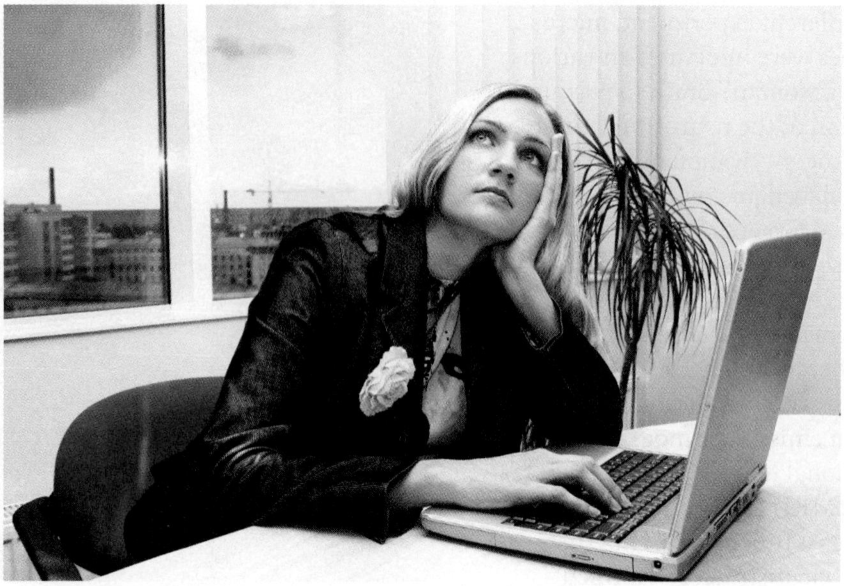

Sexually fantasizing is very common. Fantasies can be diversions from everyday reality or used to heighten sexual arousal.

the content of sexual fantasy-facilitators violates socially acceptable sexual standards and norms, it is referred to as *pornography.*

In surveys of young adult American college students, nearly all male and female respondents report having sexual fantasies. These fantasies occur spontaneously during the day with no particular external stimulus (at least, none that are recalled by survey respondents), or they are triggered by something seen or read. Sexual fantasies may be a diversion from everyday reality and/or a means to heighten sexual arousal during masturbation and sexual activity with a partner. Because the function of sexual fantasy is arousal, the content of sexual fantasies often represent themes of novelty, risk taking, and even dangerous or bizarre sexual experiences that a person would never desire or do in real life.

Sexual fantasies among American adults generally involve conventional sexual imagery with past, present, or imaginary lovers who are known to the person; scenes imitating sexual power or irresistibility (including seduction scenes and multiple partners); scenes involving somewhat varied or "forbidden" sexual situations, settings, practices, and partners; and submission/dominance in which some physical force or sadomasochistic activity is involved or implied.

Some people contend that sexual fantasies are harmful because they substitute for real-life experiences. Another contention is that imaginings of harmful or unusual practices may encourage individuals to engage in rape or sexual abuse. While not denying that on occasion fantasy—especially sexual fantasy that links sex with violence—may be harmful, it is apparent that sexual fantasy is a normal aspect of human sexuality that can positively augment sexual experience.

## Sexual Activities

Sexual partners may engage in a variety of activities to increase sexual arousal and pleasure, including the following.

### Oral Stimulation

Kissing as a form of sexual stimulation may involve deep or French kissing, in which the tongue is inserted into the mouth of the kissing partner in order to stimulate the inner surfaces of the partner's mouth and tongue. Oral sexual stimulation may also include sucking, nibbling, or biting the partner's lips, mouth, neck, and ear lobes.

### Breast Stimulation

The female breasts can respond sexually to gentle fondling, licking, kissing, or sucking by enlarging and becoming firmer. The nipples may become erect and the color of the region around the nipples (*areola*) may darken. Sexual stimulation of the breasts triggers the release of the brain hormone oxytocin, which produces feelings of emotional warmth and closeness. Some men are sexually aroused by stimulation of their breasts and nipples.

### Genital Stimulation (Manual and/or Oral)

A male's partner may rub, stroke, lick, or suck the penis (*fellatio*). A female's partner may explore with a hand and/or mouth her entire genital region, including the vagina, vaginal lips, and the clitoris (*cunnilingus*). Sex partners may participate in simultaneous oral–genital stimulation (*69* or *soixante-neuf*).

### Intercourse

There are a variety of positions:

- Partners face each other with the female on her back (*female supine position*). The male supports his weight on his knees and elbows. Being face to face allows the partners to hug, kiss, and gaze into each other's eyes.
- Partners face each other with the male on his back (*female superior position*). The female sits astride the male, generally facing her partner. Being on top provides the woman more control over the pace and rhythm of stimulation than is possible in other positions. If desired and not irritating, oral and manual stimulation of the breasts and manual stimulation of the clitoris by either partner may occur.
- Partners face each other while lying on their sides (*lateral position*). This position is sometimes preferred when partners desire less vigorous sexual interaction—for example, during pregnancy.
- Partners face each other while sitting or standing.
- Partners *do not* face each other (*rear entry* or *doggie style*). The male partner enters the partner from behind while both stand, sit, or lay.
- Anal intercourse, where the penis is inserted into the partner's anus while partner stands, kneels, or lies down.

## Sexual Response

During vigorous exercise, the brain automatically coordinates changes in several physiological processes. The exerciser need not think "heart, beat faster; lungs, take in more air; blood vessels, deliver more oxygenated blood to the muscles." Once exercise begins, the brain automatically brings about what is physiologically required.

Similarly, when a person is sexually aroused, the brain coordinates a patterned **sexual response cycle** consisting of increased heart rate, respiratory rate, blood pressure, and a general level of excitement; the tightening of many skeletal and some smooth muscles (*myotonia*); and changes in the pattern of blood flow resulting in engorgement of certain tissues (*vasocongestion*) (FIGURE 10.3). In men, vasocongestion in the pelvis results in penile erection (see Chapter 2). In women, vasocongestion produces vaginal lubrication, swelling of the clitoris, enlargement and darkening in color of the vaginal lips, and enlargement of the breasts (see Chapter 3).

**sexual response cycle** a patterned biological response to sexual arousal

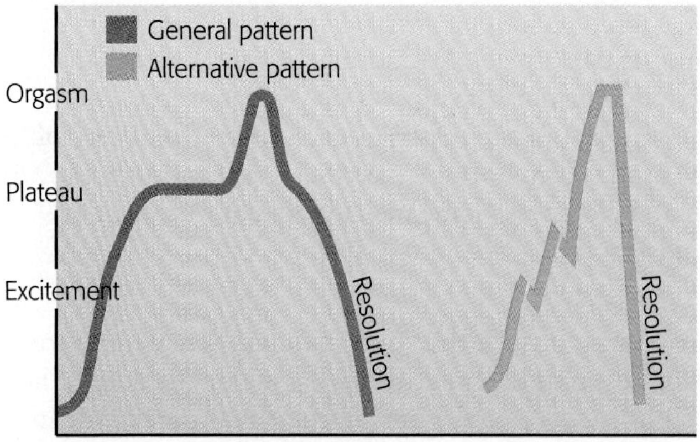


FIGURE 10.3 **The Sexual Response Cycle.** Regardless of the type of sexual stimulation, the physiological response in both men and women is similar and generally follows a four-phase pattern called the *sexual response cycle*: (1) Excitement, in which the person experiences sexual arousal from any source and the body responds with specific changes: erection of the penis in males; vaginal lubrication and swelling of the clitoris and genitalia in females. (2) Plateau, in which the physiological changes of the excitement phase level off, although subjective feelings of sexual arousal may increase. (3) Orgasm, in which the tensions that build up during the excitement and plateau phases are released. (4) Resolution, in which the body returns to the physiologically nonstimulated state.

There is considerable variation in the extent and duration of the sexual response cycle among individuals of either sex. There is even variation in the nature of the response in the same person, for not every sexual encounter is identical to every other.

## Orgasm

**orgasm** release of sexual tensions

When sexual arousal builds to a certain point, the associated sexual tensions can be released in a brain-centered response called **orgasm**. Sexual orgasm in both women and men is frequently associated with rhythmic contractions of the pelvic muscles; tightening of the muscles of the face, hands, and feet; and feelings of pleasure. Also, orgasm may involve a near-total loss of awareness of one's surroundings and body, giving rise to expressions describing orgasm such as *petit mort* ("little death"). Most commonly, men ejaculate during orgasm, although it is possible for males to experience orgasm without ejaculation and vice versa. Some women release fluid from the urethra and possibly the vagina during orgasm. Although referred to as "female ejaculate," it does not contain sperm, nor is it seminal fluid. This fluid is likely produced by tissue in the vaginal wall (*Skene's glands* or *G-spot*), transported via small tubules to the urethra, and expelled from the body by pelvic muscle contractions at orgasm.

Orgasm experience varies greatly from person to person and from time to time in the same person. There may be "big orgasms" or "little orgasms," and if a person is not sufficiently aroused, no orgasm may occur. Female orgasm is shrouded in many myths (**Table 10.2**). The media particularly perpetuate the myth that when a woman has an orgasm, bells ring, the earth shakes, lights flash, and she moans and groans—often, female orgasms are quiet.

Some individuals are capable of more than one orgasm during a sexual episode, whereas others feel satisfied and complete having experienced one. Although some individuals *can* experience more than one orgasm, setting the expectation that someone *should* have more than one is likely to increase performance anxiety and thus minimize sexual pleasure and the likelihood of having any orgasms at all.

As in other aspects of life, learning and experience may affect orgasmic response. With practice, men can learn to modulate their degree of sexual arousal

**Table 10.2** Orgasm Myths

| Myth | Fact |
|---|---|
| Simultaneous orgasm is the goal. | Any goal regarding orgasm turns sex into work, which risks lessening pleasure and creates performance pressure on partners and a risk to self-esteem. |
| Orgasms are intense and explosive. | Some orgasms are intense, some are quiet, and some are gentle. |
| The goal/purpose of sex is orgasm. | See the first fact in this list. Also, one or both partners may not feel a desire for orgasm. Furthermore, there are many reasons to have sex. Many outcomes besides orgasm suggest that sexual goals have been attained. Good sex is defined as a pleasurable experience. Following sex, you should feel good about yourself and good about your partner. |
| There is a "right way" to bring about and experience orgasm. | Physiologically, orgasm is the consequence of substantial sexual arousal. A person can reach orgasm by oral, manual, fantasy, or other means prior to or after intercourse. |
| Sexual activity stops after one partner has an orgasm. | Lovemaking can continue for as long as both partners desire, even if one has had an orgasm. |

at a high level without triggering ejaculation/orgasm. This is called ejaculation control; it is practiced in many cultures. With practice, women can learn the nuances of their unique sexual patterns to facilitate reaching high levels of sexual excitement and orgasm.

## Sexual Resolution

At the completion of a sexual episode, people transition from the erotic back to an everyday state of being. This is called **sexual resolution**. The brain and body return to an unaroused state, and for some period of time, called the **refractory period**, which can last from minutes to days, a person may not desire sex and may even be biologically incapable of responding sexually.

The end of a sporting event or concert is very specific. However, the end of a sexual episode may not be. One partner may feel "finished" before the other but may accompany and facilitate the partner's continued sexual arousal. And even when both partners no longer desire to be sexually aroused and responsive, they may nevertheless desire "together time" involving talking, cuddling, and feeling close. This experience is called *afterglow*. Depending on the situation, it can be a prelude to a subsequent sexual episode, a transition to sleep, or resuming everyday activities.

**sexual resolution** after sex, the return of the brain and body return to their usual non–sexually aroused state

**refractory period** after sex, a period of time during which a person may not desire sex and may be biologically incapable of, and even averse to, responding sexually

## Evaluation

Because human consciousness is highly evaluative, individuals evaluate nearly every sexual experience (**Table 10.3**). Evaluations generally include how well the sexual experience met one's personal goals for it, how it affected one's attitudes about oneself and one's partner, its effects on the development of one's sexual skills, communication, sexual preferences, and synchronizing sexually with the sexual partner. Individuals also evaluate the effects of sexual activities on their sexual relationship.

**Table 10.3** Some Criteria By Which Sexual Experience Is Evaluated

| |
|---|
| **Men** |
| How comfortable you feel with your partner |
| How you feel about yourself during/after sex |
| Amount of fun experienced during sex |
| Level of affection expressed during sex |
| How often you experience orgasm |
| Degree of privacy for sex |
| Degree to which you feel sexually aroused/excited |
| Degree of emotional intimacy (sharing feelings) |
| How your partner physically treats you during sex |
| Physical sensations from caressing and hugging |
| **Women** |
| How your partner physically treats you during sex |
| How comfortable you feel with your partner |
| Being with the same partner each time you have sex |
| Degree of consideration your partner shows for you |
| Partner being naked/seeing your partner naked |
| Physical sensations from caressing and hugging |
| How your partner responds to your sexual advances |
| Degree of emotional intimacy (sharing feelings) |
| How you feel about yourself during/after sex |
| Extent to which your sexual relations make you feel secure about total relationship with partner |

Adapted from Lawrence, K., & Byers, E. S. (1995). Sexual satisfaction in long-term heterosexual relationships. *Personal Relationships, 2*, 267–285.

## Sexual Difficulties

Surveys show that one-third to one-half of adults report occasional or persistent problems with sexual arousal and response. In some situations, a sexual problem emerges early in adulthood and may persist for many years. In others, sexual problems are intermittent, resulting from life situations that produce a temporary loss of interest in sex, the ability to become sexually aroused, and/or the ability to engage in or experience pleasurable sex. Some sex problems are situational, occurring in a particular circumstance (e.g., when angry, stressed, vulnerable to interruption) or with a particular partner. Temporary sexual difficulties are normal and generally resolve in time.

Long-term sexual difficulties may result from illness or disability, fear of not meeting one's own or a partner's expectations for sex, negative attitudes about sex, guilt about experiencing sexual pleasure, psychological defensiveness against erotic pleasure, relationship problems, and simply not knowing how to become sexually excited (Table 10.4). Sometimes, adjusting one's sexual expectations, attitudes, or techniques will lessen sexual problems. In contrast, consulting a health practitioner could be helpful if one has persistent sexual difficulties.

**Table 10.4** Beliefs Inhibiting Sexual Arousal and Response

| |
|---|
| **Male** |
| If a man lets himself go sexually, he is under a woman's control |
| In sex, the quicker/faster, the better |
| I am going to fail |
| I am not satisfying my partner |
| I must achieve an erection |
| She doesn't find my body attractive |
| This kind of sex is disgusting |
| I am not turned on |
| **Female** |
| Sex is all he thinks about |
| He is violating me |
| I'm not getting turned on |
| I'm only doing this because he asked me to |
| He only loves me if I am good in bed |
| These movements and positions are unpleasant |
| My body doesn't turn him on |
| I'm not physically attractive |
| When will this be over? |

Adapted from Nobre, P. J., & Pinto-Gouveia, J. (2003). Sexual Modes Questionnaire: Measure to assess the interaction among cognitions, emotions, and sexual response. *Journal of Sex Research, 40,* 368–382.

## Common Sexual Difficulties

### Insufficient Sexual Arousal

A variety of factors can prevent a person from becoming sexually aroused, including illness, fatigue, stress, depression, having ingested high amounts of alcohol and/or other drugs, and taking medications such as selective serotonin reuptake inhibitors (SSRIs) and oral contraceptives. Sexual arousal also can be inhibited by anxiety about being interrupted (roommates or children walking in; mobile phone or Internet messaging), not protecting against unintended pregnancy or STDs, the possibility of genital pain, not meeting one's own or the partner's expectations, and loss of personal or emotional control. Boredom with a predictable sexual routine or a partner's sexual difficulty can forecast an unpleasant sexual experience and thus lessen arousal.

### Vaginal Lubrication Problems

Vaginal sexual activity, particularly penis–vagina intercourse, can be painful when vaginal lubrication is minimal or absent (*vaginal dryness*). In some instances, vaginal lubrication is minimized by infection, medications (including antidepressants), alcohol and drug ingestion, long-term cigarette smoking, taking oral contraceptives, and low levels of estrogen in the body, which can occur at the beginning of a menstrual cycle, after pregnancy, or after menopause. Minimal or absent vaginal lubrication also can result from not feeling sexually excited because of insufficient nongenital stimulation (communication, expressions of closeness and intimacy), ineffective tactile stimulation, sexual performance anxieties, body image anxieties,

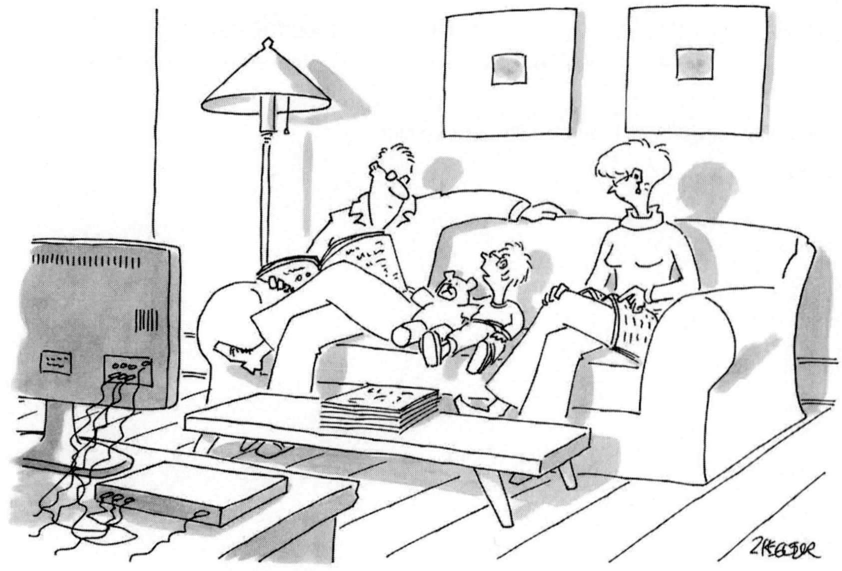


*"Once this commercial is over, I'll have a number of questions on erectile dysfunction."*



and disharmony in the relationship with the sexual partner. Vaginal lubrication problems are best managed by consulting a health professional who can identify biological, psychological, and relationship factors that contribute to them and recommend appropriate interventions.

### Erection Problems

**erectile dysfunction (ED)** difficulty in getting or maintaining an erection

**rapid (premature) ejaculation** characterized by not being satisfied with the ability to control the timing of ejaculation during sexual intercourse; ejaculation generally occurs within seconds or a minute or two after beginning intercourse

About 25 million American men have difficulty getting or maintaining an erection (clinically called **erectile dysfunction [ED]**). Erection difficulties can result from nonsexual factors including aging; injury or disease of the nervous or vascular systems; the ingestion of drugs such as alcohol, heroin, and some medications for high blood pressure; tobacco smoking; overweight; an inactive lifestyle; guilt; depression; and loss of self-esteem (e.g., following job loss). Sexual factors that contribute to erection problems include fear of performing sex poorly (including inability to get an erection) or not wanting to be sexual with a particular partner.

Medical examinations can identify biological causes of erection difficulties. Drugs that dilate pelvic blood vessels, called PDE-5 inhibitors (Viagra, Levitra, Cialis), can be prescribed when erection difficulties are the result of limited blood flow to the penis due to a medical condition. Individual and couple counseling can identify and help change thoughts, attitudes, and behaviors that block sexual arousal and hence inhibit erections.

### Rapid/Premature Ejaculation

**Rapid (premature) ejaculation** is characterized by not being satisfied with the ability to control the timing of ejaculation during sexual intercourse; ejaculation generally occurs within seconds or a minute or two after beginning intercourse. Sexuality experts generally do not prescribe how long sexual intercourse should last; the desired length of sexual intercourse depends on the needs and wants of sex partners. Rapid ejaculation may often be a normal variant in human sexuality, resulting, for example, from a high level of sexual arousal coupled with limited ejaculation control. Alternatively, it may be due to a malfunction in one or more of the biological mechanisms that produce ejaculation. It is also possible that a man's rapid ejaculation developed as a pattern to reduce anxiety associated with prolonged sexual activity—for example, the fear of being discovered.

Men seeking clinical help to slow the onset of ejaculation may be prescribed drugs that alter brain levels of the neurotransmitter *serotonin* (called *selective serotonin reuptake inhibitors [SSRIs]*). They may also use topical anesthetics that are applied to the erect penis to reduce sensation; certain condoms may serve this same purpose. Some men learn to control the timing of ejaculation by becoming aware of the bodily sensations that signal the approach of ejaculation and modulating their sexual arousal in response to these feelings.

### Painful Intercourse

In women, painful intercourse (**dyspareunia**) often is caused by a vaginal infection, insufficient vaginal lubrication, and anxiety-produced spasms of the muscles surrounding the vagina, which makes vaginal penetration painful if attempted (**vaginismus**). Women experiencing painful intercourse should consult a health professional.

**dyspareunia** painful intercourse in women
**vaginismus** anxiety-produced spasms of the muscles surrounding the vagina that make vaginal penetration painful if attempted

Another source of pain associated with sexual activity, which can affect both women and men, is a deep, aching sensation in the pelvis or scrotum caused by the congestion of blood in the pelvic region brought about by sexual arousal. This is called *pelvic congestion syndrome*. Orgasm often reverses the congestion; lack of orgasm can cause blood to remain in the pelvis, causing discomfort and pain.

### Orgasm Difficulties

Both men and women can have difficulty experiencing orgasm. Besides rapid ejaculation, in men, orgasm problems include retarded or absent ejaculation, or ejaculation without a concomitant experiencing of pleasure and/or the release of sexual tension. In women, orgasm difficulties consist of lack of orgasm or orgasm in certain circumstances and not others (for example, during masturbation but not sexual intercourse). Orgasm difficulties generally result from not becoming sufficiently sexually aroused, not wanting to be with a particular partner, fear of pregnancy or acquiring an STD, fear of psychologically letting go, lack of trust in one's sexual partner, having negative attitudes about sexual pleasure, and using ineffective sexual techniques. If medical reasons for orgasm difficulties can be ruled out, then education and counseling in effective sexual technique and developing orgasmic responsiveness through masturbation may help resolve the issue. Many women who do not experience heterosexual intercourse orgasms frequently, or at all, report not being concerned about it for themselves, but they have a strong desire to experience intercourse orgasms for the sake of their male partners.

## Managing Sexual Difficulties

Sexual difficulties may be overcome through experience and/or with help from a health practitioner. In general, managing sexual problems rests on the belief that satisfying sexual experiences are "natural" biological outcomes to sufficient sexual arousal. In other words, one does not "manufacture" satisfying sexual experiences; one "lets them happen."

Based on this premise, many sexual difficulties can be ameliorated through lifestyle and attitude changes. For example, because satisfying sexual functioning is facilitated by physical and mental health and well-being, individuals with sexual problems may benefit from attending to any problematic health issues. Sexual problems can sometimes be lessened by changing sex-negative values and thought patterns. In other situations, learning how one's body and mind respond to sexual excitement can eliminate anxiety-arousing unrealistic performance expectations. Also, sexual problems may lessen by learning new methods and techniques for enhancing sexual pleasuring, including communication skills.

Some sexual problems, particularly lack of sexual interest and desire, are often manifestations of an individual's or a couple's nonsexual issues. For example, sexual problems may be associated with fear of emotional closeness; lack of trust due to prior physical, sexual, or psychological abuse; or relationship disharmony. Psychological counseling may help resolve these issues.

## Sexual Communication

Communicating about sex can be difficult. Many people are shy about taking about sex, often because as children they were not exposed to open and easy conversation about the subject. Also, individuals may lack a sexual vocabulary; they are uncomfortable using medical/scientific words or slang/dirty words to discuss sex with partners. Because many people believe that men should take the lead in sexual relations, a man who talks about sex with a partner may fear being perceived as unmanly; a woman who talks about sex with a partner may fear being perceived as sexually aggressive or "slutty." Furthermore, sex can involve deeply felt emotions, which some people find difficult to express. Another reason partners do not discuss sex is belief in the widely held myth that true love makes sexual communication unnecessary.

Sexual communication can be both nonverbal and verbal. Nonverbal communication occurs as movements, gestures, touches, glances, and even certain kinds of dress. Often moving a hand or a face is effective and preserves an erotic mood. Whereas nonverbal sexual communication is often preferred to communicate one's sexual feelings and preferences, verbal communication of sexual desires and feelings carries less risk of misunderstandings.

If talking about sex is difficult, partners may disclose their feelings about talking about sex. They might feel comfortable sharing humorous aspects of their childhood experiences with sex education in school or at home. And they might laugh over misconceptions about sex that they learned from peers while growing up. They might share how their parents' relationship affected their attitudes about sex and love. Individuals can talk about sex-related books, articles, television, films, and even what is learned in a human sexuality course.

Most sex partners want to please each other. However, despite what one may have learned from media, friends, and prior sexual experiences, there is no way to know what pleases a partner because individuals' sexual needs, desires, and responses vary widely. A person's desires may change from one sexual episode to another. Wanting to be sensitive, someone may ask a sex partner, "Was it good?" or "Do you like it this way?" However, *yes-or-no* questions such as these can prohibit the responder from offering more details. Furthermore, a question such as "Am I doing it right?" may not elicit an honest answer because the partner fears hurting the asker's feelings. Even *either-or questions*, such as "Do you prefer this or that?" may not give the partner an opportunity for a complete response. *Open-ended questions*, such as "How would you like to be touched?" may provide the best opportunity for a partner to express her or his thoughts and feelings.

HEALTHY SEXUALITY

### Enhancing Sexual Experience

- Create pleasure by stimulating the whole body, not just the genitals.
- Vary the manner and intensity of stimulation. Allow sensations to build and wane.
- Try not to make sex = work.
- Set aside time that is free of intrusions and distractions. Turn off the phone; lock the door to ensure privacy.
- Make yourself an open, effective channel for sexual arousal before sexual activity begins. Satisfying sex is not a mechanical activity involving only bodies but a blending of mind–body energies. Remove sex-negative energies such as hunger, fatigue, and anger, and focus your energy on sex through deep breathing or other relaxing activity.
- Be aware of differences between you and your partner in the state of readiness for sexual activity. Try to synchronize your and your partner's states of sexual arousal through talking, light touching, dance, or massage before sexual activity begins.
- Address concerns about birth control and STDs.
- Take your time. Consider going slowly.
- Communicate likes and dislikes to your partner either verbally or nonverbally.
- Forget about orgasms. Learn to appreciate the many sexual sensations from touching all parts of the body.

At times, individuals may agree to have sex when they don't want to because they are not comfortable asserting themselves, feel guilty, or fear an angry response. When saying "no" to a request for sex, try to give the reason for saying no. Emphasize that the "no" is about sex right now and not a personal rejection. Be firm so as not to confuse the partner. Acknowledge that hearing "no" can be disappointing and that the partner may have taken an emotional risk. By discussing the reasons for the request for sex, an alternate activity can sometimes be found.

Occasionally a partner wants to suggest a change in the couple's usual sexual routine. There may be a specific activity that he or she wants to try, modify, or discontinue. Or, there may be general feelings of dissatisfaction with the sexual relationship. Being silent, however, for fear of offending or angering the partner is probably not helpful to the future of the relationship.

## Drugs and Sexual Experience

Drugs, teas, elixirs, potions, and magic charms intended to alter sexual desire are called **aphrodisiacs**, a word derived from the name of the mythological Greek goddess of love, Aphrodite. Besides increasing sexual desire, *aphrodisiac* also refers to a substance that eliminates sexual problems or increases sensations during sexual activity, either of which might increase sexual desire.

**aphrodisiacs** drugs, teas, elixirs, potions, and magic charms that are intended to alter sexual experience

Ancient Chinese, Indian, Arabic, Greek, and Roman cultures employed a variety of plant and animal substances as aphrodisiacs. For example, to increase a man's sexual vigor, the *Kama Sutra*, written in India 1500 years ago, prescribed a drink made of milk, honey, and the testicle of a goat, ram, or other animal. Ancient Chinese writings prescribed a variety of plant extracts to enhance erections in men and increase the amount of semen expelled at ejaculation.

Some ancient aphrodisiacs are still used today, particularly in cultures with an herbal tradition. These concoctions include extracts from the roots of ginseng and mandrake, dried and pulverized blister beetles ("Spanish fly"), and the horn of rhinoceros, which is perhaps the origin of the term "horny."

Drugs that increase brain levels of the neurotransmitter dopamine, such as cocaine, amphetamine, and methamphetamine, can produce feelings of sexual desire. Sedatives and tranquilizers generally reduce sexual desire, although they may produce relaxation to the point that a tense or anxious individual can engage in sex. Psychiatric medications called selective serotonin reuptake inhibitors (SSRIs) can lower sexual desire. Drugs such as marijuana and alcohol alter centers in the brain that govern patterns of social behavior and may "disinhibit" sexual reticence and thereby foster sexual desire. Ecstasy (MDMA, 3,4 methylene-dioxy-methamphetamine), which affects brain levels of the neurotransmitters dopamine and serotonin, can increase feelings of emotional closeness and thereby facilitate sexual desire.

Alcohol and other drugs that are reputed to be aphrodisiacs may enhance sexual desire and behavior through social expectation rather than actual biological effects. For example, in an experiment, men at a party were given drinks that contained either alcohol and tonic or tonic alone (the tastes of the drinks were masked so that the men could not tell which drink they were getting). The subjects were told that their drinks did or did not contain alcohol, but what they were told was not necessarily true. Some subjects given alcohol-containing drinks were told that they were drinking only tonic, and some receiving only tonic were told that their drinks contained alcohol. Subjects who thought they had received alcohol, regardless of whether alcohol was actually in their drinks, were more sexually aroused by erotic photos and videos than were those who thought that they had received only tonic.

Many drugs are used in social settings as symbols or "props" to help establish both the purpose of an activity and expected behaviors for individuals engaged in that activity. For example, the presence of beer at a party signifies that the event is a recreational activity at which participants are expected to display certain behaviors (dancing, talking with others, hooking up sexually). Although they are not insignificant, a drug's biological and behavioral effects often are not particularly important to establishing an event's purpose and expected behaviors. Indeed, in large doses, a drug's biological and behavioral effects (weird, unacceptable behavior, nausea, vomiting, loss of consciousness) may be the opposite of what participants desire.

## Alcohol and Sexual Experience

The effects of alcohol on sexual experience have been noted for centuries, as described 2500 years ago by the Greek poet Euneus:

> The best measure of wine is neither much nor very little;
> For 'tis the cause of either grief or madness.
> Then too, 'tis most suited for the bridal chamber and love.
> And if it breathe too fiercely, it puts the Love to flight.
> And plunges men in a sleep, neighbor to death.

Probably the most often-quoted comment about alcohol and sex comes from Act Two of Shakespeare's *Macbeth*: "It provokes the desire, but it takes away the performance."

The effects of alcohol on sexual desire and performance depend on the blood alcohol content (BAC), the grams of alcohol per deciliter of blood. One 5-ounce glass of wine, one 12-ounce bottle of beer, and one jigger of distilled alcohol (e.g., whiskey, vodka) contain the same amount of alcohol, about 0.6 ounces. In most

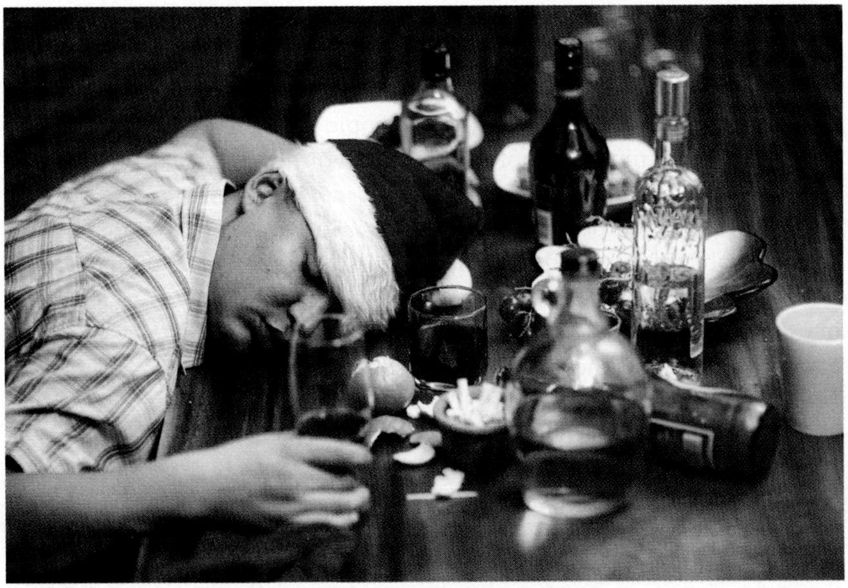

Alcohol can impair sexual arousal and sexual responsiveness.

individuals, one drink of any kind per hour increases the BAC to 0.02, enough to manifest the "loosening up" effects of alcohol. Increasing alcohol consumption to four or five drinks per hour in men or two or three drinks per hour in women raises the BAC to near 0.10, the level at which driving is illegal in most countries and states. At this BAC, erection, vaginal lubrication, and orgasm can be impaired. Even at lower BACs, some individuals are too intoxicated to give and receive sexual pleasure effectively or even be aware of what they are doing. A person might have sex with someone not otherwise considered to be a suitable sex partner. This increases the risk of unintended pregnancy (by not using fertility control correctly or at all) and acquiring an STD, and it creates a situation for sexual assault.

Many people use alcohol to quell shyness about going to parties or other social gatherings. Some use alcohol to lessen their natural inclination to be sexually cautious. Remember that accepting one's anxiety as a message to protect oneself from potential emotional or physical danger is healthy.

## Masturbation

**masturbation** self-stimulation to produce erotic arousal usually to the point of orgasm

**Masturbation** (from the Latin *manus*, meaning hand) is self-stimulation to produce erotic arousal, usually to the point of orgasm. People masturbate to experience erotic pleasure, relieve physical tensions, and transition to sleep. Some psychologists recommend masturbation as a way to learn about one's sexual responses and to become more skilled at creating various kinds of erotic experiences. Masturbation may occur during partner-sex as a mutually arousing practice or on occasions when one partner desires greater sexual stimulation and orgasm than the other, who may not want a full sexual experience but wishes to share in the partner's excitement and perhaps to create feelings of intimacy and bonding.

Whereas social and religious attitudes in many cultures consider it improper or immoral, masturbation is nevertheless practiced throughout the world. Among Americans, over 90% of males and 70% of females masturbate. Negative attitudes regarding masturbation can stem from beliefs that the purpose of sex is reproduction, that restraining one's "pleasurable" impulses is noble, and that sexual expression (especially in men) can sap vitality and produce weakness.

The most common masturbatory techniques employed by both men and women involve manual manipulation of the genitals. For males this usually means rubbing or stroking the penis, whereas for females it means rubbing or stroking the entire mons region, the clitoris, and/or the labia minora. Deep vaginal insertion with fingers or objects intended as penis-surrogates (*dildos*) is an uncommon variation. Stimulation of the breasts, nipples, and anal region are additional masturbatory techniques.

Masturbation is frequently accompanied by sexual fantasies. Approximately 75% of males who masturbate and nearly 50% of females who masturbate report that sexual fantasy occurs regularly with masturbation. The themes of such fantasies include being sexual with the usual sex partner, being sexual in unusual locales, being sexual with a celebrity or a stranger, and participating in a sexual activity that one would not actually do. Some individuals facilitate fantasy production during masturbation by reading erotic literature, viewing erotic images, or watching erotic videos.

A number of personal harmful effects have long been rumored to result from masturbation. Among them are loss of hair, insanity, pimples, warts, unhappy personal relations, and the inability to have children. None of these concerns is true. Masturbation is harmless as long as it is not injurious to the stimulated organs and the practice does not interfere with other aspects of life.

## Sexual Abstinence

Although they may feel interested in and desirous of sexual experience, some people choose to abstain from sexual activity. For example, some individuals practice lifelong sexual abstinence (called celibacy, which literally means remaining unmarried) for religious convictions. Some individuals refrain from sexual interaction, particularly sexual intercourse, until they marry. Still others refrain from sexual interaction because they fear the emotional closeness and intimacy implied by sex or they have strong negative attitudes regarding sex.

Individuals not wishing to practice lifelong sexual abstinence may nevertheless benefit from an occasional "time out" from sexual activity. For example, sexual abstinence is a certain way to avoid an unintended pregnancy or contracting a sexually transmitted disease such as HIV/AIDS. Some people find abstaining from sex helpful while recovering from an illness or the breakup of a love relationship.

Sexual abstinence can also provide the opportunity to change one's customary social behavior and permit new personal and relational experiences. By not inviting intimacy and the emotional bonding that often accompanies sex, abstinence provides a way to learn autonomy and one's boundaries and limits in interpersonal relationships. Without the diversion of sex (or looking for sex partners), an individual can focus on self-development, career, or school, and put energy into friendships. New romantic relationships can develop without the pressure for sex early in the relationship, thus permitting the partners to establish a friendship and to develop trust and caring before becoming sexual.

For some, sexual abstinence may seem a hardship because needs for sexual and physical contact and emotional closeness may not be met. During a period of sexual abstinence, needs for being touched can be met through professional (nonsexual) massage. Masturbation can relieve sexual tensions. And intimacy and bonding can be met by deepening one's ongoing friendships, giving of oneself to others through volunteer work, putting energy into increasing one's level of self-awareness and self-development, and engaging in spiritual and/or religious activity.

## SEXUALITY IN REVIEW

- Sexual interest and desire foster sex seeking, sex receptivity, and sexual experience.
- Sexual desire is influenced by personal health, feelings about the sex partner, and other factors.
- Sexual experience is often a unique experiential state in which a person's attention is focused on sexual sensations to the exclusion of other thoughts and behaviors.
- Erotic arousal produces specific changes in the body via the nervous and endocrine (hormone) systems.
- Sexual difficulties are often the result of anxieties and inhibitions regarding sexual experience.
- People employ erotica (e.g., stories, films), fantasy, and certain drugs and alcohol to increase sexual desire and pleasure.
- Communication between sexual partners can enhance sexual experience.
- Masturbation and sexual abstinence are viable alternatives to partner-sex.

## CRITICAL THINKING ABOUT SEXUALITY

1. Since becoming very serious, John and Evelyn have been having sex exclusively with each other a few times a week. Although it seems to John that Evy enjoys their lovemaking, he isn't sure whether she is having orgasms. John is very concerned about this. On several occasions he has wanted to ask Evy about her sexual response, but so far he hasn't.
   a. List at least two possible reasons for John wanting to know if Evy is having orgasms during their lovemaking.
   b. Should John ask Evy if she is having orgasms during their lovemaking? Why or why not?
   c. Assuming that John has decided to ask Evy if she has orgasms during their lovemaking, write in your own words how John should find out what he wants to know. When should John bring this up? Where? Under what circumstances?
   d. Whether or not Evy experiences orgasm in lovemaking with John, how is she likely to feel about being asked about this particular aspect of her sexuality?
2. When the topic of talking about sex came up in her human sexuality course, Susan dismissed it for her own relationship; she knew that she could never talk to Tom about their sex life, especially about her desire to make love more often. They rarely discussed their feelings, and they almost never talked about sex. Susan had tried a few times; however, the words just

wouldn't come out. Tonight she had arranged to meet Tom at a restaurant, hoping it would be easier to talk there than at home.

As she drove to the restaurant, she rehearsed what she would say and imagined how Tom would react. How would she begin? Would he be angry? Would he think she was too aggressive? Why did she feel guilty about asking for this change?

a. How should Susan start the conversation about sex with Tom?
b. What do you think Tom's reaction will be? Why?
c. If Tom does not want to change their frequency of sexual interaction, could they reach a compromise?
d. How, if at all, might addressing this issue change Susan's and Tom's relationship?

3. Explicit sexual still and moving images are prevalent throughout the media. What effect, if any, does exposure to these images have on young people as they develop into adult sexual persons?

## REFERENCES AND RECOMMENDED RESOURCES

### References

Davis, M. S. (1980). *Smut: Erotic reality/obscene ideology.* Chicago: University of Chicago Press.

George, W. H., et al. (2006). Post-drinking sexual perceptions and behaviors toward another person: Alcohol expectancy set and gender differences. *Journal of Sex Research, 43*, 282–291.

Leitenberg, H., & Henning, K. (1996). Sexual fantasy. *Psychological Bulletin, 117*, 469–496.

Marnach, M. L., & Casey, P. M. (2008). Understanding women's sexual health. *Mayo Clinic Proceedings, 83*, 1382–1387. Available at: http://www.mayoclinicproceedings.com/content/83/12/1382.long. Accessed on October 24, 2010.

Masters, W. H., & Johnson, V. E. (1966). *Human sexual response.* Boston: Little, Brown.

McCall, K., & Meston, C. (2007). Differences between pre- and postmenopausal women in cues for sexual desire. *Journal of Sexual Medicine, 4*, 364–371.

Palha, A. P., & Esteves, M. (2008). Drugs of abuse and sexual functioning. *Advances in Psychosomatic Medicine, 29*, 131–149.

Pfaus, J. G. (2009). Pathways of sexual desire. *Journal of Sexual Medicine, 6*, 1506–1533.

Ridley, C. A., et al. (2006). The ebb and flow of marital lust: A relational approach. *Journal of Sex Research, 43*, 144–153.

### Recommended Resources

Cornell University Weill Medical College, Sexual Medicine Program. (2010). Disorders of ejaculation. Available at: http://www.cornellurology.com/sexualmedicine/disorders. Information on disorders of ejaculation.

Ellison, C. R. (2004). Facilitating orgasmic responsiveness. In: S. Levine (ed.), *Handbook of Clinical Sexuality for Mental Health Professionals.* Westport, CT: Guilford. A noted sex counselor clarifies female orgasm.

MedlinePlus. (2010). Sexual problems overview. Available at: http://www.nlm.nih.gov/medlineplus/ency/article/001951.htm. Information on sexual problems.

Nobre, P. J., & Pinto-Gouveia, J. (2008). Cognitions, emotions, and sexual response: Analysis of the relationship among automatic thoughts, emotional responses, and sexual arousal. *Archives of Sexual Behavior, 37*, 652–661. Research showing that sexual performance thoughts and fears inhibit sexual arousal.

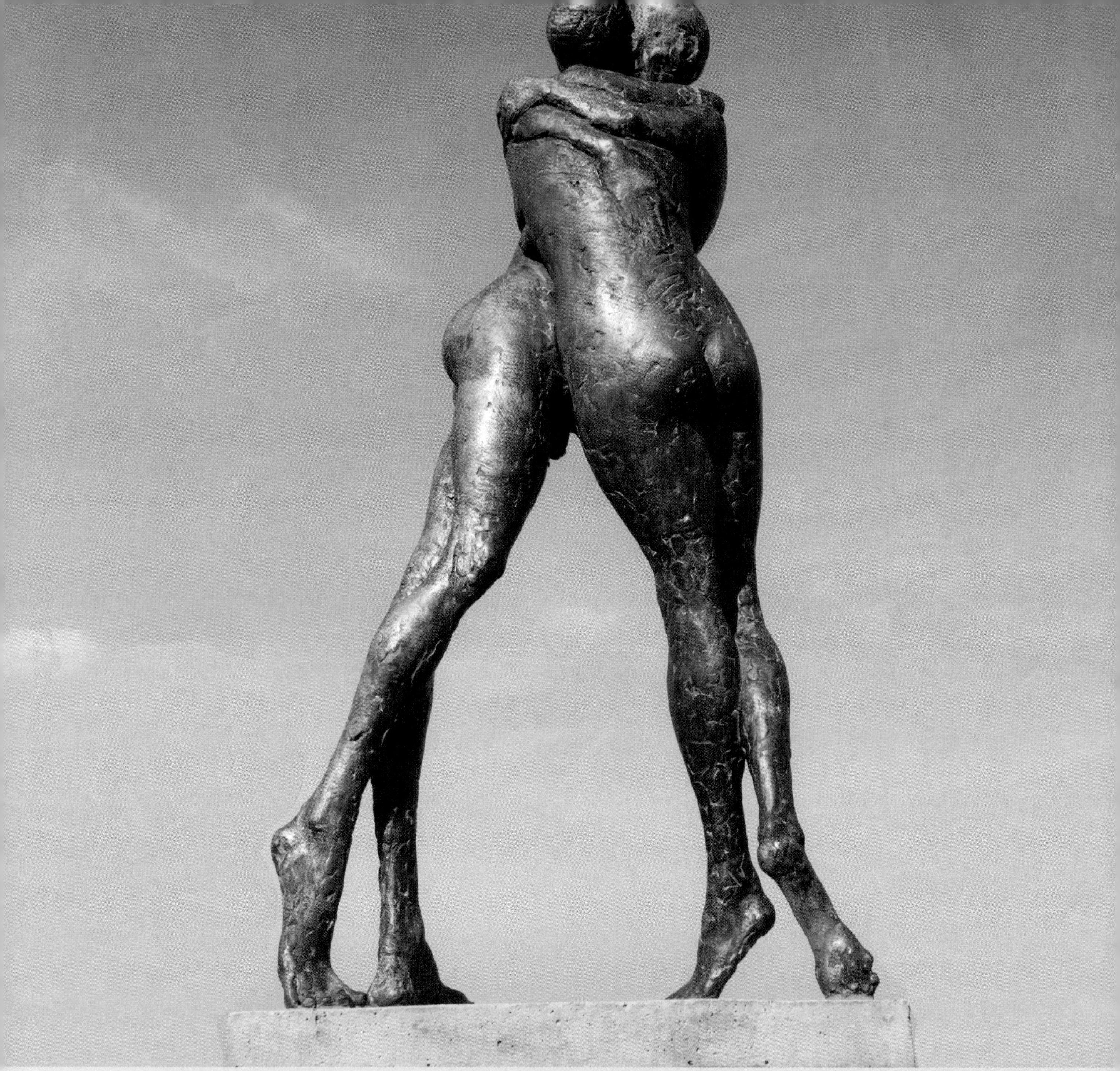

*Love is giving someone the space to be the way they are—and the way they are not.*

— Edmund Burke

CHAPTER 11

# Love and Intimate Relationships

## Student Learning Objectives

1 Describe the Triangular Theory of Love

2 Compare passionate and companionate love

3 Describe the four attachment styles

4 Define intimacy and explain its development via self-disclosure

5 Describe sexual and emotional jealousy

6 Describe loneliness and list ways people cope with it

7 List and describe the stages by which intimate relationships develop

8 Explain factors in communicating clearly

9 Discuss the reasons that intimate relationships end

Although safer sex with strangers, acquaintances, and friends can be exciting and physically pleasurable, most North American adults consider emotionally close relationships with peers to be their preferred contexts for sexual experiences. Perhaps after some sexual experimentation in adolescence and early adulthood, people conclude that sex can feel empty and meaningless when it is only for physical gratification or social rewards. They find that sex is much more gratifying when it expresses one's passion and love for another and fosters a sense of intimacy, emotional closeness, and security. Because sexual experience is integrally related to them, in this chapter we discuss love, intimacy, emotional attachment, jealousy, loneliness, relationship development, clear communication, and, alas, relationship endings.

## Love

Nearly everyone wants the feelings of closeness, acceptance, understanding, and appreciation that our culture associates with being loved. Indeed, most people believe that satisfying love relationships are primary factors in their overall health, happiness, and well-being.

Most people say they know what love is, because of either personal experience or identifying with feelings of love expressed by other adults or fictional lovers in books, films, and other media. However, love is difficult to define; dictionaries list over 20 definitions of the word. One reason that love is hard to define is that people apply the word *love* to a variety of things. People say they love baseball, music, beer, food, dogs, dolls, movies, ideas, sweethearts, spouses, and God. When a person says "I love your new car," surely something else is meant than when that same person says to someone "I love you very much." Although precise definitions may be unattainable, most people would agree that love involves a positive attitude about the beloved or loved object, affection and feelings of warmth, and wanting to interact with the beloved or loved object.

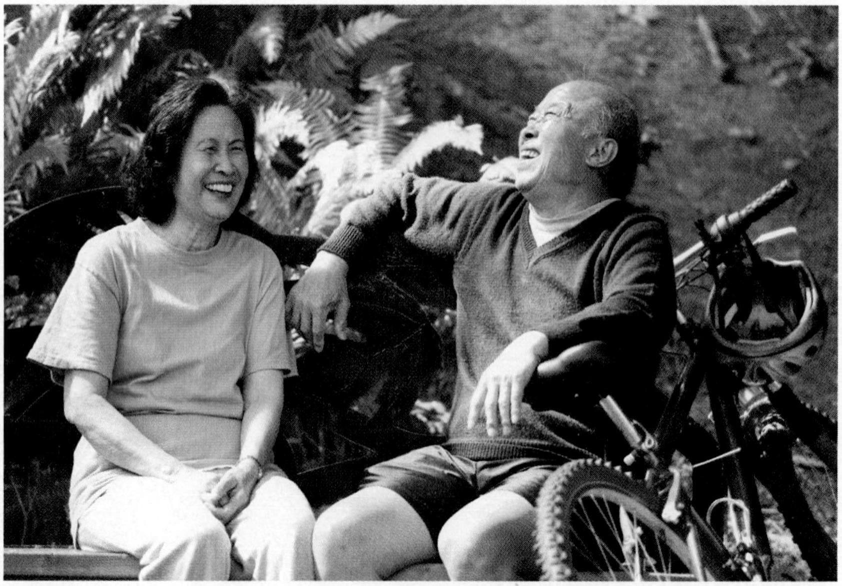

Satisfying love relationships make people happy and healthy.

**Table 11.1** Some Characteristics of the Triangular Theory of Love

| Passion | Intimacy | Commitment |
|---|---|---|
| Pounding heart | Support | Committing to each other |
| Butterflies in the stomach | Understanding | Putting other first |
| Sexual passion | Honesty | Need for each other |
| Physical attraction | Trust | Missing other when apart |
| Gazing at each other | Forgiveness | Devotion |
| Wonderful feelings | Respect | Loyalty |
| Excitement | Closeness | Protectiveness |
| Energy | Feeling relaxed | Longevity |
| Touching | Empathy | Dependency |
| Euphoria | Interest in other | |

## Scientific Studies of Love

For centuries, philosophers, poets, writers, musicians, and many others have attempted to describe the nature of love. More recently, social scientists have used survey methods and modern statistical analysis to understand love. One such approach, referred to as the **Triangular Theory of Love**, describes love as consisting of the following (**Table 11.1**):

- *Intimacy:* feelings of emotional closeness, warmth, and bondedness
- *Passion:* physical attraction and sexual excitement and desire
- *Decision/commitment:* deciding to love someone and committing to maintain that love

Various combinations of intimacy, passion, and commitment give rise to different kinds of love (**FIGURE 11.1**).

Another scientific approach to studying love has produced six **love styles (attitudes)** (**Table 11.2**), which are given the following Greek names:

1. *Eros:* passionate, romantic, often sexual love ("romantic love")
2. *Ludus:* efforts to keep romantic partner(s) emotionally off-balance ("game-playing love")
3. *Storge* (pronounced "store-gay"): a quiet love involving trust, rapport, companionship, and caring ("best friends love")
4. *Mania:* intense dependency, wanting to possess and be possessed by the lover ("possessive love")
5. *Agape* (pronounced "ag-a-pay"): unconditional caring, nurturing, giving, self-sacrifice ("unselfish love")
6. *Pragma:* a practical comparing of a lover's qualities against a predetermined list of desirable attributes ("pragmatic love")

**Triangular Theory of Love** a scientific model of love consisting of intimacy, passion, and decision/commitment
**love styles (attitudes)** six types of love (eros, ludus, storge, mania, agape, and pragma)
**passionate love** intensely consuming, and often highly sexual, love

## Passionate Love

**Passionate love** is an intense, exciting, consuming, and frequently sexual state. It is our culture's ideal of "true love." Nearly all the great love stories are about intensely emotional lovers who are consumed by thoughts about their beloved, who imagine their beloved to be perfect in every way, who crave physical contact with

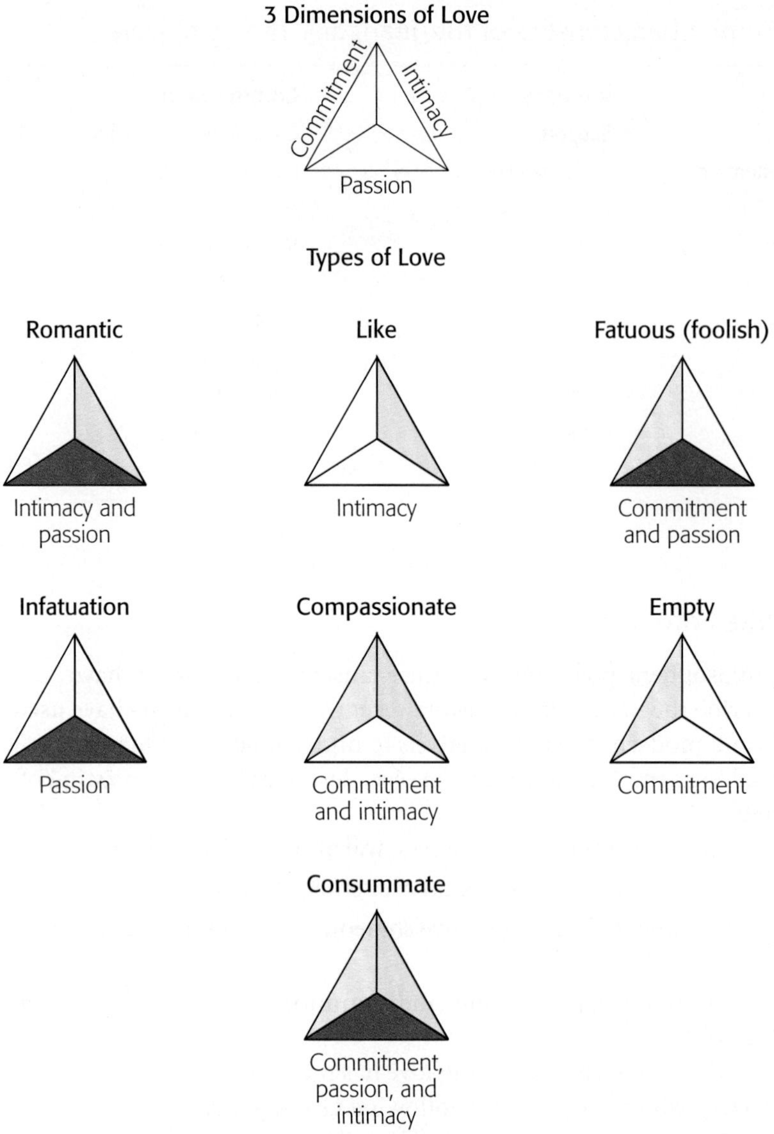


FIGURE 11.1 **The Triangular Theory of Love.** Love has three basic dimensions, each represented by a corner of the triangle. Mixing basic dimensions produces other kinds of love.

Adapted from Sternberg, R. J. (1986). A triangular theory of love. *Psychological Review, 93*, 119–135; and Beaumont, L. R. Emotional Competency: Love. Available at: http:/www.emotionalcompetency.com/love.htm. Accessed October 8, 2010.

the beloved, and who would do just about anything—overcome any obstacle—to be with the loved person. Indeed, the word *love* comes from the Sanskrit word *Lubh*, meaning *to desire*. Passionate love occurs in nearly every human culture.

Passionate love is intricately intertwined with sexual attraction, desire, and activity, which is why it also is called erotic love. Passionate lovers find each other highly sexually attractive; they touch, kiss, fondle, embrace, and have sex to express their intense passion for one another and to experience emotional union.

So mentally and sexually consuming is passionate love that it is sometimes likened to a state of addiction or temporary insanity. Some researchers have suggested that passionate love's obsessive, consuming, compulsive aspects enable lovers to take the psychological risks required to become attached and committed.

Passionate lovers experience heightened energy and ecstasy when their relationship is going well and despair when it is not. Lovers change their priorities and

**Table 11.2** Love Styles

| Style | Description | Characteristic Attitude |
|---|---|---|
| Eros (Romantic Love) | Passionate, romantic, and sexual | My lover and I have the right "chemistry" between us.<br>My lover and I were meant for each other. |
| Ludus (Game-Playing Love) | Keeps partner(s) emotionally off-balance | What my partner doesn't know about me won't hurt her/him.<br>I try to keep my lover a bit uncertain about my commitment. |
| Storge (Best Friends Love) | Quiet, trusting, caring, and companionate | The best love relationship grows out of a good friendship. |
| Mania (Possessive Love) | Characterized by intense dependency and wanting to possess and be possessed by the lover | When I am in love I have trouble concentrating on anything else.<br>I feel sick when my lover doesn't pay attention to me. |
| Agape (Unselfish Love) | Characterized by unconditional caring and nurturing, giving, and self-sacrifice | My happiness is placing my lover's happiness before my own.<br>I sacrifice my own wishes to let my lover have her/his own. |
| Pragma (Pragmatic Love) | Characterized by evaluating a lover's qualities against a predetermined list of desirable attributes | Factors important in choosing a partner are how well she/he will be as a parent or reflects on my family and career. |

Adapted from Hendrick, C., & Hendrick, S. (1986). A theory and method of love. *Journal of Personality and Social Psychology, 50*, 392–402.

routines—for example, they may skip class or work to be together. When barriers to togetherness heighten romantic passion, the condition is called "frustration attraction" or the "Romeo and Juliet effect." Lovers experience a host of sympathetic nervous system symptoms, including sweating, a pounding heart, and a feeling of "butterflies in the stomach" when with the beloved, and they experience longing and separation anxiety when apart. Passionate love has been found to be associated with activation of brain regions associated with sensations of pleasure, arousal, focused attention, and motivation to pursue specific goals and acquire rewards.

One of the ironies of passionate love is that despite the sincere belief that theirs is a lasting love, lovers' passionate feelings eventually wane or even vanish as abruptly as a bursting balloon. One reason that passionate love can be fragile is that most people cannot sustain the intensity of passionate romance for longer than several months. Other aspects of life, such as school, job, family commitments, and personal interests, require attention, and the amount of time and conscious energy spent in passionate fervor must inevitably decrease.

Another reason passionate love is fragile is that passionate lovers tend to idealize their partners. Passionate lovers revel in the partner's perceived perfections. Sometimes the loved one's actual personality characteristics are not important, as he or she is perceived as the embodiment of a fantasy love—perhaps a "knight in shining armor" or "the woman of my dreams." This is what is meant by the phrase "love is blind." As partners get to know one another better, however, their real personality characteristics become more apparent, and if the relationship is to deepen and possibly continue, the lovers must be desired for real-life reasons.

Many people use the term *infatuation* to refer to intensely passionate, abruptly ending relationships in order to distinguish them from the ideal of everlasting "true love." It should be noted, however, that while in the raptures of passion, lovers rarely refer to their experience as *infatuation*; this term is applied in retrospect when passionate feelings have waned and the romantic relationship has ended.

## Companionate Love

**companionate love** deep, low-key, committed love

Passionate love receives so much attention that it is easy to overlook **companionate love**, which embodies the qualities of trust, intimacy, commitment, durability, interdependence, a sharing of pleasures and sorrows, a willingness to make sacrifices, and an appreciation of the beloved's individual qualities. Companionate love is what people mean by "loving someone" as opposed to "being in love."

In contrast to passionate lovers, who are consumed by emotional and erotic intensity, companionate lovers are likely to have deep, low-key, tender feelings toward each other and a sense that their lives are deeply entwined. Sexual experience in companionate love, while including sexual excitement and pleasure, is likely to center on developing and experiencing intimacy, emotional bonding, and maintaining the relationship. This does not mean that companionate love cannot be passionate. Longtime love partners can and do experience intense, erotic passion, sometimes more easily when on vacation or after children have grown and left home.

## The Biology of Love

Scientists postulate that the capacity and desire to experience love in all its forms are manifestations of basic human biology, the purposes of which are promoting reproduction and health and well-being. The fact that passionate and companionate love are found in all cultures and that they are associated with specific emotional and physiological states supports this view. Love serves reproduction by motivating individuals to seek and find suitable (to them) mating partners and to establish and maintain lasting emotional bonds with them, which facilitates childrearing, a 15- to 20-year period of parental investment. Love serves health and well-being by being a basis for emotional support in times of stress and engendering feelings of joy, happiness, and hope at other times.

Many of the signs of passionate love result from increased activity of the brain chemical dopamine (a type of neurotransmitter). Dopamine facilitates focused, often obsessive attention (in this case, on the beloved), euphoria and idealization, loss of appetite, sleeplessness, and nervousness in the presence of the partner, which may be fear of rejection. Dopamine also strengthens the pleasure associated

HEALTHY SEXUALITY

### Relationship Wants and Needs

What are your wants and needs in a love relationship? Choose the three most important items from the list below. Can you choose only one? (What does your partner choose?)

I want someone to . . .

- Love me
- Confide in me
- Show me affection
- Respect my needs
- Appreciate what I wish to achieve
- Understand my moods
- Help me make important decisions
- Stimulate my ambition
- Look up to
- Give me self-confidence
- Stand by me in difficulty
- Appreciate me as I am
- Admire my ability
- Make me feel that I count for something
- Relieve my loneliness
- Support me and our children
- Accept my need to be self-sufficient and independent

with interactions with the love partner and creates a strong desire to repeat such interactions. Norepinephrine, another brain neurotransmitter, aids the establishment of memory so that positive experiences with the beloved are remembered.

Compassionate love also is thought to involve the brain chemicals serotonin, endorphins, and oxytocin. Serotonin and endorphins contribute to the sense of calm, peacefulness, and security associated with a secure emotional attachment. Oxytocin, the hormone involved in mother–infant and infant–mother attachment, in adults fosters a sense of trust and feelings of love for one's love partner.

## Attachment

**attachment** a neuropsychological system that emotionally bonds individuals to one another

**Attachment** is a neuropsychological system that fosters the emotional bonding of one person to another. In infancy and childhood, the attachment system bonds child to caregiver, called the *attachment figure*. A reciprocal attachment system, the *caregiver system*, bonds parent to child. Among adults in a love relationship, each partner becomes the attachment figure for the other, creating a reciprocal attachment/caregiver relationship. The bondedness that is characteristic of attachment is maintained by powerful emotions, including anxiety and distress from prolonged, undesired separation from the attachment figure (*separation anxiety*). Attachment also is maintained by joy and other positive emotions resulting from reunion after separation and playful interaction, shame at perceived rejection by an attachment figure, and anger, grief, sadness, and depression at the loss of the attachment figure. There are four basic attachment styles.

### Secure Attachment

Secure attachment is believing that an attachment partner is reliably available and willing to provide safety, security, love, and positive interactions. The partner is approached with a confident expectation of a rewarding relationship experience. Having a responsive, loving, and supportive partner confirms the belief that one is worthy of love and the expectation that relationships are rewarding. The secure attachment style is associated with being comfortable with depending on others for support, seeking intimacy and closeness in relationships, confidence in one's abilities to manage stress and anxiety, and a sense of self-worth that is not particularly dependent on others' approval. Regarding sexual interaction, secure attachment is associated with positive attitudes about sex, minimal sexual guilt, comfort with relating sexually, and favoring sex in the context of love relationships rather than casual sex.

### Anxious–Ambivalent Attachment

Anxious–ambivalent attachment is believing that an attachment figure is potentially loving and caring but is unreliable. This fosters fears of abandonment (especially when in need of support) and doubts about one's lovability and worth. This leads to an exaggerated desire for closeness and intimacy, dependence on others' approval for one's sense of self-worth, and preoccupation with attachment relationships, which can lead to emotional highs and lows. Anxious–ambivalent attachment is associated with using sex to feel emotionally close and to maintain attachment by focusing on pleasing the partner rather than on mutual pleasure, and succumbing to a partner's sexual advances and wishes regardless of one's own desires (including not attending to pregnancy and STD prevention). Acceptance as a sex partner becomes a symbol of one's worthiness.

### Dismissive–Avoidant Attachment

Dismissive–avoidant attachment is believing that attachment figures are likely to be unloving, uncaring, and unresponsive, and that close relationships will be disappointing. This belief fosters a desire to be independent, emotionally invulnerable, dismissive of the value of close relationships, and emotionally distant and detached. This attachment style is associated with a lack of intimacy or commitment in relationships. Dismissive–avoidant attachment also is associated with a focus on sexual activity as a way to gain social power and status and to experience physical sexual pleasure rather than emotional closeness and intimacy. Avoidance of commitment fosters a propensity to engage in casual sex.

### Fearful Avoidant Attachment

Fearful avoidant attachment is believing that others will be rejecting, unloving, and unreliable. This leads to emotional distancing and avoidance of closeness—even if desired—to avoid the expected pain of rejection. Fearful avoidant attachment is associated with negative attitudes about and low interest in sex in order to maintain emotional distance from a partner and to avoid possible rejection as a lover. Although sex may be sought primarily for pleasure rather than intimacy and closeness, sexual experience is also used to lessen feelings of loneliness and personal inadequacy.

## Intimacy

**intimacy** deep knowledge of another associated with feelings of closeness, trust, and self-validation
**self-disclosure** expressing private information about oneself to another

**Intimacy** is a characteristic of human relationships in which individuals experience feelings of closeness, trust, and self-validation. Intimacy inspires confidence that one's innermost self can be shared without fear of rejection or emotional hurt. The English word *intimacy* is derived from the Latin *intimus*, which means "within." Most dictionaries provide several definitions of intimacy, including "inmost," "most private," "closely associated," "familiar," and "very close." The word *intimacy* is sometimes used as a euphemism for sexual intercourse, although people with some degree of sexual experience know that intimacy and sexual activity, while sometimes related, are not the same; it is possible to have one without the other.

Whereas intimacy is generally construed to occur within adult relationships, its qualities of familiarity, acceptance, liking, and closeness are found in other kinds of relationships, including those between children and parents, siblings, and same- and other-sexed peers of any age. Each intimacy has unique and distinctive features that reflect the histories, desires, and psychological needs of the people involved.

Individuals have different needs for intimacy. Some regard intimacy as a positive experience, particularly when the intimate other reciprocates and is nonjudgmental. Others prefer less intimacy, valuing self-reliance and emotional privacy and eschewing support-seeking.

Intimacy in adult peer relationships relies on the partners' sharing information about their most important, private, sometimes secret aspects of themselves. This includes goals, aspirations, strengths, weaknesses, prior transgressions, fears, shame, conflicts with others, and current and past emotional hurts. The sharing of such private information is called **self-disclosure**. Most people are very cautious about revealing their innermost selves to others, as doing so can heighten concerns about the possibility of being rejected, evaluated negatively, being out of control or

## Dear Penelope . . .

***I've noticed a pattern in my relationships and those of many of my friends. The relationship starts off really well, but after a while I begin to feel tied down and that the other person is infringing on my freedom. At that point I back off. Why does this happen? Should the other person let go or continue to follow the deep feelings about me?***
***— Confused About Relationships***

*Dear Confused About Relationships,*

A satisfying relationship requires a balance of intimacy and autonomy, and it takes some practice to know how to do that. It may be that you are contributing to your feelings of being tied down by not attending to being an autonomous person.

At the beginning of a relationship, there's a tendency to blend with the partner—to become dedicated to the relationship and what your partner needs. After a while, however, you can begin to lose contact with yourself. Being with your friends, doing your own hobbies, saying "no," and keeping and stating your own opinions are just as important in maintaining a healthy relationship as are doing things for and with your partner.

When you feel tied down, instead of letting go of the relationship, arrange with your partner to give yourselves some space to be a self. This doesn't mean you no longer care for each other, and it doesn't mean you've lost interest being together in the relationship. It only means that relationship partners need to be individuals, too.

Courtesy of the UC Davis *Aggie*

being controlled, or losing one's individuality. The fears associated with intimacy are reduced by a sense of trust, the confidence that no physical or psychological harm will come from the intimate other's knowledge. It is assumed that the intimate other has one's best interests in mind at all times, and that one is accepted for oneself.

Although feeling intimate can occur between strangers who meet on an airplane or online, or who hook up for a few hours at a party or a few days while on vacation, intimate adult relationships develop most often over an extended period of time through a series of personal disclosures. One partner, desiring to share something private and personal, takes a risk and discloses intimate information to another. If the other is empathic and kind, the person feels accepted and understood and trust deepens. Moreover, the other person feels trustworthy and may view the partner as such, which can lead to reciprocal risk taking. Intimacy develops via cycles of intimate exchanges.

Verbal communication is the primary means of self-disclosure. However, nonverbal communication (e.g., postures, gestures, gazes, facial expressions that communicate emotions) also affects intimacy. Touching, sitting close, making eye contact, leaning forward, and smiling communicate attentiveness, interest, and caring. As it tends to be spontaneous, involuntary, and more effective at communicating affection and warmth, nonverbal communication often is a more reliable gauge of another's attitude than what is said.

## Jealousy

Love relationships tend to be governed by implicit and explicit rules, which often are social, religious, cultural, and legal expectations for partners' behaviors. Moreover, partners may establish their own rules for the relationship that fit their needs. Irrespective of their sincere promises, however, partners occasionally violate the rules of their relationship. Violating a relationship expectation or rule can be a breach of trust and can engender feelings of hurt, shame, and rage.

Jealousy is the feeling associated with the perception that the trust and intimacy of a relationship are threatened or may have been lost. Jealousy is an amalgam of anger, fear, and sadness. It is generated by the fear of loss of gratification of sexual, intellectual, emotional, and other needs. Jealousy also includes loss of status or face and primacy in the partner's life.

Sexual jealousy occurs when the beloved's interaction with a nonpartner is primarily sexual. Emotional jealousy occurs when the beloved becomes emotionally attached and/or in love with a nonpartner, even if the relationship is not sexual; a relationship with a close friend can sometimes elicit a partner's jealousy. Almost everyone can become jealous when a beloved is sexually and emotionally involved with someone else.

Jealousy can be helpful or harmful. Jealousy is helpful when it exposes a relationship situation that requires attention ("early warning signal"). Jealousy can be harmful when it alienates, antagonizes, and estranges partners and is based on unrealistic possessiveness and overdependency (**Table 11.3**). One of the most damaging outcomes of jealousy is interpersonal violence (see Chapter 12).

Some individuals intentionally induce jealousy in their partners to control the partner's behavior and test the partner's commitment. For example, a partner may devote more time to friends, work, or hobbies instead of the romantic partner. Another strategy is to talk about past or potential relationships. Whereas jealousy induction may serve to retain a mate, it may also backfire and drive a partner away.

**Table 11.3** Jealousy-Related Behaviors

| Goal | Strategies |
|---|---|
| Restricting Access to Rivals | Calling the partner at unexpected times<br>Taking the partner from social gatherings at which a potential rival may be present<br>Spying on the partner |
| Manipulating Partner's Behavior | Flirting with another person in the partner's presence<br>Crying or looking hurt<br>Making the partner feel guilty<br>Asking the partner for marriage; getting pregnant |
| Harming/Threatening Rivals | Hitting or fighting with rivals<br>Vandalizing a rival's property<br>Warning rival to "stay away" |
| Punishing the Partner | Hitting or threatening to harm the partner<br>Breaking dishes, slamming doors<br>Expressing anger for flirting with others<br>Threatening to break up<br>Withdrawing affection (sex) |
| Enhancing Attractiveness | Giving expensive gifts or flowers<br>Enhancing appearance/sexiness<br>Saying "I love you" more than usual<br>Giving in to partner's demands |

## Loneliness

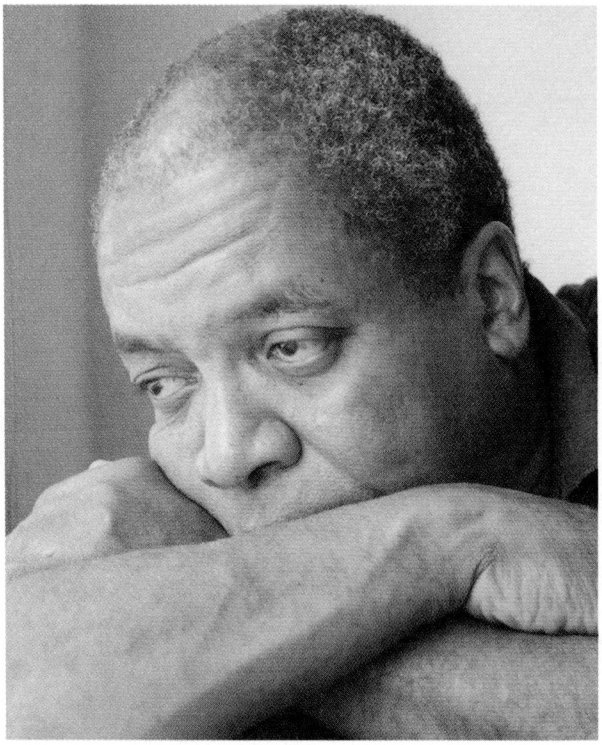

At some time or another, just about everyone feels the desperation, hopelessness, desolation, emptiness, and feelings of "not belonging" that characterize loneliness. Loneliness is the result of not having social ties that provide emotional attachment and feeling loved and valued. Loneliness may occur because a person is shy or has a history of social isolation and abuse. Perhaps someone has moved away from a familiar locale and is separated from family and friends and has not yet established new relationships. If loneliness has a purpose, surely it is to motivate seeking rewarding social ties with others.

Loneliness is not the same as being alone. People who are surrounded by others virtually all day and night may frequently feel lonely, whereas individuals who live or work in solitude may rarely feel lonely. The distinguishing feature of loneliness is not the quantity of interpersonal relationships but how closely one's relationships match one's needs and expectations for intimacy and attachment.

Because our culture values marriage and pairing, those not in close relationships can feel despairing and lonely. They wonder (especially on Valentine's Day), "When am I going to find someone?" Unfortunately, being in a love relationship is not a sure way to avoid loneliness. The severest form of loneliness often occurs in a relationship when the expectation of receiving love, caring, and acceptance is not met.

People cope with loneliness in a variety of ways. There may be a tendency to blame oneself for the situation ("I am unlikable/unlovable"). This can lead to self-imposed isolation and make loneliness worse. It is more helpful to realize that it takes time and effort to establish supportive social connections. Psychological counseling can often help identify and resolve the causes of one's loneliness.

## The Development of Intimate Relationships

Intimate relationships generally develop through the stages of readiness, finding and choosing a partner, falling in love, developing intimacy and closeness, commitment, and maintenance.

Relationship readiness is the desire or willingness to be involved in an intimate relationship. Generally, relationship readiness implies that a person is not already emotionally involved with someone else. Relationship readiness also means being desirous of an intimate relationship. For example, a history of troubled relationships can leave an individual fearful of, or ambivalent about, being in intimate relationships. Many college students say that the demands of school and work provide little time or energy for intimate relationships. Also, someone may anticipate geographic relocation and may not want to "get something started" that later might become difficult to maintain because of distance. Someone may want to live autonomously for a period of time—for example, when recovering from the breakup of a love relationship.

Those who are "relationship ready" face the challenge of finding and choosing a partner from the "pool of eligibles." In general, partners are found within the local environment or the virtual environment of the Web. One of the most powerful influences on partner choice is the belief that a potential partner is attracted to oneself. Other factors include shared interests, compatibility, certain physical attributes, and the personal characteristics of warmth, trustworthiness, kindness, expressiveness, and a good sense of humor (**Table 11.4**). Physical attractiveness includes appearing young, healthy, and vital. Social status includes ambition, job opportunities, and either possessing or in the process of attaining money and prestige.

Because people tend to associate with those who are like themselves ("birds of a feather flock together"), a variety of similar social characteristics facilitate partner selection, such as age, religion, race, educational attainment, and social background. Social similarity also helps partners conform to norms for permissible relationships. Colleges and universities foster matchmaking by bringing together unmarried individuals of similar age, intelligence, social background, values, goals, and expectations for the future. Also, people assume that physically attractive people are kind, interesting, poised, sociable, sexually warm, and sensitive ("what is beautiful is good") even if they are not.

The beginning stages of a love relationship tend to involve intensely passionate love. During the passionate stage, partners tend to idealize each other, and actual knowledge of the other is minimal. Although the lovers may say they trust one another, this sense of trust is little more than hope that risking one's heart will not end in rejection and failure. Although they may wish otherwise, new lovers usually have considerable uncertainty about the fate of the relationship.

**Table 11.4** Preferred Traits for Dating and Marital Partners

American college students were asked to rate on a scale from one to nine their preference for each trait.

| Trait | Dating Partner | Marital Partner |
|---|---|---|
| Warmth and Kindness | 8.17 | 8.32 |
| Expressiveness and Openness | 7.81 | 7.90 |
| Sense of Humor | 7.77 | 7.76 |
| Sexual Passion | 7.56 | 7.64 |
| Exciting Personality | 7.55 | 7.44 |
| Ambition | 7.36 | 7.40 |
| Intelligence | 7.24 | 7.27 |
| Similar Values/Attitudes | 7.15 | 7.48 |
| Similar Interests/Activities | 7.11 | 7.07 |
| Physical Attractiveness | 6.91 | 7.06 |
| Similar Social Skills | 6.69 | 7.04 |
| Money/Earning Potential | 6.49 | 6.68 |
| Similarity of Background | 6.39 | 6.67 |
| Social Status | 6.13 | 6.37 |
| Complementarity* | 4.51 | 4.58 |
| Prior Sexual Experience | 3.95 | 3.77 |

*Partners' differing personality characteristics balance (complement) rather than conflict.
Adapted from Sprecher, S., & Regan, P. C. (2002). Liking some things (in some people) more than others: Partner preferences in romantic relationships and friendships. *Journal of Social and Personal Relationships, 19*, 463–481.

Although falling in love sometimes involves passionate sexual interaction, most lovers expect their relationship to develop beyond sex to something more emotionally intimate. If the lovers were friends first, they are likely to have developed some degree of trust and intimacy already. If they are strangers at first, they will probably be wary while assessing if the relationship has the potential to become "serious."

As a love relationship develops, the lovers disclose more and more private information about themselves. This leads to appraisals of personal similarities and differences to determine if the relationship has the potential to develop a deeper level of intimacy. If the relationship continues, the level of trust generally increases. Sexual passion may be high at this stage of the relationship as it reinforces feelings of closeness, togetherness, and trust. Also, mutual satisfaction in sex confirms feelings like "we belong together." The excitement of the new and sense of emotional risk also heightens sexual arousal.

After appraisals of the other's suitability as a long-term partner and the development of emotional closeness, partners may sense that their relationship has progressed to a state of "us-ness," which is the sense of belonging to something—the relationship—that it is larger than oneself. Moreover, one recognizes that one's self-interests are served by the relationship. Often the state of "us-ness" is accompanied by a sense of commitment, which is the intention to continue the relationship into the future. This may entail a promise to the partner, and perhaps others, that "we are a couple."

*Relationship maintenance behaviors* enable couples to manifest their commitment to remain together indefinitely (**Table 11.5**). Generally, relationship maintenance behaviors include being positive and cheerful, offering assurances of one's love, commitment to the relationship, faithfulness, telling the partner one's feelings about the relationship, sharing couple tasks and responsibilities, spending time with family members and mutual friends, offering emotional support of the partner when facing problems in her or his life, and being positive in relationship conflict situations.

**Table 11.5** Some Relationship Maintenance Behaviors

| Behavior | Example |
|---|---|
| Being Positive | Acting nice and cheerful; not criticizing; asking how the day has gone; being complimentary |
| Being Assuring | Stressing one's commitment to the partner<br>Communicating that the relationship has a future |
| Being Open | Encouraging the partner to disclose thoughts and feelings<br>Wanting to discuss the quality of the relationship |
| Sharing Tasks | Helping equally with tasks that have to be done |
| Sharing Friends | Spending time with same friends and family |
| Giving Advice | Telling the partner what to do in problem situations |
| Giving Support | Giving advice<br>Being comforting when partner is in need |
| Arguing Positively | Apologizing when wrong<br>Being patient and forgiving |
| Sharing Activities | Sharing special rituals, routines, and time |
| Being Religious | Attending church together, praying about the marriage |

Adapted from Dindia, K., & Baxter, L. A. (1987). Strategies for maintaining and repairing marital relationships. *Journal of Social and Personal Relationship, 4*, 143–158.

## Communication in Intimate Relationships

**literal message** the literal meaning of a communication

**metamessage** the implicit meaning about the context and relationship conveyed in a message

Clear communication fosters development and maintenance of intimate relationships Communication enables partners to make each other aware of their thoughts, feelings, and experiences. It enables partners to coordinate behaviors and helps partners resolve relationship conflicts.

Communication is the process of sending and receiving messages (**Table 11.6**). A message begins in a sender's mind as an idea, wish, feeling, intention, or combination of these. Then, the sender transforms the message into symbols that can be perceived by the recipient, such as spoken or written words, images, posture or body language (gaze, touch, smile, physical proximity), objects (flowers, gifts, food), and behaviors (doing a favor, giving a kiss, ignoring an appointment). Having perceived the symbols, the recipient transforms them into interpretations or "understanding," which may or may not closely match what the sender had it mind.

Every communication has two parts, literal messages and metamessages. A **literal message** is conveyed by the symbols themselves. For example, "It's raining, better take your umbrella" is a literal message about the weather. The **metamessage** (*meta* is the Greek word for "beyond," "additional," or "transcendent") carries implicit meanings about the reason for the communication, how the message is to be interpreted, and the nature of the relationship of the communicators. When one intimate partner says to the other, "It's raining, better take your umbrella," the metamessages can be interpreted as "I care about you" and "An expectation in our relationship is that we help each other out." By saying, "Thanks, honey, for looking out for me," the partner responds to the metamessages in the communication.

**Table 11.6** Factors Affecting Communication

| Factor | Explanation |
|---|---|
| Ability to Send and Receive Symbols | With spoken messages, the ability to speak and hear or to speak and hear a particular language. If the symbol is a dozen roses on Valentine's Day, it might be the ability to grow them or pay for them. |
| Interpretation of Symbols | The outcome of communication depends on how the sender and receiver interpret the symbols in the message. If symbols are interpreted in exactly the same way, communication is facilitated. However, if the sender uses symbols with which the receiver is unfamiliar or that the receiver may interpret in a totally different way than the sender intended, then miscommunication may occur. |
| Communication Rules | Communication is governed by rules about using certain symbols and the appropriateness and conduct of the communication itself. For example, it would be improper to address the President of the United States by his first name. |
| Expectations | Communication is affected by expectations of its outcome. Senders choose symbols that they deem to have the best chance of bringing about their intentions. |
| Attributions | In the role of sender, someone may comment to themselves about their performance and may alter their communication accordingly. In the role of receiver, someone may make assumptions about the sender's character, motives, feelings, and intentions, which can affect the interpretation of the message. |
| Vulnerability and Fear | Communication in emotionally close relationships can feel risky for fear of being hurt, hurting the other, or damaging the relationship. Some common fears are being ridiculed, disliked, insulting another, violence, making a promise, losing status, setting a precedent, losing love, change, losing control of emotions, and losing control over the relationship. |

## Clear Communication

Clear communication is one in which the symbols represent as closely as possible the communicators' thoughts, feelings, and intentions. Clarity can be achieved by using *I-statements*—sentences that begin with (or have as the subject) the pronoun "I." Clarity is jeopardized by using *You-statements*—sentences that begin with (or have as the subject) the pronoun "you," as in "You always . . . ," "You never . . . ," "You are . . . ," or the interrogatives, "Why don't you . . . ?" or "How could you . . . ?" Recipients of You-statements often respond to the metamessage they generally convey, which is criticism. Very often, You-statements lead to hurt feelings and counterattack or withdrawal.

A major obstacle to clear communication is *going off beam*. In this instance, the conversation moves from one unrelated topic to another without addressing the sender's original message. *Cross-complaining*, a type of off beam, involves partners hurling a series of often unrelated complaints at each other, generally as You-messages. Another obstacle to clear communication is assuming what another person is thinking or feeling (*mind reading*).

*Follow the leader* is being drawn into an exchange of criticism–countercriticism or blame–accuse–blame–accuse because the other person is using that style of communication.

## Effective Listening

Clear communication is based not only on sending clear messages but also on listening effectively. Effective listening means being attentive not only to what a person is saying but also to what the person is feeling. Effective listening as based on **empathy**, which is the state of putting yourself in the other person's experience and experiencing the situation as she or he does. This is different than general discourse, which proceeds as I talk–you talk–I talk–you talk. Thus, while the other person is speaking, the recipient, instead of listening, is focused on creating the next portion of the dialogue. Instead of driving the dialogue onward, it is more effective to focus on the content of speaker's message and accompanying emotions. This is called *active listening*; it can be demonstrated with making eye contact and gestures, nods, and vocalizations such as "uh-huh," "yes," "go on," and "I see." When the speaker has finished, the recipient offers the speaker a paraphrase (a condensed rewording of a statement) of the remarks using an emotion word that describes the speaker's feelings and a "because statement" that describes the reason for that emotion from the speaker's point of view. For example, a speaker may express concern that she has not found an occupation that seems interesting. The listener's paraphrase could be, "You seem nervous because you haven't found a job you want to do in the future." *Nervous* is the emotion word that describes the speaker's feelings and *because you haven't found a job you want to do in the future* is the reason for that emotion.

**empathy** seeing and responding emotionally to a situation as someone else does

Here are a few suggestions for being a good listener and, therefore, a good communicator:

- Give the speaker your full attention. If you cannot, say so and ask to continue when you are ready.
- Make eye contact to communicate that you're paying attention.
- Try to assume a posture similar to the other person's. Both people should sit or stand to create a sense of equal status.
- Don't speak until the other person is finished or has asked for your response. Unless asked, do not offer your advice ("You should . . . "), your

opinion ("I think . . . "), your judgments ("That's crazy/stupid/weird"), your life history ("Here's what happened to me . . . "), or your predictions ("It/he/she will . . . ").

- Praise the other person's effort for investing the time, energy, and caring to communicate with you, especially if the communication was difficult.

Effective listening is usually more than half of good communication because the listener not only receives the speaker's message but also helps establish the physical and emotional context for the communication.

## Relationship Endings

Everything in the universe (even the universe itself) has a beginning and an end. Galaxies, stars, and planets form and disintegrate, species of plants and animals arise and become extinct, societies rise and fall. Intimate relationships also have a beginning and an end. Sometimes a relationship lasts for only a few days; sometimes it lasts until one partner dies (and even then the relationship may still be "alive" in the mind of the surviving partner). Sometimes the structure of a close relationship persists but the closeness and the dynamism wane, creating a "shell" relationship without vitality.

Close relationships may end when the partners' feelings and interests are no longer shared. The relationship may also end when one or both partners are unwilling or unable to invest time, material resources, interest, love, and support in the relationship. Another reason is that one or both partners will not commit to a sexually and emotionally exclusive relationship. In some cases, a relationship ends because of hostility from the partners' social networks. Families may not accept a son's or daughter's choice of an intimate partner, and interracial, same-sex, and disabled partnerships are still highly stigmatized in American society.

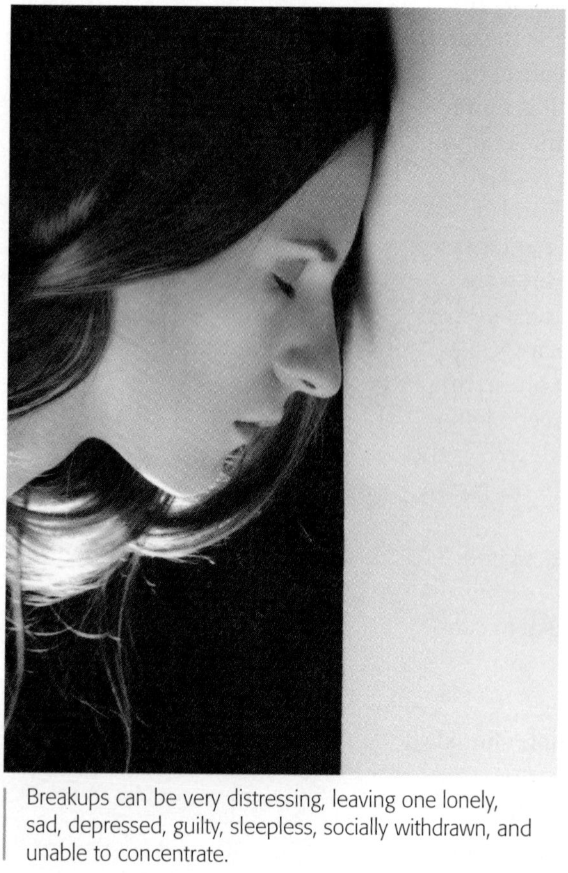

Breakups can be very distressing, leaving one lonely, sad, depressed, guilty, sleepless, socially withdrawn, and unable to concentrate.

Occasionally, the seeds of an ending are sown into a relationship at its beginning. For example, partners may seek an intimate relationship as a way to cope with personal problems. They may feel rejected and lonely because of a breakup of a previous relationship. They may fear that they cannot take care of themselves. If, as often happens, a partner or relationship does not provide the solution to a personal problem, a disappointed, angry, or frustrated individual may seek alternative ways of coping, which may be destructive to the relationship. Relationship-destroying behaviors include drug or alcohol use, extrarelationship affairs, or physically or emotionally abusing the partner.

Individuals experiencing a breakup may feel tired, lonely, sad, depressed, resentful, or guilty. They may be unable to sleep or eat and may miss classes or work. They may withdraw from friends. Concentrating on tasks may be difficult because they continually think about the former partner and dwell on reasons the relationship ended. They may feel helpless ("What will become of me?"), hopeless ("I'll *always* be alone"), or skeptical or cynical ("Love can never work out").

In contrast, some individuals feel relaxed, hopeful, and relieved that what they perceived as a bad, risky, or stagnant relationship has ended. They feel free to pursue personal goals or to seek a more rewarding relationship partner. Sometimes, individuals feel euphoric and self-confident when a relationship ends. They say that the parting was for the best, and they become more active and outgoing. However, this positive outlook may alternate with feelings of sadness and distress at the lost relationship.

Endings can be very painful, especially if the partners' lives had been intertwined for a considerable length of time. When an ending is very painful, a person may have difficulty seeing any good from their experience. But often, endings mark the start of a new and better future. And what is learned about oneself and relationships from having been in one can be assets in life and in future relationships of all kinds. As psychiatry professor Ethel Person has pointed out:

> Many loves end; some sorrowfully, some painfully, and others bitterly. Nonetheless, for many unhappy lovers, the memory of the joy that was theirs, and the legacy of change that took place within themselves as a consequence of love, imbue the experience with value that endures long after the relationship has ended. Consequently, while love may end unhappily, this does not mean that the overall effects were necessarily negative. Ultimately some loves are growth-enhancing and self-expanding while they last. Often the real impact of the experience can be evaluated only months or years after its end. In the deepest sense we come to know very few people, and so we may always treasure those few with whom we exacted those basic dramas that shaped our identities and destinies.

## SEXUALITY IN REVIEW

- Most North American adults prefer sexual relations within the context of an emotionally close (love) relationship.
- Love consists of the dimensions of intimacy, passion, and commitment. Passion tends to predominate at the beginning of a love relationship (passionate love); intimacy and commitment tend to predominate as a love relationship matures (companionate love).
- Intimacy is characterized by emotional closeness, trust, and self-validation. Intimacy develops from self-disclosure.
- Jealousy is an amalgam of anger, fear, and sadness arising from the belief that one's relationship is threatened.
- Loneliness results from not having sufficient social ties that provide feelings of being loved and valued.
- Clear communication facilitates relationship harmony.
- Love relationships can end; their endings sometimes provide opportunities for self-reflection and personal growth.

## CRITICAL THINKING ABOUT SEXUALITY

1. Write a response to each of the following:
    - What are your expectations from a love relationship? A real love relationship must include . . .
    - How do you give love?
    - What is intimacy? How does it feel to be intimate with another?
    - What is the relationship of sex and love? Is it possible to have one without the other?
    - Can romantic love be everlasting?
    - What is the best way to cope with the loss of a love relationship?

2. Describe five of the most important lessons that you have learned from recent peer-love experience(s). Indicate which lessons, if any, you wish you had known before being in love. Which lessons could have been learned by being advised by others, taking a class, or reading? Which lessons could be learned only by personal experience?
3. Beth and Ron have been married for a few years. Both work. They have no children. One evening, while Ron is checking his Facebook page and Beth writes a report for work, the phone rings and rings.

   Ron: Beth! Why didn't you answer the phone?

   Beth: I'm not your secretary.

   Ron: You don't care what happens around here, do you?

   Beth: Oh yeah, who pays for the stupid phone, anyway?

   Ron: Money, money, money. That's all you ever think about. You're as materialistic as your father.

   Beth: At least he cared about getting ahead. All you care about is playing golf with your pals.

   Ron: I'd play less golf if you were more fun to be around. All you do is work.

   Beth: If I don't, who will? You're just an irresponsible kid.

   Ron: And you're just an old nag.

   a. How do Beth's and Ron's use of "I-statements" and "You-statements" affect this conversation and their likely feelings afterward?
   b. Would you classify this communication as clear, off beam, cross-complaining, mind reading, and/or follow the leader? Explain your reasoning.
   c. Rewrite a more positive ending to this conversation beginning with Beth's line, "Oh yeah, who pays for the stupid phone, anyway?" Use empathy, feedback, and I-statements.
4. Last year, Suzanne fell head-over-heels in love with Aaron and he with her. Despite her belief that she had finally met the perfect man for her, Suzanne cannot suppress disquiet about the relationship, especially when she sees how her friend Bonnie is treated by her boyfriend, Stuart. Stuart is extremely attentive to Bonnie. He brings her flowers and little gifts, he always comments how nice Bonnie looks, and he encourages Bonnie to continue with her painting even though Bonnie knows she may never be a great artist.

   Sometimes Suzanne wishes Aaron would give her the attention that she sees Bonnie getting from Stuart. Sometimes it makes Suzanne angry, and she wonders if Aaron is really all that wonderful. Such thoughts usually make Suzanne feel guilty. Sometimes Suzanne wonders if Aaron has lost interest in her and this is his way of showing it.

   a. Do Suzanne's feelings of disquiet mean that she is not really in love with Aaron?
   b. What, if anything, should Suzanne do about her feelings?
   c. Aaron is a law student and works very hard. Is Suzanne being unreasonable to want more attention from him?
   d. One of Suzanne's friends suggested that she be more attentive to Aaron, and by doing so he would reciprocate. Is this a good strategy? Why or why not?
   e. Lately, Aaron has been suggesting that he and Suzanne get married when he finishes law school. What advice, if any, do you have for Suzanne?

## REFERENCES AND RECOMMENDED RESOURCES

### References

Aron, A., et al. (2005). Reward, motivation, and emotion systems associated with early-stage intense romantic love. *Journal of Neurophysiology, 94*, 327–333.

Cacioppo, J. T., & Patrick, W. (2009). *Loneliness: Human nature and the need for social connection*. New York: Norton.

Esch, T., & Stefano, G. B. (2005). Love promotes health. *Neuroendocrinology Letters, 26*, 264–267.

Fisher, H. E., & Thompson Jr., J. A. (2007). Lust, romance, attachment. In: S. M. Platek, J. P Keenan, & T. K. Shakelford (Eds.). *Evolutionary cognitive neuroscience*. Cambridge, MA: MIT Press.

Guerrero, L. K., Spitzberg, B. H., & Yoshimura, S. M. (2006). Sexual and emotional jealousy. In: R. D. McAnulty & M. M. Burnette (Eds.). *Sex and sexuality* (pp. 311–345). Guilford, CT: Praeger.

Jankowiak, W. J. (2008). *Intimacies: Love and sex across cultures*. New York: Columbia University Press.

Macdonald, K., & MacDonald, T. M. (2010). The peptide that binds: A systematic review of oxytocin and its prosocial effects in humans. *Harvard Review of Psychiatry, 18*, 1–21.

Regan, P. C. (2006). Love. In: R. D. McAnulty & M. M. Burnette. *Sex and sexuality* (pp. 88–113). Guilford, CT: Praeger.

Shaver, P. R., & Mikulincer, M. (2006). Attachment theory, individual psychodynamics, and relationship functioning. In: A. L. Vangesti (Ed.), *Cambridge handbook of personal relationships*. Cambridge: Cambridge University Press.

Sternberg, R. J. (1986). A triangular theory of love. *Psychological Review, 93*, 119–135.

### Recommended Resources

Baumeister, R. F., & Leary, M. R. (1995). The need to belong: Desire for interpersonal attachment as a fundamental human motivation. *Psychological Bulletin, 117*, 497–529. Explains how emotional attachment is fundamental to human life.

Boelen, P. A., & Reijntjes, A. (2009). Negative cognitions in emotional problems following romantic relationship break-ups. *Stress and Health, 25*, 11–19. Discusses how thinking patterns, including core beliefs and automatic thoughts, affect individuals' emotional reactions to relationship breakups.

Mikulincer, M., & Shaver, P. R. (2010). Attachment in adulthood: Structure, dynamics, and change. New York: Guilford. Leading relationship psychologists explain how attachment orientations affect adult romantic relationships.

Sternberg, R. J., & Weis, K. (2008). *The new psychology of love*. New Haven, CT: Yale University Press. Scientific essays on the definition and practical implications of love.

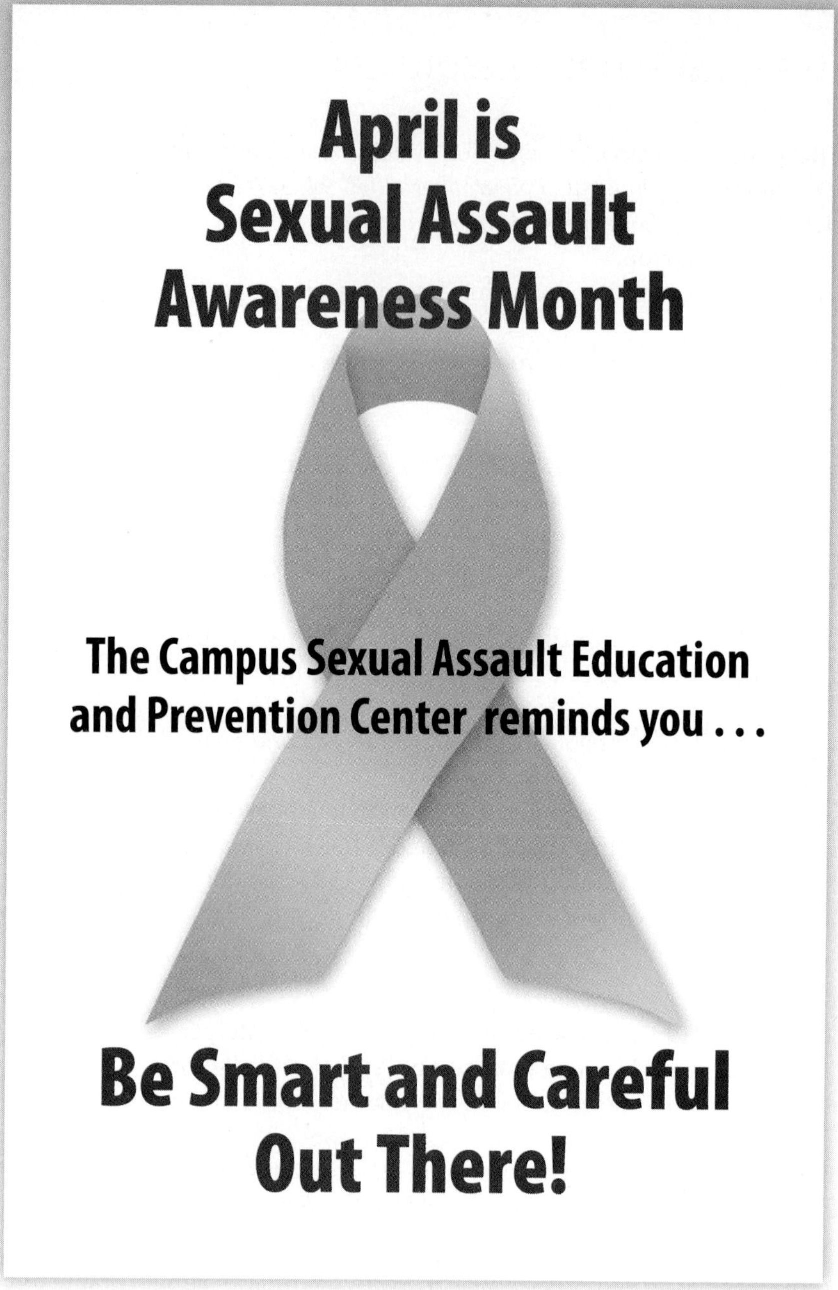
April is
Sexual Assault
Awareness Month
The Campus Sexual Assault Education
and Prevention Center reminds you . . .
Be Smart and Careful
Out There!

*"No society that feeds its children on tales of successful violence can expect them not to believe that violence in the end is rewarded."*

— Margaret Mead, anthropologist

CHAPTER 12

# Sexual Coercion and Assault

## Student Learning Objectives

1 Define rape, acquaintance rape, intimate partner violence, and child sexual abuse

2 Explain how sexual and relationship violence are affected by traditional male gender roles

3 Define rape trauma syndrome

4 Describe acquaintance rape

5 List the stages of interpersonal violence

6 Describe the consequences for victims of child sexual abuse

Violence—physical force used to inflict physical injury or death—permeates the animal kingdom. Predators use offensive violence and prey use defensive violence in their struggles for food, water, and territory, and to survive and reproduce. Humans practice violence for these same reasons and more. People use violence to assert power and control over others, to gain revenge, and as a reaction to feelings of anger, shame, and jealousy. Moreover, humans are able to imagine *potential* situations in which violence seems desirable or necessary—for example, if they believe that some person or group *might* take away their access to food, water, or shelter. Other reasons for violence include fearing harm to oneself or one's family or community, feeling disrespected, or believing that one's values and deeply held beliefs are under attack. The World Health Organization estimates that 1.6 million people in the world die each year due to violence. Because it is so destructive to individuals and social groups, all cultures regulate intragroup violence by law, religion, and cultural norm.

The World Health Organization (WHO) defines violence as "the intentional use of physical force or power, threatened or actual, against oneself, another person, or against a group or community, that either results in or has a high likelihood of resulting in injury, death, psychological harm, maldevelopment, or deprivation." Violence can be inflicted by physical, sexual, and psychological attack and by deprivation. Violence can be collective (e.g., war, genocide), self-directed (e.g., self-abuse, suicide), or between individuals, which is called interpersonal violence. Among the several kinds of interpersonal violence are sexual assault and rape, intimate partner violence, and child sexual abuse (FIGURE 12.1).

**interpersonal violence** violence between individuals including assault, battery, rape, intimate partner violence, child maltreatment and sexual abuse, elder abuse, and homicide

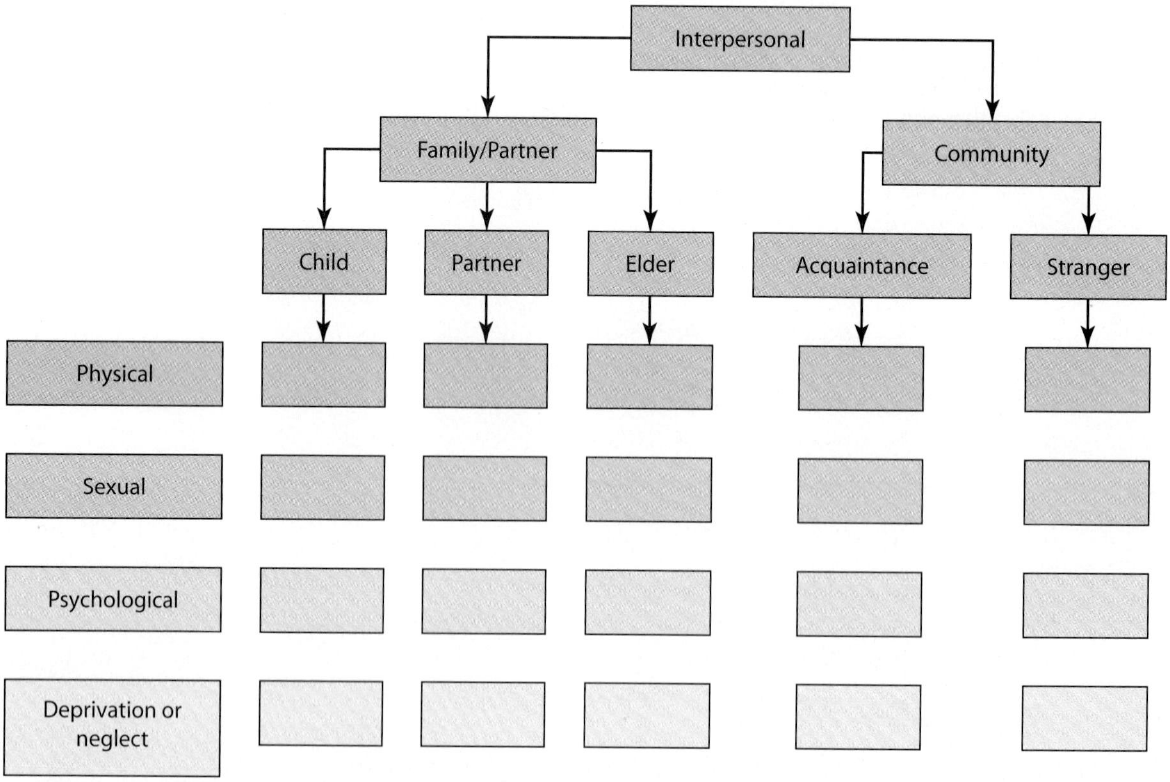


FIGURE 12.1 **Kinds of Interpersonal Violence.** Interpersonal violence—violence between individuals—takes place in families and intimate relationships and in communities. Family violence includes child maltreatment and incest, intimate partner violence, and elder abuse. Community violence includes youth violence, physical and sexual assault by acquaintances and strangers, violence related to property, and violence, abuse, and neglect in schools, workplaces, health facilities, and other institutions.

From World Health Organization, Violence Prevention Alliance. Definition and typology of violence. Available at: http://www.who.int/violenceprevention/approach/definition/en/index.html. Accessed October 5, 2010.

## Sexual Assault and Rape

The word **rape** comes from the Latin *rapere*, which means to seize or take by force. Originally, the word meant the looting and destruction of an enemy's village, town, or city and the capture of its citizens to be used as slaves. The idea that to be raped is to be vanquished persists today, as when referring to the inhumane destruction of an entire city (e.g., the Rape of Nanking, China, in 1937) or being defeated in an endeavor ("I was raped on that exam").

More commonly, the word rape refers to nonconsensual sexual behavior, generally forced penile penetration of a bodily orifice. In the conduct of a rape, a victim may also be beaten, have her or his life threatened, or be killed. The combination of forced sexual penetration and nonsexual violence is called **sexual assault**.

In the conduct of war, sexually assaulting an enemy's women and boys is often used to symbolize hatred and subjugation of "the other side." In this context, sexual assault is not committed for sexual gratification. Rather, it is motivated by the desire to control, harm, humiliate, and dehumanize the victim and her or his "side" in the war. In cultures in which women and children are considered a man's property, sexual assault can be deemed a successful attack on enemy males.

Sexual assault occurs in virtually every culture in the world. The WHO reports that, depending on the country, between 1% and 5% of adult women have been sexually assaulted in the previous five years. In some countries, almost one in four women experience sexual violence by an intimate partner, and almost one-third of young girls report that their first sexual encounter was being raped.

In North America, rape and sexual assault are crimes. Although varying by jurisdiction, rape is generally defined as nonconsensual penetration by force or threat of force of a body orifice, usually the mouth, rectum, or vagina. Penetration generally means by penis, although it also may include fingers or objects. Nonconsensual means the victim is incapable of giving legal consent because of mental development, physical disability, or being semiconscious (e.g., with alcohol or drugs) or unconscious. Types of rape include the following:

- *Date or acquaintance rape:* the victim and perpetrator know each other
- *Marital rape:* the victim and perpetrator are married
- *Stranger rape:* forced sexual contact by a stranger

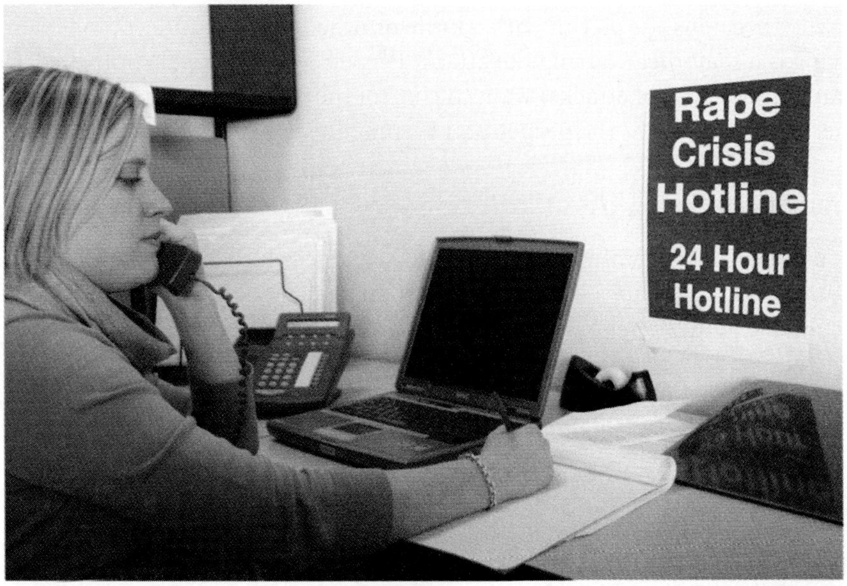


Sexual assault is the combination of forced sexual penetration and nonsexual violence.

**rape** nonconsensual sexual behavior, generally penile penetration of a bodily orifice

**sexual assault** the combination of nonconsensual sexual penetration (rape) and nonsexual violence, such as battery, the threat of harm, or homicide

- *Gang rape:* rape by two or more perpetrators
- *Statutory rape:* sexual intercourse with a legally underage person

According to the U.S. Department of Justice, more than 300,000 adult American women and 90,000 adult American men report having been raped in the previous 12 months—and because rape is largely an underreported crime, these data are thought to represent only about 40% of actual rape incidents. More than half of all rapes of women (54%) occur before age 18; 22% of these rapes occur before age 12. Among men, 75% of all rapes occur before age 18, and 48% occur before age 12.

About 80% of rapes in the United States are committed by someone the victim knows. About 52% of rapes occur on dates, at parties, or in other social situations. In their lifetimes, about 10% of American women are victims of rape or attempted rape by a husband or intimate partner, including a current or former spouse, cohabiting partner, boyfriend/girlfriend, or date. Among men who are raped, 60% know their attacker.

The vast majority of perpetrators of sexual assault are men. It is theorized that gender role attitudes and expectations facilitate the occurrence of many rapes. For example, the belief that to be masculine means one has to be aggressive encourages some men to use sexual violence to gain control over others, especially women. This leads to commonly held beliefs such as "women like a powerful man" or "women like being raped." Also, some men believe that making a sexual conquest (*scoring*) proves their masculinity. Believing that the male role is to be dominant, some men try to take what they want regardless of how their behavior may harm others. Moreover, popular media present images and messages that encourage men to see women as sex objects and objects of angry, violent control. Young men and women may not realize that these images are not intended to serve as models of appropriate behavior but instead are fictions manufactured by exploitative grown-ups to sell products.

The expectation that the male should take the lead in sex also fosters misunderstandings and violence. A woman's "no" to a sexual advance can be misinterpreted as a signal to continue until finally the woman stops or pulls away, which frustrates the male and may lead to anger-induced aggression. This gives rise to male statements like, "I didn't believe her when she said no."

Men who sexually assault women are characterized as anger motivated or power motivated (**Table 12.1**). Anger-motivated assaults (about 20% of rapes) generally manifest an intense hatred of women. They tend to be committed by a stranger who threatens the victim with a knife or other weapon. Indeed, for victims, dying is a major fear during the attack. Perpetrators of power-motivated sexual assault (about 80% of attacks) want to control the victim rather than harm or injure her or him. Usually, the perpetrator is someone the victim knows.

## Consequences of Sexual Assault

Sexual assault has many harmful and lasting consequences for victims, families, and communities. For example, being raped exposes female victims to pregnancy and acquiring a sexually transmitted disease, including HIV/AIDS. Also, a sexually assaulted woman may experience chronic pelvic pain, gastrointestinal disorders, frequent headaches, and back and facial pain. Victims also are more susceptible to alcohol and drug abuse to block out memories and anxieties associated with the attack.

**rape trauma syndrome** immediate and long-term mental health consequences from having been raped

One common psychological consequence of having been raped is the sense of having been personally violated. Victims of sexual assault face both immediate and long-term psychological consequences, referred to as **rape trauma syndrome**. Immediately following an assault and continuing for days or weeks, victims may

**Table 12.1** Types of Sexual Assault

**Power-Assertive/Power-Exploitive**

The assailant is generally described as egotistical and wanting to prove his concept of masculine power (often characterized as "macho") by overcoming and aggressively (sometimes violently) dominating and controlling a victim. The assailant's goal is primarily to humiliate and traumatize a victim (to demonstrate power) rather than to harm physically or kill. The assault often involves tying up the victim, using considerable profanity to demean and humiliate the victim, and forcing the victim to engage in various sex acts. Victims are rarely specific targets; rather, they are often age-peers who are met in bars or at parties, or hitchhiking—anywhere circumstances suggest to the perpetrator that an assault can be successfully committed. Alcohol and/or drugs are usually taken prior to committing the crime.

**Power-Reassurance**

The assailant is generally unable to develop interpersonal or romantic relationships. Victims tend to be age-peer acquaintances, neighbors, or coworkers who are spied upon or stalked prior to the crime. The assault is generally a "surprise" attack—for example, entering a victim's home while the victim is asleep. The attack may involve minimal physical force, and no weapons or threats of death, which is the reason perpetrators are sometimes referred to by law enforcement personnel as "gentleman rapists." The assailant may fantasize being the victim's lover and may force the victim to emulate foreplay. The assailant may revisit the victim's home after the rape and even make follow-up telephone contact. Also, the assailants tend to take trophies or souvenirs from the victim and keep detailed records of assaults.

**Anger-Retaliatory**

These attacks are usually impulsive, spontaneous, and brutal. The victim is rarely a specific target but instead an unfortunate and vulnerable symbol of a group the assailant hates. The assailant's goal is revenge for real or imaginary wrongs; sex is a means of punishment. Because the assailant's goal is to discharge pent-up feelings of hatred and anger, victims are often hit, and whereas the intention is not to kill, the victim may be beaten to death if she or he resists.

**Anger-Excitation**

In these attacks, commonly called "sadistic," the assailant's goal is to inflict pain and suffering upon a victim, from which the assailant is sexually aroused. Victims tend not to be specific targets, but they are thought to represent evil and powerful groups (e.g., women, "society") whose power the assailant is trying to minimize. Victims may be brutally tortured and then killed to prevent identifying the assailant or for self-gratification. Drugs and/or alcohol are usually involved.

manifest one of the following reactions: (1) frequent crying and appearing agitated, hysterical, and anxious; (2) appearing calm and emotionally in control, as if nothing happened; or (3) experiencing shock and disbelief or being disoriented, confused, and unable to carry out normal tasks.

After a while, a victim may try to adjust to having been sexually assaulted by minimizing or refusing to accept or discuss the extent of trauma ("everything is fine"; "it could have been worse"). Alternatively, a victim may respond by talking incessantly about the assault, perhaps repeatedly analyzing her or his own behaviors and guessing at the assailant's motives. Sometimes a victim may change residence, school, job, and/or appearance, or withdraw from former relationships. Also, a victim may experience emotional detachment, distrust of others, and social withdrawal; guilt and shame surrounding the assault; depression; sleep disturbances; difficulty with intimate and sexual relations even with trusted others; and various manifestations of anxiety including **post-traumatic stress disorder (PTSD)**, the symptoms of which include:

**post-traumatic stress disorder (PTSD)** long-term psychological harm from having been sexually assaulted

- Re-experiencing the rape via unbidden, intrusive images, thoughts, dreams, and "flashbacks"—having the sense of reliving the assault, including the terror and other disturbing emotions associated with the attack. As one victim explained, "a flashback is not a memory of the assault; you are *there*."
- Avoiding stimuli associated with the assault or general emotional unresponsiveness (*emotional numbing*). This can include experiencing fear when in locales that resemble the scene of the assault, being unable to recall the assault (*denial*), or being able to "make the mind go someplace else" to avoid

thoughts and memories of the assault (*dissociation*). The victim may manipulate others and the environment to keep things under control. This may include detachment and estrangement from others or being unable to have loving feelings. Victims may become compliant to avoid real or imagined potential abuse.

- Persistent arousal symptoms, such as difficulty falling or staying asleep or being edgy, jumpy, irritable, and sometimes irrationally angry. Victims may have difficulty concentrating, be hypervigilant to their surroundings, and have an exaggerated startle response.

Family members, friends, and intimates also suffer when someone they know, love, and care about has been sexually assaulted.

Recovering from sexual assault requires patience and support. Sexual assault survivors are encouraged to seek psychological counseling from rape-recovery professionals. Also, joining a support group of other assaulted individuals can be helpful in releasing the shame and horror associated with the assault. Support and understanding from family, friends, intimate partners, and the community are also valuable.

## Sexual Assault at American Colleges and Universities

**acquaintance/date rape** rape or sexual assault committed by someone the victim knows

According to the American College Health Association, each year about 6% of American college women and 2% of American college men experience attempted or completed sexual assault. Also, about 4% of college women and 2% of college men experience verbal threats for sex against their will.

Approximately 90% of sexual assaults on college campuses are committed by someone the victim knows (**acquaintance/date rape**). The attacker is usually a classmate, friend, boyfriend, ex-boyfriend, or other acquaintance. Most acquaintance rapes occur when students are in the same place (e.g., at a party, studying together in a dorm room). College students are the most vulnerable to acquaintance rape during the first few weeks of the freshman and sophomore years. Actual "date rape" tends to occur at the beginning of a dating relationship. The victim is raped in a car or residence after a date. Date rapes make up between 10% and 15% of completed rapes and nearly 40% of attempted rapes. Gang rapes, which tend to occur at parties, are much less frequent than other types of rape.

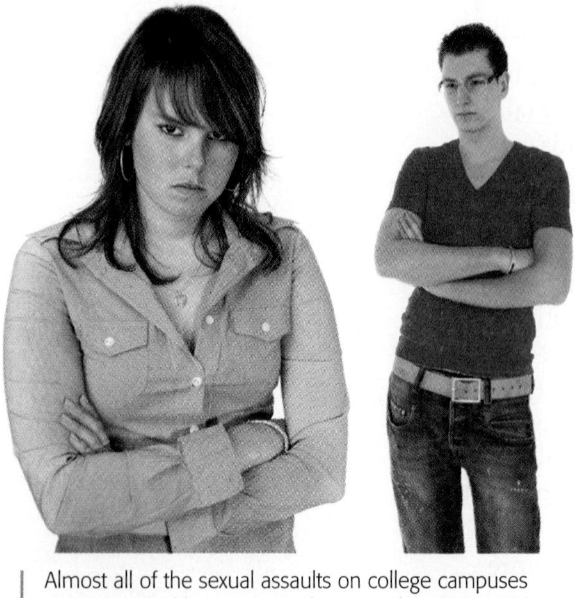

Almost all of the sexual assaults on college campuses are committed by someone the victim knows.

Acquaintance rape among college students is sometimes attributed to miscommunication between those involved. It is thought that men are socialized to believe that women initially resist sexual advances to preserve their reputation as "moral" but really prefer being overcome sexually. Thus, if a woman says no, a man thinks he is to proceed as if she said yes. In addition, some men believe that a woman perceived as a "tease" or "loose" wants sex. Men view certain cues from women as evidence that they are interested in having sex; cues include wearing revealing clothing, agreeing to go to a secluded location or the man's room, drinking alcohol, and flirting.

Alcohol and drug use among perpetrators and victims is associated with 75% of rapes among college students. Some men interpret alcohol use by women as a sign of sexual interest and availability, and some women use alcohol to justify inappropriate behaviors. College women who use drugs, attend a school with a high rate of drinking, or belong to a sorority are at greater risk for rape. Even though a woman knows that drinking and being alone with a man could be dangerous, she may deny that she is at risk herself. Also, if intoxicated on alcohol or on drugs, a woman may not notice efforts to get her into an isolated location. Furthermore, alcohol and drugs can reduce one's capacity to verbally or physically resist a rapist. When alcohol or drugs are involved in acquaintance rape, the woman is generally held by others to be more responsible than the rapist.

College student victims of acquaintance rape suffer the same psychological harm as rape victims generally. However, college acquaintance rape victims may leave school for fear of facing their attacker on campus. Among the many tragedies of acquaintance rape is that many victims, perpetrators, and others do not interpret sexual assault by a victim's friend, dating partner, or intimate partner as criminal assault. Rather, many believe the myth that rape is committed only by strangers. Thus, rape by an acquaintance is something other than rape. This unfortunate misinterpretation may be reinforced by the fact that the victim may have been drinking, may have used drugs, and even may have had sex with the assailant previously. For these reasons, many victims of acquaintance rape do not report their assault to authorities, fearing violent reprisal by their assailant, blame for "not knowing better," and "revictimization" by the legal process.

## Intimate Partner Violence

Intimate partner violence (IPV) is physical, psychological, or sexual harm by a current or former intimate partner or spouse, consisting of threats of or actual use of physical force; being humiliated, insulted, continually criticized, threatened, and demeaned; and nonconsensual forced and/or abusive or degrading sexual behavior or having sexual intercourse for fear of a partner's otherwise violent behavior.

**intimate partner violence (IPV)** physical, sexual, or psychological harm by a current or former partner or spouse, ranging from one hit to chronic, severe beatings

A report from the WHO based on data collected from over 24,000 women living in 10 countries (Bangladesh, Brazil, Ethiopia, Japan, Namibia, Peru, Samoa, Serbia and Montenegro, Thailand, and the United Republic of Tanzania) showed that the proportion of women who had ever experienced physical or sexual violence, or both, by an intimate partner in their lifetime ranged from 15% to 71%.

In North America, IPV is a serious public health problem. The extent of IPV is unknown because it is grossly underreported; the U.S. Centers for Disease Control and Prevention estimates that each year in the United States IPV is responsible for nearly two million injuries and 1300 deaths (about 10% of homicide victims are killed by an intimate partner). A woman is beaten by a husband or boyfriend every 15 seconds. More women are treated in hospital emergency rooms for intimate partner battering injuries than for muggings, rapes, and traffic accidents combined. Between 4% and 8% of pregnant women are abused at least once during the pregnancy, making battering during pregnancy the leading cause of birth defects and infant mortality. According to the American College Health Association, 16% of college women and 10% of college men report emotional abuse in their intimate relationships; nearly 3% of college women and 2% of college men report physical abuse.

IPV is often associated with personal and cultural attitudes that support male dominance and aggression, and the derogation and objectification of women. In some cultures, wife beating is considered "normal," and women dare not com-

## Dear Penelope . . .

***Two years ago I had a boyfriend who was sexually abusive. He never forced me to have intercourse with him, but we did everything else. There were a lot of mind games and manipulation involved; he made me feel like I "owed" him and said that this would be "the last time" more than once.***

***So I've decided that an orgasm is hardly worth the trouble and am not interested in anything physical beyond kissing. I don't want to touch or be touched because I have fiercely negative feelings associated with foreplay activities. I think that if I did get into another physical relationship, the cons would lead the pros, with the emotional pain outweighing the physical pleasure.***

***The problem is that I don't see my attitude changing, even if I get married, which will obviously pose some problems. Do you have any suggestions on what I should do, or should I let time work on it? I talked to a counselor last year, but that didn't affect my feelings on this topic.***

***— Still Affected by the Past***

*Dear Still Affected,*

Shutting down sexually, which is what your negative feelings about sex represent, is your way of protecting yourself from further abuse, including memories and associated feelings of prior abusive experiences.

If your self-protection prevents you from even considering trusting in another relationship, then counseling should be able to help you work through your negative feelings from your previous relationship and understand how healthy, close relationships work. Your previous experience with counseling should not be taken as a sign that counseling now or in the future will not be helpful. Sometimes counseling doesn't "take" on the first try. Sometimes we are not ready to heal our emotional wounds.

Sexual relationships teach us things about ourselves and about being emotionally close that can be learned only by experience. Your prior relationship has given you many potential lessons: That you can care about your well-being, that you have needs, that you have boundaries and limits, that you want and believe that sexual experiences can be positive and pleasurable, that you do not always want to serve the other person at the expense of yourself, and that you know when you are being abused. Seeking health and wholeness by processing these lessons is apparently on your personal and relationship agendas right now, which is why you wrote your letter to me. Be patient and compassionate with yourself.

Courtesy of the UC Davis *Aggie*

plain. IPV also may be a manifestation of a loss of impulse control exacerbated by alcohol or drug use.

An episode of intimate partner violence often occurs in the following stages:

*Stage of Calm:* Interaction in the relationship consists of "normal," even kind and loving behavior. There may be minor incidents of "acting out," such as a harsh critical remark, slamming a door, or demanding sex from a partner.

*Stage of Tension Building:* This stage involves minor incidents of abuse (e.g., threats, pushing, slapping, outbursts of intense anger, harsh criticism, blaming) with a noticeable rise in the level of tension. The victim may become fearful ("be walking on eggshells") and may try to placate or avoid the abuser. The victim may keep tight control of feelings of anger and fear, and try to "fix" the situation/relationship. Arguments may increase in both frequency and intensity.

*Trigger:* The tension-building phase ends when something—almost anything—triggers a violent episode of IPV. For example, the abuser may want to dominate an argument or punish the partner for arguing at all ("whip the partner into shape," "teach the partner a lesson"). Sometimes the trigger consists of the partner talking to a friend, wearing the "wrong" clothes, pursuing a hobby or career, or criticizing some aspect of the abuser's behavior, such as alcohol use. If the abuse is a recurring theme in the relationship, the victim may withdraw from arguments as a means of self-protection or sometimes precipitate the violence to break the tension. If the violent episode is the first in the relationship, the victim may be shocked and confused and wonder and even ask the abuser what she or he did to trigger the attack.

Whatever the specific behavior, and no matter how innocent or justified, the trigger is often something perceived by the abuser as a threat to the relationship or dominance. This can manifest as extreme jealousy and intense anger, which motivates some form of physical, emotional, or sexual abuse to control the partner.

Another common trigger is stress—such as work, school, family problems, finances, and performance pressure—which causes a buildup of anxiety and tension. The stressed partner may blame the other ("It's all your fault!"), a falsehood that in the abuser's mind establishes the partner as a logical and justifiable target for a violent outburst.

*Violent Stage:* Violence can be one way or mutual. Victims of violence may be afraid to hit back, fearing enraging the abuser even more and putting themselves (or their children) in greater jeopardy. Some victims do not fight back because they do not believe in violence. However, in some relationships both partners engage equally in violence, but in most instances there is a clear aggressor and a clear victim, who retaliates in order to preserve a sense of dignity and self-respect even at the risk of enduring greater physical harm.

*Honeymoon Stage:* In the immediate aftermath of a violent episode, the abuser may cry and be contrite, apologetic, guilty, and ashamed. The abuser may promise never to act violently again. The abuse may be followed by acts of love and gifts. The abuser may act loving and kind. The partner may feel sympathetic, happy that the abuse is ended, and hopeful that it will never reoccur. Alternatively, the abuser may act as if the violence did not take place, or minimize its consequences. Also, the abuser may blame the victim for precipitating the abuse, a contention with which the victim may concur.

*Repetition Stage:* The cycle repeats again and again; in a long relationship, the violence may worsen until the victim feels forced to do something and end the relationship. Violent episodes end only when the victim leaves the relationship or one or both partners seek professional help. Sometimes the violence ends when criminal charges are brought against the abuser after a beating.

About 40% of women and 20% of men sustain physical injuries during their most recent victimization. These include scratches, bruises, welts, broken bones, and knife wounds. Long-term victims of IPV experience physical and psychological consequences similar to those of sexual assault, including substance abuse, alcoholism, disordered eating, suicide attempts, and PTSD.

Children also suffer when exposed to IPV. Some become physically injured themselves during IPV between their parents. Also, observing parental IPV is frightening and traumatic to children, raising the risk of subsequent attachment problems, stress, and physical and emotional problems. Children who grow up

**Table 12.2** Risk Factors for IPV Victimization

| |
|---|
| **Individual Factors** |
| Prior history of IPV<br>Being female<br>Young age<br>Heavy alcohol and drug use<br>High-risk sexual behavior<br>Witnessing or experiencing violence as a child<br>Being less educated<br>Unemployment<br>For men, having a different ethnicity from their partner's<br>For women, having a greater education level than their partner's<br>For women, being American Indian/Alaska Native or African American<br>For women, having a verbally abusive, jealous, or possessive partner |
| **Relationship Factors** |
| Couples with income, educational, or job status disparities<br>Dominance and control of the relationship by the male |
| **Community Factors** |
| Poverty and associated factors (e.g., overcrowding)<br>Low social capital—lack of institutions, relationships, and norms that shape the quality and quantity of a community's social interactions<br>Weak community sanctions against IPV (e.g., police unwilling to intervene) |
| **Societal Factors** |
| Traditional gender norms (e.g., women should stay at home and not enter workforce, should be submissive) |

in physically violent environments are more likely to find themselves in violent relationships as adults.

There is no single cause of IPV, but there are risk factors for both victimization (Table 12.2) and perpetration (Table 12.3). In both women and men, alcohol problems contribute to physical and psychological abuse. Those who are most susceptible to IPV often have been exposed to IPV and/or child abuse. Exposure to IPV as a child may cause psychological harm that increases the risk of IPV as an adult.

Ways to prevent IPV include providing shelters, safe houses, and other protective environments for abused women; reducing unemployment, poverty, and racism; holding abusers accountable for their actions; training law enforcement and healthcare professionals to recognize and intervene in cases of IPV; training everyone in nonviolent conflict resolution; and reducing the amount of violent imagery on television, in films, and in popular music.

## Child Sexual Abuse

**child sexual abuse (CSA)** sexual contact or other sexual behavior between an adult (or late teen) and a child
**incest** sexual abuse of a child by an older relative or emotionally close adult

**Child sexual abuse (CSA)** is sexual contact or other sexual behavior between an adult (or late teen) and a child. CSA includes sexual kissing, touching breasts, fondling of genitals, and oral, anal, or vaginal intercourse. Noncontact child sexual abuse includes genital exposure ("flashing" or masturbation), verbal pressure for sex, and sexual exploitation for purposes of prostitution or pornography. **Incest** is sexual abuse of a child by a relative. The relatedness can be kinship (e.g., biological parent, sibling, extended family member) or someone identified as a family member (e.g., in-law, stepsibling, stepparent, close family friend). Because incest is a betrayal of trust and a violation of the self, it can also refer to any relationship in which the

**Table 12.3** Risk Factors for Perpetration of Sexual Assault

| |
|---|
| **Individual Factors** |
| Alcohol and drug use |
| Coercive sexual fantasies |
| Impulsive and antisocial tendencies |
| Preference for impersonal sex |
| Hostility toward women |
| Hypermasculinity |
| Childhood history of sexual and physical abuse |
| Witnessing family violence as a child |
| **Relationship Factors** |
| Association with sexually aggressive and delinquent peers |
| Family environment characterized by physical violence and few resources |
| Strong patriarchal relationship or familial environment |
| Emotionally unsupportive familial environment |
| **Community Factors** |
| Lack of employment opportunities |
| Lack of institutional support from police and judicial system |
| General tolerance of sexual assault within the community |
| Settings that support sexual violence |
| Weak community sanctions against sexual violence perpetrators |
| **Societal Factors** |
| Poverty |
| Societal norms that support sexual violence |
| Societal norms that support male superiority and sexual entitlement |
| Societal norms that maintain women's inferiority and sexual submissiveness |
| Weak laws and policies related to gender equity |
| High tolerance levels of crime and other forms of violence |

child is emotionally bonded to the abuser or acknowledges that the abuser has authority.

Child sexual abuse is *always* for the benefit of the abuser, generally without regard for the reactions or choices of the child and the effects of the behavior on the child. In the United States, the annual number of reported cases of CSA is about 90,000. However, it is thought that 90% of cases go unreported because children are afraid to tell anyone what happened to them and the legal procedure

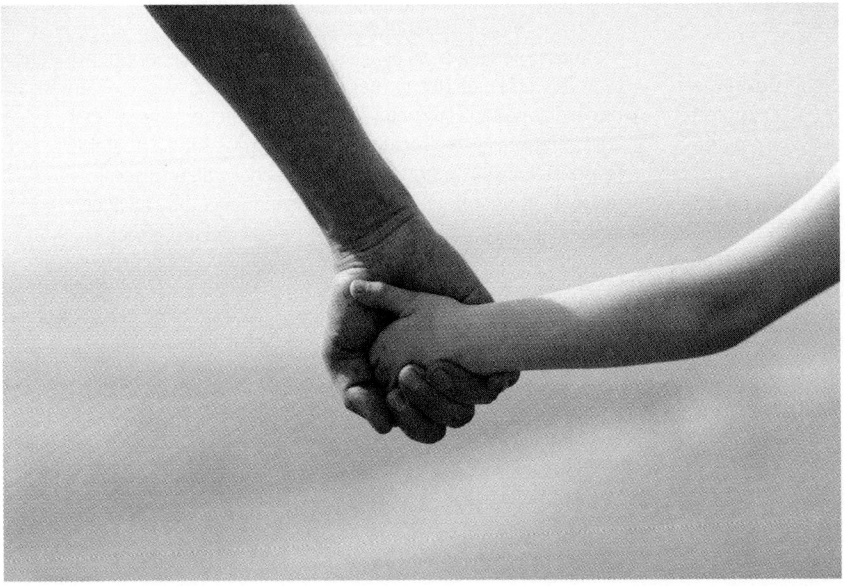

Recovery from child sexual abuse is facilitated by caring and emotional support.

for validating CSA is complex. Child sexual abuse has been reported by 20% of women and 10% of men surveyed worldwide. About 60% of perpetrators of CSA are nonrelative acquaintances of the child, such as a friend of the family, a neighbor, a childcare person, or a teacher or coach. About 30% of perpetrators of CSA are relatives of the child, such as a parent, stepparent, grandparent, sibling, cousin, or other relative. Strangers are perpetrators in about 10% of child sexual abuse cases. Most often, men are perpetrators, regardless of whether the victim is a boy or a girl. Women are perpetrators in about 12% of cases reported against boys and about 6% of cases reported against girls. Contrary to common belief, homosexual men are *not* more likely to sexually abuse children than other men are.

Perpetrators of CSA who know their child victims often use the child's affection, loyalty, and trust as weapons of abuse. To maintain a child's compliance, they may threaten a child with violence or loss of love. If the abuser is a family member, a child victim may not expose the truth because of fear of the abuser's anger, disbelief from family members, shame, and fear that the family will break up. Even children too young to understand sexual activity may nevertheless have a sense that what is happening is wrong. They may be torn between wanting to comply with the older, more powerful person and wanting the abuse to stop.

Children who experience CSA may develop low self-esteem and a feeling of worthlessness. They may become withdrawn and mistrustful of adults, and/or become depressed and suicidal. Some children may show symptoms of PTSD, including agitated behavior, frightening dreams, and repetitive play in which aspects of the abuse are expressed. Because of CSA, children may develop sexual behavior(s) or seductiveness that is inappropriate for their age. Alternatively, vic-

HEALTHY SEXUALITY

### Profiting from Violence

Mass media, defined as television, radio, film, music, the Internet, video games, magazines, books, and newspapers, is a massive business. Whereas people turn to it to become informed and entertained, it's no secret that the principal aim of much of the mass media is providing the "eyes and ears" of potential buyers to sellers of products and services. For example, MTV's "Value to Advertisers" Web page (http://www.cabletvadbureau.com/02Profiles/MTVProf.htm) points out the following:

- "No other channel can deliver the young adult demographic like MTV."
- "Young adults 15–17 are excited consumers and extremely impressionable. Now is the time to influence their choices."
- "When it comes down to shelling out money, this crowd wields a lot of influence and spending power . . . persons aged 12–34 account for 41% of all retail shopping dollars spent. MTV viewers aged 18–34 spend $8 billion on clothes, $845.5 million on video game systems, $2.2 billion on fine jewelry, $5.5 billion on major household furnishings, $885 billion on audio equipment, $5.3 billion on foreign vacations, and $21.6 billion on personal computers."
- "MTV is (consistently) the top rated basic cable television network. MTV can take you where you need to be."

Of course, before any mass medium can sell people something, it must get their attention. A tried and true way to do that is to present content that contains a significant amount of interpersonal violence, including not only physical violence but also coercion, threats, put-down humor, and disrespect. The U.S. Federal Trade Commission reported that about 60% of television programs contain violence. An hour of prime-time television includes about five violent acts. An hour of children's programming includes about 20 violent acts. The average American child will witness 12,000 violent acts on television each year, amounting to about 200,000 violent acts by age 18. A vast majority of video games involve intentional violence.

Numerous studies have shown that exposure to violence in the mass media fosters aggressive behavior. While not denying the prevalence of violence in media, industry executives and content providers are quick to point out—and researchers agree—that it is scientifically incorrect to assert that mass media content is responsible for all manner of interpersonal violence because the potential for interpersonal violence is influenced by a variety of individual and social factors. Nevertheless, what does it say about a society in which:

- A song lyric refers to a woman as a "ho"?
- A young woman's pink T-shirt has the word "BITCH" emblazoned in silver glitter across the front?
- Women in popular music, video games, and films are portrayed as sex objects whose sole purpose is another's sexual gratification?
- A song lyric expresses a man's violent, homicidal rage at a woman?

tims of CSA may avoid anything of a sexual nature. They may believe their bodies are dirty or damaged and are uncomfortable with their genitals.

If a child reveals sexual abuse to an adult, it is vital that the child's disclosure be taken seriously. Not doing so or trying to minimize the child's discomfort and distress only reabuses the child. It often is very painful for an adult to acknowledge that a child has been sexually abused or exploited. Parents and caretakers may need to seek professional help to deal with their own feelings about the abuse so that they are able to provide support to a child.

Parents and caretakers who have been told or suspect that a child has been sexually abused should try to remain calm, as displays of anger and anxiety may frighten the child even more and add to the feelings of guilt and shame. A child should be reassured that what happened is not his or her fault. The abuse should be reported immediately and a medical examination and psychological consultation sought. With professional guidance and the support of loving and caring parents and other family members, children can recover from sexual abuse.

Because the vast majority of instances of CSA are unreported, many adults carry the wounds of their abuse as children into adulthood. Dramatic examples of this are the thousands of people worldwide who have accused priests and clergy of sexually abusing them in childhood. Some of the common long-term effects of CSA include PTSD and/or anxiety, depression and thoughts of suicide, sexual anxiety and sexual disorders, poor body image and low self-esteem, the use of alcohol and other drugs, self-mutilation, and disordered eating. Also, victims of CSA are at a higher risk for experiencing rape and intimate partner violence as adults.

Recovering from CSA can be facilitated by the support of family, friends, and intimates. Getting rid of guilt and shame stemming from the abuse is very helpful. This can be accomplished by attending workshops and conferences on adult victims of child sexual abuse, learning about CSA, getting counseling, and participating in support groups of other CSA victims. Suggestions for preventing child sexual abuse are presented in **Table 12.4**.

**Table 12.4** Lessening the Risk of Child Sexual Abuse

| |
|---|
| Tell children that if someone tries to touch their body and do things that make them feel uncomfortable, they should say NO to the person and tell a parent or other trusted adult about it right away. |
| Teach children that they have the right to forbid others to touch their bodies in any way. |
| Tell children that respect does not always mean doing what an older person tells them to do. |
| Do not tell children to do everything the baby sitter or group leader tells them to do. |
| Do not tell children to give relatives hugs and kisses. Let them express affection in their own way (or not). |
| Instruct children never to get into a car with a stranger without a parent's permission. |
| Never leave children unattended in public places. |
| Alert children that perpetrators may use the Internet. Monitor children's Internet usage. |
| Encourage professional prevention programs in the schools. |
| Provide a safe, caring environment so children feel able to talk freely about sexual abuse. |

Adapted from American Academy of Pediatrics. Parenting Corner Q&A: Sexual Abuse. Available at: http://www.aap.org/publiced/BR_SexAbuse.htm. Accessed October 5, 2010.

## SEXUALITY IN REVIEW

- Sexual and relationship violence consists of rape, intimate partner violence, and child sexual abuse.
- Rape is nonconsensual forced sexual behavior.
- Rape is motivated by the desire to dominate and harm rather than sexual release.
- Rape Trauma Syndrome is a consequence of having been raped.
- Intimate partner violence is physical, psychological, or sexual harm by a current or former intimate partner.
- Child sexual abuse is sexual contact or other sexual behavior between an adult and a child.
- A variety of personal and community efforts can reduce the incidence of sexual and relationship violence.

## CRITICAL THINKING ABOUT SEXUALITY

1. The United States has more forcible rapes, more battered women, and more homicides than any other industrialized country. Offer hypotheses to explain reasons that U.S. society is so sexually violent and what might be done to change the situation.
2. For over 20 years, a woman had experienced pelvic pain, the cause(s) of which no physician could diagnose. At age 43, after relocating to a new community, the pain became severe and she visited a new doctor for relief. Unlike any other doctor, the new doctor inquired about prior sexual abuse. The women freely admitted to this experience, but dismissed it as a possible cause of her symptoms as she believed she had worked through the experience in counseling soon after it happened. Just to be sure, the physician referred her to a psychologist who specialized in recovering from prior sexual abuse. The issue eventually resolved. Offer an explanation for how prior sexual abuse could lead to undiagnosable chronic pelvic pain?
3. How often do you carry out the U.S. Center for Substance Abuse Prevention's suggestions for preventing sexual assault? Use this scale: N = Never, I = Infrequently, F = Frequently, A = Always. Offer yourself suggestions for moving any items from "N" and "I" to "F" and "A"

| | |
|---|---|
| N I F A | When going out, always tell someone where you are going and with whom, take a cell phone, and $20 to $30 for emergency transportation. |
| N I F A | Do not leave a party, concert, game, or other social occasion with someone you just met or do not know very well. |
| N I F A | Investigate a first date or a blind date with friends. Insist meeting the person in a public place such as a movie, sporting event, or restaurant and meet the person there. |
| N I F A | If someone is coming on to you forcefully, say "NO" firmly. Don't smile or otherwise try to protect that person's feelings. Use the word "rape" to show what is really going on. Get away or scream if you assess it is safe to do so. Lie if you must. Say you have herpes, gonorrhea, or some other transmissible disease. |

N I F A When drinking, do not leave your drink alone on the table or bar, consume drinks out of large, open containers, such as punch bowls, trade or switch drinks with others, continue to drink something that looks or tastes "different." Watch for signs of drug effects in friends and help them.

4. Describe the strengths and weaknesses of your campus sexual assault prevention program. With other students in your class, write a "feedback report" to the college administration that includes suggestions for improving the program.

## REFERENCES AND RECOMMENDED RESOURCES

### References

Campbell, R., et al. (2009). An ecological model of the impact of sexual assault on women's mental health. *Trauma, Violence and Abuse, 10*, 225–246.

Reddington, F. P., & Kreisel, B. S. (2009). *Sexual assault: The victims, the perpetrators, and the criminal justice system*. Durham, NC: Carolina Academic Press.

Stuart, G. L., et al. (2008). The role of drug use in a conceptual model of intimate partner violence in men and women arrested for domestic violence. *Psychology of Addictive Behavior, 22*, 12–24.

Testa, M., & Livingston, J. A. (2009). Alcohol consumption and women's vulnerability to sexual victimization: Can reducing women's drinking prevent rape? *Substance Use and Misuse, 44*, 1349–1376.

U.S. Department of Justice. (2006, June 29). National Crime Victimization Survey (NCVS). Available at: http://bjs.ojp.usdoj.gov/index.cfm?ty=dcdetail&iid=245. Accessed July 5, 2010.

World Health Organization. (2002a). World Report on Violence and Health. Available at: http://www.who.int/violence_injury_prevention/violence/world_report/en. Accessed July 11, 2010.

World Health Organization. (2002b). World Report on Violence and Health. Available at: http://www.who.int/violence_injury_prevention/violence/global_campaign/en/chap6.pdf. Accessed July 12, 2010.

### Recommended Resources

Littleton, H. L. (2010). The impact of social support and negative disclosure reactions on sexual assault victims: A cross-sectional and longitudinal investigation. *Journal of Trauma and Dissociation, 2*, 210–227. Discusses the role of social support in posttrauma adjustment.

MedlinePlus. (2010). Sexual assault. Available at: http://www.nlm.nih.gov/medlineplus/sexualassault.html. Information on sexual assault from the National Library of Medicine.

National Sexual Assault Hotline. 1-800-656-HOPE. Free, confidential services.

Ohlone College. (2010). Preventing sexual assault/rape. Available at: http://www.ohlone.edu/org/security/preventsexualassault.html. Tips from the college's campus security.

Rape, Abuse, and Incest National Network (RAINN), http://www.rainn.org. The largest antisexual assault organization in the United States, leading national efforts to prevent sexual assault, improve services to victims, and ensure that rapists are brought to justice.

World Health Organization. (2005). Multi-country study on women's health and domestic violence against women. Available at: http://www.who.int/gender/violence/who_multicountry_study/en/index.html. A report based on interviews with 24,000 women from 10 countries documenting the widespread prevalence of intimate partner violence, nonpartner violence, sexual abuse during childhood, and forced first sexual experience.

# Glossary

**abortion** the intentional, premature termination of pregnancy

**acquaintance/date rape** rape or sexual assault committed by someone the victim knows

**acquired immune deficiency syndrome (AIDS)** a variety of infectious diseases related to weakening of the immune system due to infection with human immunodeficiency virus (HIV)

**adolescence** the stage of life when individuals transition from childhood to adulthood

**agents of socialization** social and cultural groupings that instill in members group-specific beliefs, values, attitudes, and rules of behavior

**amenorrhea** not menstrating

**amniocentesis** procedure for removing fetal cells from the uterus of a pregnant woman and examining the cells for inherited disorders or diseases

**amnion** a saclike structure in which the fetus develops

**anabolic steroids** testosterone-like substances

**androgen insensitivity syndrome (AIS)** also called testicular feminization; an inherited disorder in which individuals are genetically XY males but, because their cells are insensitive to male hormones, develop female sexual anatomy

**androgens** hormones that promote the development and maintenance of male and some female sex characteristics

**aphrodisiacs** drugs, teas, elixirs, potions, and magic charms that are intended to alter sexual experience

**areola** the pigmented region of the breast surrounding the nipple

**assisted reproductive technologies** medical procedures that involve removing ova from a woman's body, combining them with sperm in the laboratory, and returning them to the woman's body or that of another woman

**attachment** a neuropsychological system that emotionally bonds individuals to one another

**attitudes** beliefs that are associated with a positive or negative judgment or evaluation of an idea, person, object, or group

**autosomes** the 22 pairs of human chromosomes except for the sex chromosomes

**bacterial vaginosis** a vaginal infection, often caused by *Gardnerella vaginalis*

**barrier methods** contraceptive methods that physically or chemically block the pathway of sperm into or inside the female reproductive tract

**beliefs** thoughts and ideas you assume to be true

**breasts** milk-producing organs that can also be sexually sensitive

**calendar rhythm** method of estimating the "safe days" for sexual intercourse by charting menstrual cycle length on a calendar

**case study methods** drawing scientific conclusions from the study of one or more individuals

**cause-and-effect relationships** predictable patterns and outcomes in scientific investigations

**cervical cap** a rubber, thimble-shaped contraceptive that fits on the cervix (lower part of the uterus)

**cervix** the lower part of the uterus

**cesarean section** surgical delivery of the fetus via incision in the mother's abdomen

**chancre** a painless sore that is one of the first signs of a syphilis infection

**child sexual abuse (CSA)** sexual contact or other sexual behavior between an adult (or late teen) and a child

**chlamydia** a sexually transmitted bacterial infection of the genitals, anus, mouth, eyes, and occasionally the lungs

**chorionic villus sampling (CVS)** a procedure for testing fetal cells during pregnancy for inherited defects

**chromosomes** structures in the nuclei of cells that contain DNA and genes

**circumcision** surgical removal of the foreskin of the penis

**clinical case study** drawing scientific conclusions from observations made of one or more individuals who seek help for medical problems

**clitoris** a sexually sensitive organ located near the urethra

**colostrum** a yellowish precursor to mature mother's milk

**combination hormonal contraceptives** contraceptives containing estrogen and progestin

**companionate love** deep, committed love

**congenital adrenal hyperplasia (CAH)** also called adrenogenital syndrome; an inherited disorder of sexual development in which an individual is born with ambiguous genitalia and cannot visibly be classified as either male or female at birth

**congenital (birth) defect** any abnormality in a newborn observable at birth

**conscious beliefs** beliefs one is aware of

**contraceptive sponge** a nonprescription contraceptive device that is inserted into the vagina

**Cowper's (bulbourethral) glands** a pair of male glands that produce lubricating fluid

**cremaster** a thin muscle that raises and lowers the scrotum relative to the body

**cystitis** infection of the bladder

**deoxyribonucleic acid (DNA)** a large molecule in chromosomes that carries all the genetic information of an organism

**diaphragm** a dome-shaped, latex cup that is coated with a spermicide-containing gel or cream and placed in the vagina to cover the cervix

**douching** rinsing the vagina with fluid (e.g., water, diluted vinegar, commercial douches)

**dysmenorrhea** abdominal pain during menstruation ("menstrual cramps")

**dyspareunia** painful intercourse in women

**ejaculation** the release of semen

**ejaculatory duct** a straight tube that connects the vas deferens to the urethra

**embryo** the earliest stage of intrauterine development, from fertilization to week 10

**emergency contraception** either drug or IUD methods to prevent pregnancy if fertilization might have occurred

**emission phase** the movement of semen to the back part of the urethra

**emotions** patterns of brain activity that generate a sense of pleasantness or unpleasantness, which help evaluate as positive or negative an anticipated or actual experience and the outcome of a planned or actual behavior

**empathy** seeing and responding emotionally to a situation as someone else does

**endocrine disruptors** industrial chemicals that disrupt the functions of sex hormones

**endometrium** the inner lining of the uterus responsible for nurturing the fetus

**epidemiological study** comparing two or more groups in their natural setting

**epididymis** a coiled tube connected to the testis that stores and matures sperm

**episiotomy** an incision in the perineum from the vagina to the anus

**erectile dysfunction (ED)** difficulty in getting or maintaining an erection

**erogenous zones** body regions that are highly sexually sensitive, including the lips, glans penis, glans clitoris, the outer third of the vagina, the nipples, and the anal region

**estrogen** a sex steroid hormone that is predominant in females

**ethnographic study** observations of an entire community in which the observer lives for a period of time

**experimental study** scientific results derived from comparing a test or experimental group with a matched control group

**expulsion phase** the release of semen from the penis

**external female primary sex characteristics** mons veneris, labia minora, labia majora, and clitoris

**failure rate** a measure of contraceptive effectiveness, given as the percentage of women who are likely to become unintentionally pregnant using a particular method during the first year of use

**fallopian (uterine) tubes** a pair of structures responsible for transporting eggs from the ovaries to the uterus

**female condom** a polyurethane sheath that fits into the vagina

**female secondary sex characteristics** female-specific body structures not involved in the production or delivery of eggs or maintenance of pregnancy

**fertility awareness methods** contraceptive methods that rely on estimates of when an ovum is fertilizable or when ovulation has occurred

**fertilization** the union of a sperm and egg (ovum) to form a zygote

**fetus** the stage of intrauterine development from about the tenth week after fertilization to birth

**follicle** a bed of nutrient- and hormone-producing cells in the ovary in which an egg matures

**follicle-stimulating hormone (FSH)** facilitates maturation of ova

**foreskin** a fold of skin that covers the glans penis

**gender** classifying individuals socially, psychologically, behaviorally, and even morally according to their biological sex

**gender identity** the sense of oneself as being biologically male or female

**gender roles** socially desirable behavioral expectations of men and women

**gender stereotypes** beliefs about the "natural" or "typical" characteristics of men and women

**genes** chemical sequences in DNA that direct the synthesis of proteins in cells or which control other functions

**genetic testing** testing for abnormal genes and chromosomes in cells taken from adults and fetuses

**genital duct system** a four-segment biological tube for transporting sperm and seminal fluid

**gonadotrophin releasing factor (GnRF)** stimulates follicle-stimulating hormone (FSH) and luteinizing hormone (LH) production

**gonorrhea** a sexually transmitted bacterial infection of the genitals, anus, mouth, and eyes

**hepatitis B** a viral disease of the liver caused by hepatitis B virus (HBV) infection

**hereditary (genetic) disorders and diseases** disorders or diseases that result from inheriting an abnormal chromosome or gene from one or both parents

**herpes** a sexually transmitted viral infection of the genitals, anus, mouth, and eyes, characterized by the appearance of wet, open, painful sores at the site of the infection

**human chorionic gonadotropin (hCG)** a hormone produced by the embryo that signals the mother's body that a state of pregnancy exists

**human immunodeficiency virus (HIV)** the cause of AIDS

**human papilloma virus** the cause of anogenital warts and often cervical cancer

**hymen** tissue that partially covers the opening of the vagina

**hypothalamo-pituitary-gonadal (HPG) system** a "team" of hormone-producing structures responsible for sperm, egg, and hormone production

**hysterectomy** surgical removal of the uterus

**incest** sexual abuse of a child by an older relative or emotionally close adult

**infertile** inability to conceive a child after one year of trying

**internal female primary sex characteristics** ovaries, fallopian tubes, uterus, and vagina

**interpersonal violence** violence between individuals including assault, battery, rape, intimate partner violence, child maltreatment and sexual abuse, elder abuse, and homicide

**intimacy** deep knowledge of another associated with feelings of closeness, trust, and self-validation

**intimate partner violence (IPV)** physical, sexual, or psychological harm by a current or former partner or spouse, ranging from one incident to chronic, severe beatings

**intrauterine device** a small, plastic T-shaped object placed in the uterus as a fertility control method

**labia majora** the outer fleshy folds that cover the vagina

**labia minora** the inner fleshy folds that cover the vagina

**labor** the expulsion of the fetus from the mother's body

**laboratory observation study** observations derived in laboratory settings rather than clinical or real-life ones

**literal message** the literal meaning of a communication

**love styles (attitudes)** six types of love (eros, ludus, storge, mania, agape, and pragma)

**lowest observed failure rate** the effectiveness of a contraceptive method when used properly

**luteinizing hormone (LH)** a hormone produced by the pituitary gland that is responsible for releasing the egg from the ovary and stimulating the production of progesterone

**male condom** a latex rubber sheath that covers the erect penis

**masturbation** self-stimulation to produce erotic arousal usually to the point of orgasm

**menarche** first menstrual period

**menopause** the cessation of ovulation and menstrual periods

**menstrual (fertility) cycle** the period of time from one menstruation to another

**menstruation** the near-monthly discharge of uterine tissue debris and blood from the vagina

**metamessage** the implicit meaning about the context and relationship conveyed in a message

**molluscum contagiosum** a virus-caused STD

**mons veneris** a mound of fatty tissue covering the vulva

**naturalistic observation** studying many people at one time in their natural setting

**norms** rules of appropriate behavior that result from a group's shared beliefs and values

**orgasm** release of sexual tensions

**ovarian (graffian) follicle** an egg and its surrounding nutrient and hormone-producing cells

**ovaries** a pair of organs in the pelvic cavity in which eggs and sex hormones are produced

**ovulation** release of a mature, fertilizable egg from the ovary

**Pap smear** a diagnostic test for cancer of the cervix

**passionate love** intensely consuming, and often highly sexual, love

**penile withdrawal** withdrawing the penis from the vagina before ejaculation in order to prevent insemination

**penis** the male organ of copulation and urination

**perineum** the region between the lower part of the vagina and the anus

**placenta** an organ unique to pregnancy that transports oxygen and nutrients from the mother to the fetus and waste products from the fetus to the mother

**posttraumatic stress disorder (PTSD)** long-term psychological harm from having been traumatized, including sexually assaulted

**preimplantation genetic diagnosis (PGD)** used during in vitro fertilization to screen for the presence of genetic (inherited) diseases before an embryo is transferred into the uterus

**premenstrual dysphoric disorder (PMDD)** premenstrual symptoms severe enough to impair personal functioning

**primary sex characteristics** body structures directly involved in the production and delivery of sperm or eggs, fertilization, and pregnancy, as well as sexual activity

**progesterone** a sex steroid hormone involved in the maintenance of pregnancy

**progestin-only contraceptives** contraceptives for women that contain only a synthetic version of the natural hormone progesterone

**prostate gland** an organ at the base of the bladder that produces part of seminal fluid

**puberty** specific biological changes that transform a child's body into a sexually and reproductively capable adult's

**pubic lice** insects that live on the hair shafts in the pelvic region

**rape** nonconsensual sexual behavior, generally penile penetration of a bodily orifice

**rape trauma syndrome** immediate and long-term mental health consequences from having been raped

**rapid (premature) ejaculation** characterized by not being satisfied with the ability to control the timing of ejaculation during sexual intercourse; ejaculation generally occurs within seconds or a minute or two after beginning intercourse

**refractory period** after sex, a period of time during which a person may not desire sex and may be biologically incapable of, and even averse to, responding sexually

**safe days** when using fertility awareness methods, the days in the menstrual month when fertilization is unlikely

**sample** a small number of observations assumed to represent accurately all possible similar observations

**sampling** making a small number of observations from a large group

**sampling bias** drawing conclusions from samples that do not accurately represent the larger group from which they are drawn

**scabies** an infestation of the skin by mites

**scientific method** a way to gain knowledge of the world utilizing observations, measurements, and experiments

**scrotum** the sac of skin that contains the testes

**secondary sex characteristics** body structures associated with each sex that are not involved in the manufacture and delivery of sperm or eggs, fertilization, or pregnancy

**self-disclosure** expressing private information about oneself to another

**semen** the mixture of seminal fluid and sperm that is ejaculated

**seminal fluid** fluids produced by the seminal vesicles and prostate

**seminal vesicles** a pair of glands near the bladder that manufacture part of seminal fluid

**seminiferous tubules** small tubules in the testes in which sperm are produced

**sex chromosomes** the X and Y chromosomes in human cells; an XX constitution directs female development, and XY constitution directs male development

**sex determining region Y (SRY) gene** a gene on the Y chromosome that controls development of a fetus as a male; in the absence of this gene, development proceeds as female

**sex typing (sex assignment)** the assigning of a gender to newborns, generally based on the appearance of genitals

**sexual assault** the combination of nonconsensual sexual penetration (rape) and nonsexual violence, such as battery, the threat of harm, or homicide

**sexual desire** an urge to experience sexual pleasure and/or sexual intimacy

**sexuality** aspects of one's personhood that are involved with sexual classification, sexual activity, and creating erotic experiences

**sexually transmitted disease (STD)** an infection or infestation caused by a biological agent (e.g., virus, bacterium, insect) that is transferred from person to person by sexual interactions

**sexual orientation** the propensity to be sexually attracted to and generally desirous of emotional attachment to members of a particular biological sex

**sexual resolution** after sex, the return of the brain and body to their non–sexually aroused state

**sexual response cycle** a patterned biological response to sexual arousal

**sexual scripts** norms of preferred sexual behavior

**sexual self** a sense of oneself as a sexual being

**smegma** a white, cheesy substance that can accumulate under the foreskin

**socialization** the process by which individuals learn the behavioral rules of the social group(s) to which they belong

**social role** a position or status within a group

**spermatogenesis** the process by which sperm cells mature

**spermicide** a chemical capable of killing sperm

**sterility** the condition of being biologically incapable of having children; permanently infertile

**sudden infant death syndrome (SIDS)** the sudden unexpected death of an infant for no known reason

**survey methods** asking people to report their observations, generally of their own thoughts, feelings, attitudes, and behaviors

**syphilis** a sexually transmitted bacterial infection caused by the bacterium *Treponema pallidum*

**teratogen** any environmental agent that causes abnormal fetal development and birth defects

**testes** the pair of male reproductive organs that produce sperm cells and steroid sex hormones

**testicular ferminization** also called androgen insensitivity syndrome; individuals with this inherited disorder are genetically XY, but, because their cells do not respond to androgenic hormones, they often develop female-appearing anatomical structures

**testosterone** the principal male sex steroid hormone

**transgenderism** gender identity not congruent with the biological sex

**transitioning** a progressive mental and physical "letting go" of the everyday so that a full sexual experience can occur

**Triangular Theory of Love** a scientific model of love consisting of intimacy, passion, and decision/commitment

**trichomoniasis** vaginal infection caused by the protozoan *Trichomonas vaginalis*

**tubal ligation** the cutting or blocking of the fallopian tubes so a woman can no longer get pregnant

**typical user failure rate** the effectiveness of a contraceptive method that takes into account all of the errors when in general use in a population

**ultrasound scanning** use of sound energy to obtain an image of a fetus in the uterus of a pregnant woman, as well as determine the presence of multiple fetuses, the orientation of the fetus, and the location of the placenta

**umbilical cord** a structure that transports blood from the fetus to and from the placenta

**unconscious beliefs** beliefs one is unaware of

**unsafe days** when using fertility awareness methods, the days in the menstrual month when fertilization is likely

**urethra** the tube that courses through the penis and through which urine and semen pass

**urethritis** infection of the urethra

**urinary tract infection (UTI)** urethritis and/or cystitis

**uterus** an organ in the pelvic cavity in which a fetus develops

**vagina** a tube extending from the uterus to the outside of the body

**vaginal spermicides** foams, gels, creams, and suppositories that contain a spermicide

**vaginismus** anxiety-produced spasms of the muscles surrounding the vagina that make vaginal penetration painful if attempted

**vaginitis** yeast or bacterial infection of the vagina

**values** beliefs pertaining to concepts of right and wrong, good and bad, moral and immoral

**vas deferens** a tube that transports sperm from the scrotum into the body

**vasectomy** the cutting or blocking of the pair of vas deferens to make a man incapable of fertilization

**vulva** the lower part of the female pelvis and between the legs where the external genitalia are located

**xenoestrogens** chemicals in the environment that mimic the actions of human hormones

**zygote** a fertilized egg

# Index

## C



## D

## E



## F

## T



## U



## V



## W



## X



## Y



## Z

# Photo Credits

## Chapter 1

**Opener** © Andresr/ShutterStock, Inc.; **page 2** © AbleStock; **page 10** © David Buffington/Photodisc/Getty Images; **page 12** © Nicholas Sutcliffe/Dreamstime.com

## Chapter 2

**Opener** © Karin Hildebrand Lau/ShutterStock, Inc.; **2.3A** © Daniel Sambraus/Photo Researchers, Inc.; **page 32** Courtesy of J01 Mark D. Faram/U.S. Navy; **page 33** © Katrina Brown/Dreamstime.com

## Chapter 3

**Opener** © AVAVA/ShutterStock, Inc.; **page 40** © ASTIER/age fotostock; **3.3 (left)** © JPD/Custom Medical Stock Photo; **(middle)** © Daniel Sambraus/Photo Researchers, Inc.; **(right)** Courtesy of Anna Swisher; **page 46** © Geoff Caddick/PA Wire/AP Photos; **page 49** © Diego Vito Cervo/Dreamstime.com

## Chapter 4

**Opener** © Bendao/Dreamstime.com; **page 56** © Jill Lang/Dreamstime.com; **4.3** © David M. Phillips/Science Source/Photo Researchers, Inc.; **page 62** © attem/ShutterStock, Inc.; **page 63** © Natalie Shmeliova/Dreamstime.com; **page 65** © Photos.com; **4.7** Courtesy of Susan Schultz; **page 73** © Tim Osborne/ShutterStock, Inc.

## Chapter 5

**Opener** © Christy Thompson/ShutterStock, Inc.; **page 95** © Robert Crum/Fotolia.com

## Chapter 6

**Opener** © Corbis; **6.2 (photo)** Courtesy of Library of Congress, Prints & Photographs Division, National Photo Company Collection [reproduction number LC-DIG-npcc-19687]; **page 108** © www.imagesource.com/Jupiterimages; **page 110** © Nyul/Dreamstime.com

## Chapter 7

**Opener** © Billy Lobo/ShutterStock, Inc.; **page 124** U.S. Department of Energy Genome Programs. Available at: http://genomics.energy.gov. Accessed December 28, 2010; **7.1** Courtesy of Lisa G. Shaffer, Signature Genomic Laboratories; **7.2A** © Phototake, Inc./Alamy Images; **page 129** © Andres Rodriguez/Dreamstime.com; **7.5** © Simon Pederson/ShutterStock, Inc.

## Chapter 8

**Opener** © Monkey Business Images/ShutterStock, Inc.; **page 143** © Astroid/Fotolia.com; **page 144** © sergei telegin/ShutterStock, Inc.; **page 150** © LiquidLibrary; **pages 152, 156** © Photos.com

## Chapter 9

**Opener** © oliveromg/ShutterStock, Inc.; **page 168** © Miguel Villagran/AP Photos; **page 171** © Pachot/Dreamstime.com; **page 173** © Douglas C. Pizac/AP Photos

## Chapter 10

**Opener** © Elena Elisseeva/ShutterStock, Inc.; **page 185** © Yuri Arcurs/ShutterStock, Inc.; **page 186** © Mircala/Dreamstime.com; **page 197** © Nazar Niyazov/Dreamstime.com

## Chapter 11

**Opener** © Bernhard Richter/ShutterStock, Inc.; **page 204** © Supri Suharjoto/ShutterStock, Inc.; **page 213** © Oscar C. Williams/ShutterStock, Inc.; **page 218** © Victoria Alexandrova/ShutterStock, Inc.

## Chapter 12

**Opener (ribbon)** © Arnien/Dreamstime.com, **page 228** © Ivonne Wierink/Dreamstime.com; **page 233** © BlueOrange Studio/ShutterStock, Inc.